Healthy Work

Healthy Work

An Annotated Bibliography

Namir Khan
Nina Nakajima
Willem H. Vanderburg

with the collaboration of Ken Jalowica,
Esther Vanderburg, and David Vanderburg

The Scarecrow Press, Inc.
Lanham, Maryland • Toronto • Oxford
2004

SCARECROW PRESS, INC.

Published in the United States of America
by Scarecrow Press, Inc.
A wholly owned subsidiary of
The Rowman & Littlefield Publishing Group, Inc.
4501 Forbes Boulevard, Suite 200, Lanham, Maryland 20706
www.scarecrowpress.com

PO Box 317
Oxford
OX2 9RU, UK

British Library Cataloguing in Publication Information Available

Library of Congress Cataloging-in-Publication Data
Khan, Namir, 1955–
Healthy work ; an annotated bibliography / Namir Khan, Nina Nakajima, Willem H. Vanderburg ; with the collaboration of Ken Jalowica, Esther Vanderburg, and David Vanderburg.
p. cm.
Includes bibliographical references and index.
ISBN: 978-0-8108-5285-3
1. Industrial hygiene—Bibliography. I. Nakajima, Nina, 1974–
II. Vanderburg, Willem H. III. Title.

Z6675.I5K48 2004
[RC967]
016.6136'2—dc22 2004017712

The paper used in this publication meets the minimum requirements of American National Standard for Information Sciences—Permanence of Paper for Printed Library Materials, ANSI/NISO Z39.48-1992.
Manufactured in the United States of America.

Contents

Preface

The evidence from socio-epidemiology is solid: human work has become one of the primary sources of physical and mental illness. Not long ago it was reported that the primary supplier of General Motors was Blue Cross. The Surgeon General of the United States has warned that expenditures on mental illness are rising at the alarming rate of 7 percent per year. Even if the correlation between this rate of increased expenditure and the actual rate of increase of mental illness is a weak one, it is clear that much more attention needs to be paid to what is happening to human work and how these changes spill over into human lives, communities and nations.

The purpose of this annotated bibliography is to bring together diverse bodies of literature related to human work in a manner that supports preventive approaches to work design and organization. Such approaches ensure that the design and decision making regarding human work examine how these affect human life and society, in order to make use of this understanding in a negative feedback mode. Adjustments could then be made to these designs and decisions in a way that achieves the desired results while simultaneously preventing or greatly reducing undesired and harmful effects. Such approaches are both diagnostic and prescriptive and have the promise of reshaping work according to a triple bottom line: economic, social and environmental. This bibliography is part of a series documenting the possibility of preventive approaches in the areas of materials and production, energy, work and cities, the conceptual framework of which has been developed in my book *The Labyrinth of Technology*.

The diagnosis of what is happening to human work is relatively straightforward. Our research began by examining what people who are likely to shape tomorrow's workplaces (including engineers, managers, business administrators and accountants) learn about how technology in general, and workplace technology in particular, influences human life, society and the biosphere. We then examined to what extent they learn to make use of this knowledge to adjust decision-making processes so as to obtain the desired results while simultaneously preventing or greatly minimizing undesired effects. The answer was: almost nothing. They collectively learn to "steer" workplace technologies into the future by relying primarily on performance values such as efficiency, productivity, profitability and cost-benefit ratios, which measure the desired outputs that can be derived from the requisite inputs but are entirely mute on the question of how any improvements may be realized at the expense of increasing harmful effects. It is as if they were driving a car by concentrating on the performance of the vehicle as indicated by the gauges on the dashboard, only occasionally glancing out of the windows to see where they are heading in order to safely reach their destination. Preventive approaches teach future practitioners to look out of their "professional windows" to see where human work is heading and to adjust design and decision making accordingly, much as they would drive their vehicles. The conventional wisdom has it that operating to higher social, health and environmental standards is necessarily more expensive. However, this is the case only if these matters are dealt with by not looking beyond a practitioner's domain of specialization, which institutionalizes end-of-pipe approaches. Each time the standard is raised, additional devices and services must be added to the "system," and this raises costs dramatically. However, if we educate future practitioners to be not only technically competent in their areas of specialization but also to have a certain social and environmental literacy, it opens up the possibility that with a few additional hours of thinking and adjusting their designs and decisions, a substantially superior ratio of desired to undesired effects may emerge. Such preventive approaches are therefore often economically, as well as socially and environmentally, superior to their conventional counterparts.

To facilitate the task of the reader and user of this annotated bibliography, I will set out a few of the basic linkages between human work and the remainder of human life, communities and societies. It is essential to recognize that our relationships with our surroundings are necessarily reciprocal ones. For workplaces, this means that as we shape our work, this work simultaneously shapes us, our lives and our communities. It is part of a fundamental reciprocity of which I will briefly outline three dimensions: physical, social and spiritual. On the physical level, we depend on a constant throughput of matter and energy to live, and to replace or repair our body cells. Such throughputs of matter and energy contribute to our body load insofar as they contain toxic substances, bacteria and viruses. If this body load exceeds our immunological resources, it threatens our physical integrality and could make us ill or even cause our death. On the social level, each experience of our surroundings in a small way modifies the organization of our brain-minds. Our nervous systems depend on a reciprocal exchange of experiences as well as the nurture, love and support of others. Excessive monotony, sensory deprivation, an upbringing in isolation or by animals, the withholding of nurture and love during infancy, a lack of emotional and social support, a want of love or belonging, dilemmas from which there appear to be no way out—all these and more can impair the development of our social selves and consequently our relationships with others, which, in the extreme, may lead to substance abuse, nervous breakdown, multiple personalities, or suicide. On the spiritual level, we belong to communities that cannot know all of reality and hence must live as if the reality they have come to know is reality itself. Moreover, these communities do not know the Good and hence must live as if the very best thing in their individual and collective life is that Good. Together with our communities, we are thus plunged into a spiritual world of make-believe and culturally-created religious absolutes. Anomalous experiences, contacts with other ways of life, and socio-economic or political crises can, in the extreme, lead to anomie or suicide in the lives of individual members of these communities or to a decline or collapse of the group or society itself. All this is well known from cultural anthropology and history.

A crisis in one dimension can trigger crises in the others. Toxic substances can affect people's personalities and behavior patterns. Disease can make it impossible for our bodies to respond to us, effectively cutting us off from others and the world. Malfunctions of the brain-mind can reduce our lives to little more than isolated moments of existence, as we see in Alzheimer's patients, for example. In the course of our lives we encounter many situations that produce contradictions between particular moments and our lives, which may not necessarily lead to crises but which can undermine the integrality of our lives. We embody a constant tension between our lives and the disorder within or without. Living our lives involves a constant weaving and repairing of relationships in the face of illness and death. All three dimensions come together in the way we learn to symbolize our lives by means of our community's culture.

The reciprocal relationships between ourselves and our surroundings compel us to live our lives in a dialectical tension between freedom and alienation, depending on whether or not the influence we exert over our surroundings is greater than the influence our experiences of these surroundings "possess" the organization of our brain-minds and thus our lives. In the same way, we live a tension between health and illness, and moral integrity and chaos.

Our relationships with our workplaces are a microcosm of this reciprocal interdependence between us and our surroundings. Hence, workplaces can be alienating if their effects spill over into the remainder of our lives and thereby exercise a decisive influence. Similarly, workplaces can lead to both physical and mental illness. If the spillover effects onto the remainder of people's lives are substantial, hiring someone for a wage may lead to a condition of significantly possessing his or her life, which raises moral and ethical concerns.

As a consequence, our relationships with our work and work settings may be classified along the following spectrum. On the one extreme, we find relationships in which the demands work places on us far outstrip our resources. Such resources include education, experience, creativity, imagination, motivation and commitment. On the other extreme, we encounter relationships in which our resources far outstrip the demands. Either extreme can crush our humanity through unbearable stress or destructive boredom. In the middle of this spectrum we encounter work that slightly stretches our resources, thus leading to creative responses through which we learn new things, expand our resources and grow. In addition, these jobs provide a great deal of satisfaction derived from having successfully met new challenges.

Superimposed on this spectrum is the issue of control over our resources. These may be of little value if the work is so organized as to depend on the most minimal subset of these resources, as exemplified by the traditional assembly line and the emerging intellectual assembly line. Hence, a lack of control over our resources can further narrow the spectrum of healthy relations between ourselves and our work.

All this must be further assessed over time. Work experiences are the uninvited guests to the remainder of our lives. However, if after work we can replenish our resources and recover our energy by relaxing, eating and sleeping, our work will not "mine" these resources. If, on the other hand, we cannot recover our resources, then our work may gradually mine them and our humanity. How well we can recover these resources is affected by many factors, including how supportive and socially healthy our families and communities are, the quality of our nutrition and lifestyle, and the many stressors (or lack thereof) generated by our urban habitat.

The technical division of labor paved the way for the substitution of capital for labor which, more than any other factor, has transformed work and workplaces during the last 200 years of mechanization, industrialization, automation and computerization. It dramatically improved the efficiency, productivity and profitability of labor in the following five ways. First, by rationally decomposing work into a series of production steps, workers could be assigned narrow repetitive tasks that they could readily master. No time or effort needed to be devoted to the broader context of the tasks that preceded or followed the one at hand. These constituent elements of work could then be optimized to eliminate wasted motions in order to ensure the best performance. Second, it was now possible to prepare, optimize, implement and evaluate a production plan in the form of the optimal sequence of the optimized constituent production steps. Third, as a consequence of this decomposition and rational recomposition of work, it was possible to assign production steps either to machines or to human beings, to obtain the greatest possible efficiency, productivity and profitability. This opened the road first to mechanization and later to automation and computerization. None of this was possible with traditional craft work. Fourth, the tasks assigned to human beings could be performed by those people having just the required skill level, as opposed to those able to accomplish the most difficult steps, as in craft work. This greatly reduced labor costs. Fifth, workers were isolated from one another and group structures eliminated, with the result that a great deal more time was available for production. Desired outputs were obtained from requisite inputs with a greater efficiency, labor productivity and profitability, thanks to the technical division of labor.

The technical division of labor simultaneously undermined the integrity of individual and collective human life in five ways. First, Adam Smith had already noted in 1776 that it would make human beings as stupid as they could possibly become. The monotony of carrying out the same operation over and over again atrophied human creativity, skill, problem-solving ability and a great deal else involved in living. Second, insofar as people still used skills, these had no common denominator with craft skills because they did not originate in a person's mind through the accumulation of experience, skill and creativity but according to the "one best way" determined by someone else. This arrangement required the suppression of the self in work, necessitating a great deal of mental energy and thus leading to nervous fatigue, with a range of psychosocial consequences. Normally even the most routine activities (such as handwriting) express something of a person's life and experience, as shown by the possibility of correlating the characteristics of handwriting with personality traits or the use of handwriting as forensic evidence.

Third, the more the technical division of labor was developed in conjunction with mechanization, automation and computerization, the more workers lost control over their work: the methods to be used, the time to be allocated, how work was to be paced, how problems should be looked at and what solutions attempted, what deadlines were to be set and met, how to report and when, and how to assess progress. In other words, a separation of knowing, doing and managing occurred. This separated the hand from the brain, destroyed the self-regulating character of work, and replaced it with long-ineffective negative feedback loops that barred workers from effectively dealing with problems. Those who knew and planned the production process were not the same people who did the work, which required supervisors to ensure that the work was done according to plan. Socio-epidemiology has shown that the degree of control is the primary determining variable of healthy or unhealthy work.

Fourth, as mechanization, automation and computerization advanced, greater demands were placed on workers tending and monitoring machines and performing tasks at increasing speeds, with the result that a split-second's inattention could lead to serious consequences. At the same time, problem-solving demands increased because of the gap that inevitably occurred between the ideal work plan and how all this worked out in reality, including the problems that originated upstream in the work process. Even if workers could solve some of the problems, they almost never had the authority to do so. There were other demands as well, related to being paced by machines, quotas and reporting responsibilities. All these demands coupled with little control created, as we now know, unhealthy work.

Fifth, the isolation of workers eliminated social support precisely as demands rose and control diminished. In sum, the development of the technical division of labor, first in blue collar work and later in white collar work, greatly weakened the integrity of individual and collective human life. Work was dehumanized. Excluding much of the normal expression of the self in externally organized work allowed people to participate only as a hand or a brain and reduced social relations to a minimum. The effects spilled over into people's lives, social relationships, families and communities. The operations of workers and their social interactions were now primarily technically based and only secondarily founded on experience and culture.

There were two landmarks in the development of this technical division of labor. The first was the invention of scientific management as formulated by Frederick Taylor in 1911, and the second was the invention of interchangeable parts, followed by the assembly line introduced by Henry Ford in 1913. Both of these developments removed significant barriers to the technical division of labor. The separation of the work process into a logical sequence of production steps is referred to as the horizontal division of labor; the separation of hand from brain, involving various levels of supervision and management, is called the vertical division of labor.

The assault on the humanity of workers was never well received. It initially required a draconian factory discipline, which set the stage for poor management-labor relations in the countries that industrialized first. A more progressive relationship tended to develop in the countries that industrialized later, in part because they learned from earlier mistakes.

Enormous costs have been incurred to implement end-of-pipe fixes designed to deal with the problems of production. These include industrial relations, job enlargement, ergonomics, human factors, most quality of working life movements, health services, stress-reducing therapies and counseling. All of these deal with significant symptoms but none address the root of the problem, namely the suppression of the human self in work. In other words, we have essentially optimized *gross* efficiency, labor productivity and profitability, and not *net* efficiency, labor productivity and profitability. Attempts to get at the root of the problem include sociotechnical work design and the anthropocentric approach. These can lead to a better ratio of desired to undesired effects in the organization of human work.

Karasek and Theorell have synthesized the findings of socio-epidemiology related to work by means of their demand-control model, which divides jobs into four categories according to the demands made by a work setting and the control people have over their resources in order to meet these demands. They have identified five independent variables (not of equal importance) by which work settings may be characterized: decision latitude, psychological demand, physical demand, social support and job security. Not all of the demands imposed by work organizations produce stress and lead to disease. For example, they cite the findings of a study showing that engineers experience qualitative challenges as satisfying, but quantitative challenges (such as time pressure) as stressful. The difference is not difficult to comprehend. With sufficient control, the former permit engineers to creatively apply their resources, expand them by learning from these situations, derive satisfaction from success, and thus reduce stress levels. Quantitative challenges, on the other hand, permit learning but there is little satisfaction, and stress is not reduced. The two must therefore be distinguished in a model that attempts to predict unhealthy work situations that produce disease. Thus decision latitude (which includes skill discretion and decision authority) permits learning, the expansion of one's skill set, and the reduction of stress. In the model, decision latitude was labeled as control and plotted on the y-axis, while psychological demand was labeled as demand and plotted on the x-axis. Their orthogonality was rooted in the fact that demand may represent a risk to human health while control does not. The remaining independent variables, namely physical demand, social support and job security, were found to be less important for creating healthier workplaces. This left

Karasek and Theorell with a two-dimensional demand-control model. The four kinds of work experiences they identified were labeled as active jobs (high demand, high control), low-strain jobs (low demand, high control), passive jobs (low demand, low control), and high-strain jobs (high demand, low control). The active and passive jobs had medium strain. The model predicted that these four categories of work experiences would have different effects on human health, non-work activities and community participation. This is well supported by the evidence of socio-epidemiology.

Active jobs and low-strain jobs, both characterized by positive control, are jobs in which the influence people have over work-related technology tends to be greater than the influence this technology has over them. Passive and high-strain jobs, both characterized by negative control, are generally jobs in which the reverse is the case. It is clear that mechanization, automation, and computerization push more and more jobs into the lower half of the demand-control chart. The result is higher levels of stress that, over time, translate into job strain to produce the present epidemic of work-related disease. Lean production, downsizing, business process reengineering, and the emergence of the intellectual assembly line with enterprise integration have intensified these trends even further.

There is another aspect to the reciprocal relationship between people and their work settings, which is of growing importance in an age in which computerization in many instances amounts to installing intellectual assembly lines, where human resources are treated much like natural resources, and where many jobs entail hidden risks to people's physical and mental well-being. These developments invite a sense of a lack of fairness—a feeling that one party is doing all the taking and the other all the giving. All this has profound implications for human work, as shown by the reward imbalance model.

Following the Second World War, there was a growing realization, especially in Scandinavian countries and Germany, that the substitution of capital for labor had gone too far. A great deal of experimentation occurred to achieve a better balance between the productivity of capital and the productivity of labor. A number of alternative work design approaches were developed, some of which had spectacular results. However, the experiments were short-lived. There were many factors, including the fact that many of the corporations experimenting with alternative approaches were small and were soon taken over by large transnationals that were content to export these labor problems to the south. Free trade agreements made this an attractive option. Furthermore, growing underemployment and unemployment undermined the cooperative efforts of management and labor to resolve common problems.

The fundamental problems are not likely to go away, however. It must be recalled that the Fordist-Taylorist production system evolved under the conditions of a scarcity of highly-skilled labor and an abundance of natural resources. These are opposite to those that exist in the world today. We overconsume natural resources and underconsume human work. If labor productivity grows by 2 percent in any given year, it will take 2 percent less labor to produce the same economic output the next year. In order to keep underemployment and unemployment under control, the economy must therefore grow by at least 2 percent. How much longer can this strategy continue if we are to have an economically viable, socially just, and environmentally sustainable future? How long can the stability of the global economic order resist the coming resource crises, as is evident from the fact that most nations' ecological footprints are substantially larger than their national boundaries? There is little doubt that sooner or later the balance between the productivity of capital and the productivity of labor will have to be changed by a variety of means, including a shift from labor taxes to ecological taxes. Such developments would encourage the kinds of experimentation with work design that occurred in Scandinavia and some other European countries during the 1960s and 1970s. The final chapter on this is far from being written by current management-labor and free trade agreements. Underemployment and unemployment, spiraling health costs, north–south injustices, global warming and other environmental issues will have no long-term solutions without reinventing work. This annotated bibliography is designed to be a useful tool in the hands of all those committed to finding genuine solutions to human work in the twenty-first century.

This bibliography was compiled as part of a larger research project investigating the potential of preventive approaches for building an alternative technological and economic strategy for our time. The intellectual direction of this research was my responsibility. The compiling and editing of this annotated bibliography was initially under the direction of Namir Khan but completed under the direction of Nina Nakajima. We wish to thank the student research assistants named on the title page, without whose help this project could not have been completed. We would also like to thank Mark O'Hare for helping to edit and format the manuscript. I also wish to acknowledge the support of the Social Sciences and Humanities Research Council of Canada, which funded the overall project for many years. I trust that this expenditure of public funds will make a contribution to addressing the problems faced by our industrial civilization.

Willem H. Vanderburg
Toronto

Healthy Work Bibliography

1. Abel, Emily K., and Margaret K. Nelson, eds. *Circles of Care: Work and Identity in Women's Lives*. Albany: State University of New York Press, 1990.

Keywords: women, caregivers, psychology, feminism

Along with the expansion of the service society, the nature of caregiving has changed in our society. The caregiving activities that were previously provided in the domestic domain, mostly by women, have been transferred to the wage labor force and are performed by service workers, the majority of whom are women. This book on the experience of women caregivers contains a number of essays covering different aspects of caregiving. Apart from the first two essays on the theoretical aspects of caregiving, other essays are grouped according to the location of the care that include the domestic domain, formal organizations (hospitals, old age homes, mental institutions), and the informal economy (waged home care). In these essays, the caregiving activities provided in each context are outlined and their effects on the caregiver are demonstrated. Of relevance to healthy work is the feminist perspective on caregivers' experiences that suggests that caregiving is oppressive to women. Furthermore, in the context of formal organizations, such work has been termed "emotional labor" because bureaucracies force workers to follow standardized techniques and do not allow for the use of personal knowledge.

2. Adam, Alison, J. Emms, E. Green, and J. Owen, eds. *Fifth International Conference on Women, Work and Computerization*. Manchester, UK: North-Holland/Elsevier, 1994.

Keywords: women, computers, automation, feminism

This book contains a diverse collection of papers from the IFIP International Conference on Women, Work and Computerization. A number of dominant themes are featured: "Philosophy and Information Systems," "Community, Communications, and Information Networks," "Information Technology, Flexibility, and Restructuring," "Information Systems Design and User-Centered Perspectives," "Education, Training, and Learning," and "Feminist Theoretical Perspectives on Power, Knowledge, and Technology."

The editors are concerned about several features that characterize work on gender and IT in the 1990s. "Firstly, the boundaries defining 'technology' and 'the technical' are themselves a focus for analysis, rather than being taken for granted—as are the definitions of masculinity and femininity. A number of chapters in this volume . . . explore this theme." The editors also note that there exists "an interesting co-existence of very diverse 'layers' within research on gender and computing specifically. Access itself is still a concern, as is practical support for women and girls in computing: whether in higher education or in the workplace."

Also discussed in this volume is the role of feminist theory within AI and information course design, as well as the sociology of IT in general.

3. Adler, Paul S., ed. *Technology and the Future of Work*. Oxford: Oxford University Press, 1992.

Keywords: automation, deskilling, work design, sociotechnical systems

The deskilling effects of automation are challenged in this collection. New technologies would lead to less skilled and narrower jobs, it was believed. Newer research shows, however, that higher skill levels and broader jobs result in higher productivity. Two key themes thread the articles together: competence and learning. The effective use of technology for higher productivity requires competent workers; competent workers, in turn, require new skills and new roles. Learning refers to both the ability of the organization to adapt to new technologies and to provide continuous learning opportunities for employees. The first four chapters focus on the impact of technology on job content and work organization. Strategies for education, recruitment selection, training, and development on the part of the organization to meet the new competencies are featured in the next two chapters. Desirable employee relations that contribute to effective design of new technological jobs are the subject of chapters 8 and 9. Two papers on management strategies for successful sociotechnical systems conclude the book.

4. Adler, Paul S., and Terry Winograd, eds. *Usability: Turning Technologies into Tools*. New York: Oxford University Press, 1992.

Keywords: automation, computers, work design, case study, skill, sociology, psychology

This volume begins with the premise that as the technologies embedded in our own tools have grown more complex (especially in the case of computer-based information systems, communications technologies, etc.), the challenge of designing effective tools has become more difficult. The authors argue that "for users to exploit the full range of the new tools' potential function—indeed, to use them successfully at all—'usability' must be a high priority in the process of designing these tools."

This book proposes new approaches to the "design for usability" challenge. It adds to a growing literature that considers questions of design and usability from points of view such as cognitive psychology (see the work of D. Norman) and the sociology of work and technology (see S. Zuboff and L. Suchman). The chapters in this book also reflect the research being done in computer-supported cooperative work, human-computer interaction, and work-oriented systems design.

The text is multidisciplinary and has a strong "real-world" orientation. The first section focuses on case studies that illustrate the broad dimensions of usability and the major themes of the book. The second section draws on multiple case studies to draw some general conclusions about the relationship between technology design and the nature of work and skills.

5. Aft, Lawrence S. *Work Measurement and Methods Improvement.* 3rd ed. New York: Wiley Interscience Publication, 2000.

Keywords: productivity, work methods, industrial engineering, graphical analysis, time studies, data systems, time systems, ergonomics, work sampling, labor reporting

Serving to explain the fundamental concepts and principles of the study of time and motion, this text was created mainly for managers and workers because of an increased demand for documentation, measurement, analysis, and improvement.

During the 1980s, Americans feared losing their global economic dominance to Japan, partially due to the neglect of industrial engineering by many organizations. The major function of industrial engineering was the measurement of productivity and cost, and when this basic component was lost, organizations were less able to discern if they were making or losing money. Due to the shortsighted financial view many hold in senior management, industrial engineering is too often seen as an overhead cost, and is considered disposable or unneeded.

Productivity is defined in three stages: labor, capital, and management. Without the data of cost and production, proper management cannot be possible. Moreover, industrial engineering methods provide us with ways to improve our status of labor and capital by bringing us the information we need to optimize, maximize and improve productivity.

The text covers an overview of industrial engineering's role, time studies, standard data systems, predetermined time systems, work sampling, physiological work measurement, labor reporting and ergonomics and offers practical ways to improve productivity.

6. Agrell, Anders, and Roland Gustafson. "The Team Climate Inventory (TCI) and Group Innovation: A Psychometric Test on a Swedish Sample of Work Groups." *Journal of Occupational and Organizational Psychology* 67, no. 1 (1994): 143-51.

Keywords: participation, support

The Team Climate Inventory (TCI) was developed by Anderson and West (1994) and showed that group innovation is related to the following four factors: (1) vision and group goals; (2) participation; (3) support for innovation; (4) task orientation and climate for excellence. The only contribution this article makes to the field of healthy work is that it confirms Anderson and West's research using a Swedish sample. The knowledge of appropriate conditions for fostering innovative work by groups is useful for designing a healthy work group.

7. Ainger, Andrew, Rukesh Kauia, and Richard Ennals. *Executive Guide to Business Sources through Human-Centred Systems*. Berlin: Springer-Verlag, 1995.

Keywords: group work, computers, TQM, anthropocentric, skill, industrial democracy

The role of "human-centered" work systems is explored from a business/management perspective. Examples of the practical application of appropriate strategies demonstrate how executives and decision makers can begin to implement such systems. The authors suggest that "human-centered systems build upon core skills of the workforce within a rich, emancipatory environment, utilizing the benefits of technology. Change can be embraced to achieve competitive advantage and mutual benefit."

The fundamental premise of the book is that "the human resource has been under-appreciated by management, in both manufacturing and the service sectors . . . and that managers have traditionally been reluctant to take the risk of trusting the workforce." Overcoming this reluctance is seen as "the new entrepreneurial challenge."

See chapter 2 for an overview of various theories related to human-centerdness, "designing tools for skilled workers," "technocentric vs. human-centered approaches," and industrial democracy principles. See also chapter 5 on "Empowerment," chapter 6 on "Teamworking," and chapter 7 on "Skill and Competence."

8. Alex-Assensoh, Yvette M. *Neighborhoods, Family, and Political Behavior in Urban America*. Contemporary Urban Affairs 3. New York: Garland Publishing, 1998.

Keywords: urban poor, political behavior, community development, urban, marginality, social, neighborhood

In poor neighborhoods, where well over 40 percent of the residents live below the poverty line, the growth of single parent households, antisocial behavior, and social isolation has increased dramatically over the past two decades. Inner-city poverty in recent years has, according to scholars, become far worse than in the past.

While many individuals in the urban ghettos are poor, ill-educated, and poorly housed, they are invisible in the eyes of policy makers, political candidates and employers. The current political inactivity of urban communities threatens political stability and democracy in the United States. The book examines the political consequences of a disenfranchised community and the political resources available to inner-city residents.

Alex-Assensoh examines the origins of contemporary urban poverty such as the decentralization of inner-city manufacturing jobs, the rise of low-wage service sector employment, and the reduction in the number of low-skilled jobs available that paid a livable wage. The book also addresses cultural and structural explanations for inner-city poverty.

9. Alfredsson, Lars, Curt-Lennart Spetz, and Töres Theorell. "Type of Occupation and Near-Future Hospitalization for Myocardial Infarction and Some Other Diagnoses." *International Journal of Epidemiology* 14, no. 3 (1985): 378-87.

Keywords: health, stress, case study

The authors' abstract of this article accurately describes the contents: "There is urgent need for studies of possible associations between psychosocial factors at work and myocardial infarction. Myocardial infarction could be regarded as a serious 'objective' illness the onset of which is influenced to some degree by psychosocial factors. If this is true, a thorough exploration of exactly which psychosocial work factors are important may give guidelines to job designers, occupational physicians, and unions who plan new worksites and need to know which factors are beneficial and harmful. Furthermore, such data may be useful for health policy makers who need to know which occupational groups should receive particular attention for the prevention of cardiovascular disease. We also need to study concomitantly other illnesses in order to learn which psychosocial factors have more general importance to illness precipitation or predisposition and which factors are specific to cardiovascular illness."

10. Alfredsson, Lars, and Töres Theorell. "Job Characteristics of Occupations and Myocardial Infarction Risk: Effect of Possible Confounding Factors." *Social Science Medicine* 17 (1983): 1497-503.

Keywords: health, stress

The authors' abstract of this article accurately describes the contents: "In this paper some previously found associations between psychosocial occupational characteristics and myocardial infarction (MI) are scrutinized regarding confounding effects. Standardized occupational characteristics were obtained for 118 occupational groups by means of a nation wide interview survey (3876 men). Possible confounding factors available were smoking, low level education, high proportion of immigrants (mainly of Finnish origin) and heavy lifting. The standardized characteristics were utilized in a case-control study of 1216 men 40-64 years of age, living in the Stockholm County. It was concluded that occupations characterized by both high demand and at the same time small possibility of control or growth ('strain') are associated with an elevated MI risk regardless of the confounding factors. Taking each of the confounding factors into account the risk of developing MI for men aged 40-54 years employed in these strenuous occupations is about twice as high as for those employed in other occupations."

11. Alic, John A. "Technological Change, Employment, and Sustainability." *Technological Forecasting and Social Change* 55, no. 1 (May 1997): 1-13.

Keywords: automation, unemployment, sustainability, work design, productivity

This article begins by noting that while in the past technological change created more jobs in total than it destroyed, this does not mean it will be the case in the future. The author suggests that "with technology—particularly computers and automated processes—reducing the direct labor context of production in almost all sectors, it is not clear that there will be enough work either for the developed or the developing countries." The transition to sustainable development, according to Alic, "requires that most people in most places achieve levels of economic security they deem adequate. Thus, creating decent jobs by the hundreds of millions poses a fundamental bottleneck to sustainability."

The relationship between technology and employment is examined; four fundamental dimensions are isolated regarding technological change, employment and productivity growth: (1) automation that is primarily computer-based, (2) work reorganization involving flatter organizational hierarchies, multiskilled work teams, etc., (3) the redesign of products so they require less labor input (e.g., semiconductor chips), and (4) the new international division of labor in which developing countries are becoming sites not only for labor-intensive production but for advanced manufacturing.

The author also speculates on the impact of information technologies on labor productivity in the future, asking "how might we create enough jobs for people to buy the goods and services that the world economy could, in principle, produce?"

12. Allen, Thomas J., and Michael S. Morton, eds. *Information Technology and the Corporation*. New York: Oxford University Press, 1994.

Keywords: computers, management

This book is intended to help organizations manage the impact of information technology (IT). Contributors describe the ways in which IT "is integral to processes internal to the firm, to product design, to delivery of services, and to interorganizational relations." The essays in this collection convey the extent to which computerized information handling has become "the lifeblood of the organization, shrinking the effects of time and distance, and altering the very nature of work."

Part 1 ("The Information Technology Revolution") deals with the present and projected implications of the information technology revolution. See especially chapter 1 "An Economic Study of the Information Technology Revolution" and chapter 3 "Electronic Markets and Electronic Hierarchies." Part 2 ("Strategic Options") explores different strategies for gaining advantage through information technology. See especially chapter 11 "Technology and Work Organization." Part 3 ("The Organization and Management Response") examines the impact of IT on people and organizations and the ways in which organizations have responded to that impact. See in particular chapter 17 "Computer-aided Monitoring: Its Influence on Employee Job Satisfaction and Turnover" and chapter 20 "Information Technology in Marketing."

13. Alterman, Tony, Richard B. Shekelle, Sally W. Vernon, and Keith D. Buran. "Decision Latitude, Psychological Demand, Job Strain, and Coronary Heart Disease in the Western Electric Study." *American Journal of Epidemiology* 139, no. 6 (1994).

Keywords: heart disease, occupational disease, stress, case study

This article offers results from follow-up epidemiological research on men who participated in the Chicago Western Electric Study (1957-1983) at the Hawthorne Industrial Works near Chicago, Illinois. The authors examine the hypothesis established by R. Karasek, T. Theorell and others, that proposes that "job strain . . . determined by psychological demand and decision latitude, contributes to the development of hypertension and coronary heart disease."

Results of this study indicate that "decision latitude was inversely associated with 25-year mortality from coronary heart disease and the association persisted after adjustment for coronary risk factors and education," however, the protective effect of decision latitude was stronger among white-collar workers. In contrast there was no association between coronary heart disease, mortality and psychological demand.

The study found that there was evidence for "a protective effect of decision latitude against mortality from coronary heart disease" but that the role of decision latitude "warrants further investigation."

The authors also note that more comprehensive results could be derived from research that studies a greater range of objective measures of the work environment and pays closer attention to subjective perceptions of workers.

14. Altman, Morris. *Worker Satisfaction and Economic Performance: Microfoundations of Success and Failure*. New York: M. E. Sharpe, 2001.

Keywords: employee motivation, job satisfaction, performance, economics

The author contends that "How workers are treated in the context of the firm's general human relations or industrial relations environment plays a fundamentally important role in determining the economic performance of the firm and, thereby, of the economy as a whole."

A manifesto of equality and fairness, the book offers a challenge to the idea that America's free market capitalism is the only possible successful way of social organization, as well as offering an optimistic alternative to its resulting inequality and injustice in the distribution of income and wealth within and among affected countries. Altman concludes that while globalization has created a great deal of economic wealth, it has created it only for a minority of the world's population.

15. Amick III, Benjamin C., and David D. Celentano. "Structural Determinants of the Psychosocial Work Environment: Introducing Technology in the Work Stress Framework." *Ergonomics* 34, no. 5 (1991): 625-46.

Keywords: stress, technology, machine-pacing

The authors' abstract of this article accurately describes the contents: "To extend current models of psychosocial work stress research into organizational structure, technology is introduced. An exploratory model is developed combining research from ergonomics, epidemiology, and organizational science. It is hypothesized that technology influences a worker's health by structuring the job, and the relationship between the job and a worker's health is mediated by attitudes at work. To test the model, data are used from a 1978 NIOSH survey of postal workers sorting mail (N=4903). Path analysis shows technology is indirectly associated with job satisfaction and psychosomatic symptoms by how it structured the job. A machine-paced technological system of work is associated with greater job demands, less control in the job, and less co-worker support but not with supervisor support. The implications of this model for prevention strategies at the workplace are discussed suggesting that influencing supervisor support is the most effective way to affect a person's job satisfaction and level of psychosomatic symptomology."

16. Andresky Fraser, Jill. *White-Collar Sweatshop: The Deterioration of Work and Its Rewards in Corporate America*. New York: W. W. Norton and Company, 2001.

Keywords: white collar workers, work environment

Andresky Fraser describes the human cost of the miracle of ever-rising stock prices and rising productivity of the white-collar workforce. The negative result of this boom cycle was the over-working of white-collar workers who can no longer escape their work because of the rise of technology, such as cell phones, pagers, and laptop computers. They also face increased job insecurity and declining pensions and health benefits. In the end, Fraser offers tentative suggestions to the solution of the white-collar sweatshop, which she believes, with the "chainsaw" school of management, does not work in the long run to improve the financial condition of a firm. Instead, she believes that with the "accumulated effect of years' worth of deteriorating workplace conditions . . . the 'sweatshop' corporations no longer seem invincible."

17. Andriessen, J. H. Erik, and Robert A. Roe, eds. *Telematics and Work.* Hillsdale, NJ: Lawrence Erlbaum Associates, 1994.

Keywords: telematics, computers, telecommunications, information technology, teleworking, teleconferencing, work organization, work design, politics, economics

The concept of telematics refers to the integration of computer, telecommunication and information technologies. This volume focuses on the application of telematics in working environments. The central questions of the book are: "How will the present and future development of telematics affect the nature and organization of work, and under which conditions will this development be optimal?" The editors suggest that: "From the various contributions it is clear that telematics is not a single direct cause or determinant of particular changes in work and organization. The development and application of telematics depend on decision making of actors at a political scene both outside and inside the work organizations. The effects of the use of these applications appear to be co-determined by many other factors. In fact, the technology interacts with political, economic, and social factors in a complex process that shapes new organizational forms and work relationships." The book consists of four sections, each of which offers a different perspective of telematics. The first section discusses the political frameworks within which the development of telematics technology takes place. The second section describes a number of work-related applications of telematics, including electronic mail and computer conferencing, and their impacts on work organizations. Section 3 looks at teleworking, computer supported cooperative work, and other work arrangements. Section 4 focuses on the question of the degree to which telematic systems require a different approach to design and implementation when compared to other technical systems. Moreover, this section stresses the importance of certain social, economic, political and technical conditions for the successful introduction of telematics.

18. Appelbaum, Eileen, Thomas Bailey, Peter Berg, and Arne L. Kalleberg. *Manufacturing Advantage: Why High-Performance Work Systems Pay Off.* Ithaca, NY: Cornell University Press, 2000.

Keywords: manufacturing industries, manufacturing, management, industrial management, performance standards, economics

Manufacturing stands at a critical juncture between improved production and pressing competition between companies. While this creates a downsizing of price, corporations themselves must constantly restructure and merge while depending on low-wage factories situated throughout a global supply chain.

A key component for companies dealing with this challenge is high-performance work systems (HPWs). Expected to improve competitive advantage as well as cut costs, these new work systems also raise questions regarding wages and important nonmonetary outcomes for workers.

Written primarily because such little hard evidence was found to prove or disprove the efficiency of these work systems, the book covers discretionary effort, market dynamics of various industries, workplace transformation and its effect on plants and workers, as well as productivity growth, performance effects, worker outcomes and effects on earnings of high-performance systems.

The premise that high-performance work systems can help firms to enhance competitive advantage by reducing costs and improving plant performance, as well as the effects that these high-performance practices have on wages and important nonmonetary outcomes for workers are examined in this book. It is these themes that are central to the question of whether the United States will succeed in maintaining a strong manufacturing base. Issues in relation to the market dynamics in steel, apparel, and medical electronic instruments and imaging and the role of workplace practices in achieving competitive advantage are also examined. Next, the authors delve into the issue of how the structure and content of work in high-performance work systems differ from the more traditional forms of work in the manufacturing field; that is then followed by these findings being documented from chapters 7 through 10. This is concluded with a discussion of the mechanisms through which high-performance work systems can affect productivity growth.

19. Appelbaum, Eileen, and Rosemary Batt. *The New American Workplace: Transforming Work Systems in the United States*. Ithaca, NY: ILR Press, 1994.

Keywords: sociotechnical, flexible

The changes in American workplace design that have been taking place and that appear impossible to ignore in the future are investigated. Part 1 "The Challenge" introduces the reader to the problems with American workplaces and explains how the framework for cumulative growth in productivity (via mass production) has disintegrated. As a result, fundamental change is necessary. The traditional American institutional framework, however, stands as an obstacle to this change. The two strategies—the American human resource model and the lowering of costs approach—are discussed. However, these are reforms of the mass production system rather than fundamental reorganizations.

In other countries during the same timeframe, alternative production systems were emerging. These systems are the focus of chapter 3 of part 2. Self-managed teams, quality circles, training, worker participation, codetermination, work councils and other approaches adopted by United States organizations are described. The authors stress that piecemeal adoptions of these strategies will not prove successful without supportive climate, institutions and polices. Chapter 4 researches four work models: Swedish sociotechnical systems, Japanese lean production, flexible specialization (Italy) and German diversified quality production. Each model is described in terms of its management methods, work organization, human resource practices and industrial relations.

Part 3 "Alternative Strategies in the United States" seeks to assess the impact and results of these imported strategies. The evidence of surveys between 1982 and 1993 is considered in chapter 5. Chapter 6 outlines the results of case studies executed between 1970 and 1992. Once again, the results show that alternatives have only been implemented on a piecemeal basis and "do not add up to a coherent alternative to mass production."

The obstacles to adopting coherent alternatives as well as how to overcome them at the organizational and policy levels are presented in the fourth and final section. However, "high-performance" workplaces do exist, the authors argue, in organizations that have combined the best features of sociotechnical and lean production systems along with American human resource and industrial relations practices.

20. Applebaum, Herbert. *The Concept of Work: Ancient, Medieval and Modern*. SUNY Series in the Anthropology of Work. Albany: State University of New York Press, 1992.

Keywords: history

The author adopts a historical and anthropological perspective to study the experience of work in ancient, pre-industrial and modern periods. The book benefits from a holistic approach that regards work as a fundamental human activity embedded in the fabric of society. "Seeing culture as if one whole," such an approach views "work as influencing and being influenced by all other basic institutions in a culture." The author also recognizes that all human activity in a society is profoundly affected by "the manner in which work is organized and the way in which it is conceptualized."

Various definitions and conceptions of work are discussed in relation to their appropriate historical context, with particular attention given to the implications of these conceptions for human well-being and the quality of life in general. In addition, the crucial role of technology to human work is extensively reviewed. See especially chapter 19 "Modern Technology and Work" for insightful data on the dehumanization of work, technology and unemployment, organizational change, deskilling, QWL, the control of work, the social impact of technologies, etc.

The conclusion and final summary of the text offer various thoughts on the future of work, proposals for ensuring a high quality of working life and the role of governments in planning and designing of healthy work environments.

Overall, this is an excellent historical overview of the conceptualization of work throughout the ages.

21. Argyle, Michael. *The Social Psychology of Work.* 2nd ed. London: Penguin Books, 1989.

Keywords: psychology, sociology, industrial democracy, QWL

This volume continues a long-established tradition of research in the social psychology of work that began with the famous Hawthorne studies of the 1930s and the Tavistock Institute of Human Relations.

The author introduces the book by outlining the weaknesses of early theories of behavior at work. Classical organization theory, for example, is criticized because it "left out any reference to groups, had an inadequate view of motivation and led to boring, repetitive jobs."

In reviewing the history of work (particularly modern industrial work) Argyle considers some of the major social problems created: alienation and low job satisfaction, low motivation and productivity, industrial and organizational conflict, and problems of technological change.

Chapter 3 provides a summary of issues related to technology and job design. Areas discussed include the following: job enlargement; flexible work groups; job enrichment; the Quality of Working Life movement; sociotechnical systems; and social organization of the workplace. The importance of working groups, social interaction, communication and problem solving is the topic of chapter 6, and organizational change in the context of industrial democracy is the focus of chapter 8. In terms of preventive and healthy work strategies, chapter 10 is of particular interest. A good summary of research results on stress and physical and mental health is provided here. See also chapter 12 "The Future of Work" for programs and policies relating to the creation of "ideal working conditions."

22. Arnesen, Eric, Julie Greene, and Bruce Laurie, eds. *Labor Histories: Class, Politics, and the Working-Class Experience*. The Working Class in American History. Chicago: University of Illinois Press, 1998.

Keywords: labor, United States, history, working class, labor movement, trade unions, labor policy

The essays in this book stem from the basic argument that class has been and remains a central category of analysis that is indispensable to the study of working people and to the history of the United States. In doing so, topics such as ethnicity, religion, migrant laborers, gender, and agricultural history are explored, demonstrating the diversity of this field.

23. Arnetz, Bengt B. "Technological Stress: Psychophysiological Aspects of Working with Modern Information Technology." *Scandinavian Journal of Work, Environment, and Health* 23, no. 3 (1997): S97-S103.

Keywords: computers, stress, telecommunications, human factors

The author argues that "the two-way interaction between the external information technology environment and bodily and mental reactions needs to be taken more into account in the design and use of modern information technology." Understandably, it is reported that "there appears to be an increased awareness of human factors when the risks and benefits of the rapid spread of information technology are discussed."

The purpose of the study presented here "was to evaluate prospectively the impact of a controlled stress-management program on psychosocial well-being, efficiency, and physiological stress indicators." The author indicates that "numerous studies have shown that the great majority of computerization projects fail to meet their deadlines with the originally specified functionality mainly because human factors are not sufficiently taken into account during the planning and implementation phase of the project. . . . In a study of the bodily, mental, and psychophysiological reactions of employees involved in the design of advanced telecommunications systems and of office employees using regular video display technology, several stress-related psychosomatic disorders have been identified." They include sleep disturbances, psychophysiological stress and somatic complaints. Controlled intervention programs aimed at enhancing organizational structures and individual coping strategies have been proved effective in counteracting the negative side effects of working with information technology.

24. Arnopoulos, Sheila, and McGill Human Resource Associates, Inc. *Participative Management in an Advanced Technology Plant: Canadian General Electric in Bromont*. Montreal: McGill Human Resource Associates, Inc., 1985.

Keywords: participation, work design, teams, case study

The Canadian General Electric jet engine blade and vane plant in Bromont, Quebec, opened in 1983, consists of self-managing teams with participative management and job rotation. The report describes the social design of the plant through Arnopoulos' uncritical praise as well as through worker interviews. The case study compliments the plant's strategies for decisions by consensus, innovative workers, network, not hierarchy, employee input into workplace design, designing a participative management workplace and gain sharing. The result is a plant with lower staff requirements, lower absenteeism, high productivity and fewer manufacturing losses.

25. Aronowitz, Stanley, and Jonathan Cutler, eds. *Post-Work: The Wages of Cybernation*. New York: Routledge, 1998.

Keywords: automation, unemployment, labor movement, general

This is a transdisciplinary series of essays that focus on issues concerning the reconceptualization of the notion and practice of work. The essays are directed at helping the reader better understand the nature of various economic, political and technological changes underway, their consequences, and what labor and other social movements might do about them. The contributors address everything from the current state of the labor movement to the impact of computerization of work, the fight for a guaranteed income, and the struggle for shorter work hours, as well as the relationship between school and work, alternative organizations of labor, and the role of welfare. After the introduction, "The Post-Work Manifesto" leads the volume with a critique of contemporary economic trends and a call to action. The manifesto concludes with suggestions that "may infuse many social movements as we edge toward the millennium."

In chapters 2, 3, and 4, Michael Lewis, William DiFazio and Lynn Chancer discuss the case for a moral right to income, a justification of the right to employment, and why there is no movement of the poor in America. Louis Weiner examines the "education to work" controversy in chapter 5—that is, "the notion that if the American workforce were more highly-skilled, adept at analytical thinking, and problem solving, the economy would be more competitive internationally, generating jobs equally well-paying as those being lost." In chapter 6 "From Chaplin to Dilbert: The Origins of Computer Concepts" Joan Greenbaum explores one of the crucial aspects of the current economic debate: the impact of computers in the white-collar workplace.

26. Aronowitz, Stanley, and William DiFazio. *The Jobless Future: Sci-tech and the Dogma of Work.* Minneapolis: University of Minnesota Press, 1994.

Keywords: computers, automation, unemployment

This volume examines the relationship between technological change (specifically computerization and automation) and joblessness. The authors suggest that "all of the contradictory tendencies involved in the restructuring of global capital and computer-mediated work seem to lead to the same conclusion for workers of all collars—that is, unemployment, underemployment, decreasingly skilled work, and relatively lower wages."

The book argues that the scientific-technological revolution of our time—largely attributable to various applications of computer-based information technologies—"is not confined to new electronic processes but also affects organizational changes in the structure of corporations. It has fundamentally altered the forms of work, skill, and occupation. The whole notion of tradition and identity of persons with their work has been radically changed."

The authors describe the way in which technological innovation is no longer episodic. Rather, "technological change has been routinized. Not only has abstract knowledge come to the center of the world's political economy, but there is also a tendency to produce and trade in symbolic significations rather than concrete products."

The full implications of this technological transformation for employment and unemployment are analyzed most closely in part 1 "Techno-science and Joblessness." See chapter 1 "The New Knowledge Work," chapter 2 "Technoculture and the Future of Work," chapter 3 "The End of Skill?", chapter 4 "The Computerized Engineer and Architect," and chapter 5 "The Professionalized Scientist."

27. Artandi, Susan. "Computers and the Post-Industrial Society: Symbiosis or Information Tyranny?" *Journal of the American Society for Information Science,* September 1982: 302-6.

Keywords: computers, post-industrial society, automation

The world is moving toward a post-industrial society in which knowledge and information are strategic resources. Central to this society are information, communication, and computer technology implying social changes that in turn imply major policy questions. There is a need to consider the present and future effect of large-scale computerization on the individual's rights, style of life, method of work, and the ways in which society and institutions operate.

28. Association for Computing Machinery. *Conference on Computers and the Quality of Life*. Washington, DC: George Washington University, 1990.

Keywords: general, computers, quality of life

This volume contains papers and abstracts of papers presented on Computers and the Quality of Life at George Washington University in September 1990. The conference, sponsored by the ACM Special Interest Group on Computers and Society, represented an experimental attempt to hold a single conference that included many diverse areas—resisting the current trend toward ever more specialized meetings.

The position argued by the contributors to this volume is that "by its very nature, study in the discipline of Computers and Society depends on computer technology, sociology, psychology, philosophy, law, management, and organization theory, as well as the many application areas affected." To this end the articles in this volume bring a diversity of perspectives on almost all relevant issues bearing on computers and society.

Topics explored in some detail include the following: "Teaching Computers and Society Courses"; "Information Systems"; "Social Transformations and Quality of Life"; "Democratic Participation and Computing"; "Computer Impacts on Work"; "Computer Ethics"; "Computer Services for the Aged"; "Computers and the Physically Handicapped"; "Information Systems and On-Line Networking"; "Expert Systems and Clinical Practice"; "Computers and Health Care"; and "New Communications Technology."

29. Avery, Christine, and Diane Zabel. *The Flexible Workplace: A Source of Information and Research*. Westport, CT: Quorum Books, 2001.

Keywords: hours of labor, flexible, part-time employment, workweek

Even though there is a large body of literature on the changing nature of work and workplace flexibility, there are but a few that synthesize the research on all aspects of this topic. The main goal of the book is to remedy this situation. The chapters explain the concepts of flexible work, trace the origin and growth of this workplace trend, and review the research on a range of flexible work arrangements. Also identified are aspects of the subject that warrant additional research, as well as strategies for locating additional information, including relevant books, databases, reports, newsletters, Internet sources, videos, organizations, and search terms.

30. Axtell, Carolyn M., and Sharon K. Parker. "Promoting Role Breadth Self-efficacy through Involvement, Work Redesign, and Training." *Human Relations* 56, no. 1 (January 2003): 113-31.

Keywords: employee empowerment, employee development, self-sufficiency, organizational behavior

The influence of organizational practices on role breadth self-efficacy (RBSE)—a person's confidence in performing proactive, interpersonal tasks that go beyond traditional boundaries—is examined. A longitudinal study showed that increased task control, membership of an active improvement group, and breadth of training were associated with increased RBSE. Providing a stronger basis for causal inference, membership of active improvement groups at time I also had a positive lagged effect on later RBSE. These findings support the proposition that RBSE can be enhanced via organizational intervention. The study also showed that, after controlling for greater involvement, job enlargement had a negative lagged effect on RBSE. This suggests the potential detrimental consequences of enlarging jobs without also expanding employees' autonomy and influence.

31. Ayres, Robert U., and Karl H. Ebel. "Human Factors in CIM." 219-44 in *Computer Integrated Manufacturing*, edited by Robert U. Ayres. The Past, the Present, and the Future 2. London: Chapman and Hall, 1991.

Keywords: CIM, skill, automation, anthropocentric

The debate over the role of humans in the manufacturing process rages on. Some argue for the importance of workers' experience and skills while others strive for the "unmanned factory." This chapter presents the debate in a clear manner, discussing various anthropocentric and technocentric strategies, and their apparent effectiveness. It is concluded that the technocentric approach to CIM cannot be effective because flexible automation requires highly qualified and motivated workers who are capable of dealing with relatively frequent equipment breakdowns and software problems. The central question investigated is, "To what extent can machines be expected to take over other (control) functions of human workers in the near future, thus becoming direct substitutes for human labor?" Different types of mental and physical tasks are analyzed in terms of how suitable machines and/or humans are at performing them. Practical guidelines for designing CIM systems with human considerations are also presented.

32. Babson, Steve. *Lean Work: Empowerment and Exploitation in the Global Auto Industry*. Detroit: Wayne State University Press, 1995.

Keywords: lean production, health, industrial relations, policy, case study, participation, comparative

This collection of essays uses a critical and comparative perspective "to address the primary questions of what a lean-flexible production system is [in the automobile industry], and how it affects work and workers." The authors also consider a number of related questions in order to determine whether lean work facilitates empowerment of workers or tends to exploit them.

The following basic questions are examined: "What . . . are the performance outcomes of lean production in terms of productivity and quality and how can these be measured? Does lean-flexible production empower workers and enhance their skills? Is it a 'fragile' system that depends on voluntary worker participation? Or can the system exploit workers and strengthen management control?" And one of the most crucial questions, "What are the appropriate tools/goals of public policy in guiding work re-structuring?"

Various components of lean production systems, such as employee involvement, flexible specialization and team or group work programs are analyzed in the context of the questions noted above. The implementation of lean work in unionized and non-unionized settings is extensively discussed, as is the extent of worker resistance to these systems. The volume also has a strong cross-cultural component, assessing the lean work experience in the United States, Europe, Mexico, Germany and Japan.

In general, the essays suggest that lean production systems work best in sociocultural settings with a history of labor-management cooperation. In other settings such systems may seem exploitative of labor. Thus, Paul Adler suggests that the Toyota production system at New United Motor Manufacturing, Inc. (NUMMI) at Fremont, California, may be viewed at best as a system of "democratic Taylorism" (chapter 11). Mike Parker and Jane Slaughter go further and offer a scathing critique of the book *The Machin That Changed the World* (that had lauded lean production unreservedly) and refer to lean production as "management by stress" (chapter 2).

33. Bacharach, Samuel B., and Edward J. Lawler, eds. *Organizational Politics.* Research in the Sociology of Organizations. Stamford, CT: Jai Press, 2000.

Keywords: organizational politics, institutional politics, social networks, interorganizational relations

There are a range of papers used in this book that try to ascertain how notions of organizational politics are currently being explored. The first paper approaches political problems in organizations by applying the principles of self-interest, of legitimacy, and of inertia. It is argued that these principles are affected by sociocultural forces, and that they work concurrently to affect politics in organizations and systems of organizations. The next paper takes the notion of paranoia and puts it within the context of organizational analysis. By linking paranoia with the personality construct and the notion of political action, specifically the political actions of leaders, its influence on tactical action within organizations is demonstrated. The third paper deals with a general assumption of organizational politics that there is a correlation between how people view politics in their organizations and their political behavior as individuals. The following paper offers the observation that organizational theorists who focus on power tend to ignore issues of structure. The fifth paper maintains that legitimacy processes are closely connected with organizational politics, meaning that the correlation between an organization and its environment affects interorganizational legitimacy processes, which are defined as the collective recognition of, and orientation to, binding rules. The next paper states that even though some organizational researchers have explored interorganizational politics and others have focused on the political behavior of organizations within the context of their environment, the fact remains that organizational politics occur inside as well as outside organizations. The final paper explores the political processes of institutional change by examining how the capital distribution system has been affected by different courses of action.

34. Bachrach, Peter, and Aryeh Botwinick. *Power and Empowerment: A Radical Theory of Participatory Democracy*. Philadelphia: Temple University Press, 1992.

Keywords: participation, democracy, comparative

This book presents an innovative interpretation of participatory democracy as a social scientific concept capable of becoming "a full-blown theory of democracy." The author argues that "the objective of participatory democracy is . . . not just to democratize the workplace for its own sake, but to have the workplace emerge as a point of leverage from which to achieve a more egalitarian redistribution of power, leading to a greater democratization of the entire political process."

The author further contends that "if participation is to develop into an effective strategy for democratizing American society, it needs . . . the support, legitimation, and guidance that social scientists could readily provide." According to the author, many democratic theorists who favor the democratization of industry have nonetheless "carefully avoided the problem of implementation."

See, in particular, chapter 2 for "A Critical Analysis and Reconstruction of Participatory Theory." See chapter 4 for a discussion of "Workplace Democracy in Europe" and chapter 5 for an analysis of "Workplace Democracy in America." Chapter 8 examines "Class Struggle: A Key Concept of Democratic Theory" and chapter 9 considers "Democracy as Praxis."

35. Badham, R. "Human-centered CIM." *Futures*, December 1991: 1047-60.

Keywords: CIM, anthropocentric

The work design philosophy embodied in the human-centered computer integrated manufacturing (CIM) approach provides a radical alternative to traditional technology-oriented and Taylorist approaches to CIM. In order to extend the work that has been done on redesigning factory production and planning tools and systems, this approach can usefully be enhanced by drawing on research on "simultaneous engineering" and the technical and organizational redesign of the design/manufacturing interface. The vision of the "informated" factory of the future embodied in this human-centered CIM vision provides a much needed challenge to traditional guiding images of the ideal automated factory.

36. Baglioni, Guido. *Impossible Democracy? The Progress and Problems of Participation in the Firm*. Aldershot, UK: Avebury, 1996.

Keywords: participation, democracy, comparative

This study "reviews the concepts and experiences that have marked employees' participation in the firm, within capitalist economies, over the last century." The author regards workers' participation as "seeking to alter or improve employment relationships, working conditions and often also workers' socioeconomic standing in society." A comparative approach is used covering European countries, the United States and Japan.

The author's aim is to evaluate the phenomenon of employee participation "free from ideological constraints, with an eye to solutions that are realistically viable."

After analyzing the different models that have shaped the notion of participation, the author "focuses on two key issues: the relationship between participation and political democracy, and that between participation and the firm's functioning."

The overall features and models of participation are presented in chapter 1. The problems involved are highlighted in the introduction, and the author's perspective is given in chapters 7 and 8. The progress of participatory experience is discussed in chapters 2 through 6 and current proposals are offered in the last part of chapter 8.

37. Bar-Hayim, Aviad, and Gerald S. Berman. "Ideology, Solidarity, and Work Values: The Case of the Histadrut Enterprises." *Human Relations* (Tavistock Institute of Human Relations) 44, no. 4 (1991).

Keywords: participation, organizational culture, equality, democracy

This research study examines various aspects of work and organizational culture in Israeli collectivist industrial enterprises known as "Histadrut" (General Federation of Labor in Israel). These economic/industrial organizations are designed with a well-functioning cooperative structure and ideology that makes them "particularly suitable for exploring organizational culture. . . . In short, the Histadrut's goal has been to create a non-exploitative free workers' society in which labor and capital are not alienated from each other." Some of the ideals of this strong collectivist culture are "employment for everyone, equality among employees, solidarity, mutual help, etc."

The authors note that with the adoption of modern industrial processes (necessary to improve productivity and competitiveness) in the Histadrut, traditional collectivist values have been strained. The article discusses the methods by which the Histadrut has attempted to resolve this dilemma and "democratize the working life in the labor economy." Strategies and methods reviewed include the following: committees, workers' representation on company boards of directors, and vocational and professional training for managers and workers.

Essentially the study reveals a growing split between the older enterprises of the Histadrut (that emphasize the "collectivist values of class solidarity, mutual help, and the importance of work and labor unions") and the newer enterprises, "where a different cultural pattern prevails (one that is indifferent to class solidarity and focuses instead on personal rewards, job satisfaction, etc.)."

38. Barker, Kathleen, and Kathleen Christensen, eds. *Contingent Work: American Employment Relations in Transition*. Ithaca, NY: Cornell University Press, 1998.

Keywords: temporary employment, part-time employment, seasonal labor, piece work, contract system, employee fringe benefits, law and legislation, labor laws and legislation

In 1997 the Teamsters went on strike against UPS. This strike, won by the Teamsters due in large part to their public support, highlighted the impact of contingent work—an umbrella term used to describe a variety of tenuous and insecure employment arrangements such as employee leasing, temping, some self employment, independent contracting, and part-time or part-year work. This book argues that contingent work represents a profound deviation from the employment relations model that dominated most of the last century's labor relations, and in doing so delineates essential features of contingent work from both the organization's and the worker's point of view. Also examined are the business forces driving contingent work, as well as an assessment of the consequences that this type of work has on the individual, the community and the family by taking issues such as race, class, and gender into account. This is then followed by questions on how current labor and employment laws need to be rewritten to provide contingent workers with the same sort of job security and protection that is offered to full-time employees.

39. Barley, Stephen R. *The New World of Work*. London: British-North American Committee, 1996.

Keywords: computers, automation, skill, hierarchy, knowledge

Barley predicts that there will be a vast increase in technical jobs and occupations in the future. Moreover, computers and other technologies will continue to introduce a technical component into non-technical jobs. Based on empirical evidence provided in the book, the author contends that these trends will lead to a shift from vertical to horizontal organization structures. He cites corporate growth, the commercialization of scientific knowledge and technological change as the main reasons for this flattening of organizations. Corporate growth is leading to professional bureaucracies (groups) that can offer more equipment and facilities and will therefore need more technicians. Similarly, the commercialization of scientific knowledge and technological change will lead to new technical jobs and occupations. The specialized nature of science and engineering makes a vertical structure very difficult, since the people in the high end of the hierarchy are expected to have the knowledge to understand the work of everybody below them.

This new world of work will include a new "class" of jobs that cannot fit into the established categories of professional/craft white-collar/blue-collar work. Because of the education, knowledge and skill required to be a technician, it will become difficult to place them at the bottom of the hierarchy, as was done until recently. How can a manager who has no understanding of the technician's work and who is perhaps less educated exercise authority over him or her? The argument for flatter organizational structures is once again supported. Barley goes on to analyze the implications of these new trends. Although he does not directly address it, the implications for healthy work are significant. An implicit conclusion of this work is that the control dimension of work will increase and the demand dimension will improve.

40. Barns, Ian. "Post-Fordist People? Cultural Meanings of New Techno-economic Systems." *Futures*, November 1991: 895-914.

Keywords: Fordism, culture, sociology

This article applies Langdon Winner's concept of technologies as "forms of life" to the task of interpreting the cultural meanings of a (possibly) emerging "post-Fordist" social order. The particular focus of interest is on the kinds of persons and communities that a post-Fordist society might produce. The four writers examined—Morton Schoolman, Stuart Hall, David Harvey, and Donna Haraway—reflect a wide diversity of views about the emancipatory potential opened up by a new order resulting from the diffusion of new technologies. Despite their differences, these writers do help us to see the importance of a form of moral discourse which on the one hand takes seriously the significance of technoeconomic changes in shaping human identities, and on the other attempts to articulate a vision of human meaning that can shape technological change for just and emancipatory social purposes.

41. Barrett, Richard S. *Challenging the Myths of Fair Employment Practices*. Westport, CT: Quorum Books, 1998.

Keywords: employee selection, employee tests, discrimination in employment, employment tests

Concerned primarily with the employment of minorities, women, and older or disabled workers, the book seeks to demystify legal, professional, and ethical issues relating to testing procedures for employment. There are three main themes that run throughout Barrett's argument. The first concerns a description of current good practice. The second deals with the validity of claims. The third is an assessment of the adverse impact of contemporary practices upon minorities, the disabled, and women.

Targeted toward human resource managers as well as other executives who deal with employment equity issues, the book covers law and regulations, test objectives and job analysis, non-cognitive selection procedures, cognitive and other kinds of tests, issues of validation, intentional discrimination and adverse impact, ethical and legal considerations, equity laws and acts, as well as statistics and various appendices.

42. Bassman, Emily. *Abuse in the Workplace: Management Remedies and Bottom Line Impact*. Westport, CT: Quorum Books, 1992.

Keywords: stress, case study, psychology, QWL, policy

This fascinating and unique book by a psychologist employed as a human resource planner probes into an area of social/behavioral research that it would appear has been largely unexplored. The author examines various forms of employee abuse in the workplace, "the causes for its increase over the past decade, organizational factors that both promote it and prevent it from coming to light and interventions necessary to prevent its occurrence or minimize the damage." Special attention is also given to "organizational development issues such as quality, employee involvement, and managing diversity for their influence in creating an environment that minimizes abusive practices."

Personal accounts and documented stories of mistreatment are effectively used to amplify and dramatize the central themes discussed in the text.

The importance of properly addressing employee abuse is underscored by an assessment of the many consequences and costs (both direct and indirect). Those noted include the following: "stress, disability claims, workers' compensation claims, medical costs, lawsuits (including wrongful discharge) . . . poor quality (of work), high turnover, absenteeism, poor customer relationships . . . sabotage . . . lowered employee commitment, etc."

The relevance and timeliness of the insights provided in this volume cannot be overemphasized. Because of the prevailing economic climate, the prevalence of overwork, and the extreme "pressures on companies today to improve performance, new stresses are introduced between manager and employee." And, as the author points out, it is the employee who is usually the victim "when these stresses cause the relationship to become dysfunctional."

In the context of preventive practices and strategies for positive change, chapters 11 through 14 are the most pertinent. Chapter 11 discusses company programs with the potential to assist employees in coping with stress in the workplace. These include employee assistance programs (EAPs), wellness programs, non-union grievance systems and employee surveys.

Chapter 12 "develops a framework for senior management to ensure that abusive management is not tolerated." The importance of building a supportive organizational culture to promote the well-being of employees is stressed.

Chapter 13 further examines organizational culture and provides a practical organizing model based on selective values, behavior and feedback.

Chapter 14 offers three fundamental suggestions for company employees who desire a transformation of the workplace that will result in "a healthier, fairer, more empowering, more productive, and more profitable enterprise."

43. Becker, Franklin, and Fritz Steele. *Workplace by Design: Mapping the High-Performance Workscape*. San Francisco: Jossey-Bass, 1995.

Keywords: work design, workplaces, health, safety, competitiveness, teams

Workplaces must be considered as systems and not as the sum of desks, computers and walls. The interrelationship between workers and their workspaces must also be recognized as having a powerful influence on the performance of the organization. These are the foundations on which the principles of the re-engineered office presented in this book are based. Part 1 "The Workplace as a Tool for Achieving Goals" introduces the concept of organizational ecology and how it can lead to a high-performance workplace. Geared toward managers and executives who are encouraged to implement office re-engineering, the incentives they are provided are *not* reduced absenteeism, more healthy and satisfied workers and thus higher productivity. Instead, the book asserts that higher productivity and competitiveness result solely out of the better use of space. Chapter 6 "Creating a Healthy Environment" is an exception to this mindset, for the importance of worker well-being is acknowledged here. This chapter discusses the history of the worker health and safety movement, sick-building syndrome, worker comfort and control, safety and security, physical fitness, natural light, employee facilities and green buildings.

In the remainder of part 1, workspace design considerations for new ways of working such as teamwork, non-territorial offices, telecommuting and cross-functional collaboration are suggested. This section is summarized by a chapter outlining various re-engineering strategies and required organizational structures. Part 2 elaborates further on leadership roles, planning processes and how to implement high-performance office strategies. Case studies of corporations are provided throughout.

44. Beder, Sharon. *Selling the Work Ethic: From Puritan Pulpit to Corporate PR*. London: Zed Books, 2000.

Keywords: work and wealth, status and success, motivating work, coercion and persuasion, conditioning, hours of work

Nowadays, society revolves around work. This raises questions such as how did paid work come to be so central to our lives? and why do so many people need their job to tell them who they are and what to do with themselves? The author examines the origins and practices of work in a culture in which the wealthy are respected and inequality is justified. However, these values are neither natural nor inevitable; they have been actively promoted—through the education system, religious preaching, socialization, and corporate propaganda—by those who benefit the most from them. This book provides an absorbing account and critique of this central aspect of modern capitalist society.

45. Beechey, Veronica, and Tessa Perkins. *A Matter of Hours: Women, Part-time Work and the Labor Market*. Cambridge, UK: Polity Press, 1987.

Keywords: part-time, labor, feminism, policy, women

Several sociological perspectives (particularly labor process and feminist theory) are used in this book to assess the issue of part-time work, especially as it relates to women's experience. Included is a detailed analysis of part-time employment in several British industrial settings. Policy implications and the development of a comprehensive theoretical framework are also emphasized.

The central argument of the authors is that "gender enters into the construction of part-time jobs and that the division between full-time and part-time work is one crucial contemporary manifestation of gender within the sphere of production."

This is a significant work, not so much for its direct contribution to preventive or health-related work strategies, but for its focus on gender as an important factor in the overall social and psychological health of the working population.

46. Beehr, Terry A. *Psychological Stress in the Workplace*. People and Organizations. London: Routledge, 1995.

Keywords: stress, health, support, psychology, stress management

In this empirically-grounded work, an organizational psychology perspective is used to study occupational stress. The importance of the subject is underscored by reference to the social psychology, health and economic costs involved. The reputed billions of dollars lost each year because of job stress are due to, among other noted factors, "increased costs of medical insurance to employers and employees, stress pressure on medical facilities and professionals . . . lost productivity due to illness," etc.

The lack of consensus that surrounds the definition of stress is discussed (and attributed largely to the variety of disciplines through which the subject is studied as well as the personal proclivities of the various researchers) along with the problems this poses for prevention and treatment.

Topics covered in the book include the following: various research techniques and models, stressors in the workplace; outcomes of occupational stress (as they pertain to both individuals and organizations); treatments of organizational stress (with a separate chapter on social support); and directions for future research.

Qualitative and quantitative methods are employed throughout the text to explain four basic approaches to occupational stress.

Two areas of special interest in this volume that are often underexplored in other treatments of the subject are (1) the role of time in mediating job stress and (2) the spillover effect of work-related stress outside of the workplace. The inclusion of both of these important factors in the text represents a significant addition to the literature on occupational stress.

47. Bell, Daniel. *The Coming of Post-Industrial Society: A Venture in Social Forecasting*. New York: Basic Books, 1973.

Keywords: post-industrial society, sociology, knowledge, technology, white-collar work, information, rationalization, forecasting

In this now classic sociological work, Daniel Bell argues that advanced industrial societies are entering a new phase in their development. He suggests that this will make them as different from what we now know as "industrial society" as such societies differed from "pre-industrial" ones. Bell believes that the characteristics of this new "post-industrial" society are be to found in the spheres of technology, the economy and the social structure. The economy undergoes a shift from being a predominantly manufacturing one to a service one; in technology, the new science/knowledge-based industries become central; and in the social structure we see "the rise of new technical elites and the advent of a new principle of stratification." The suggestion is that a new type of occupational structure develops in which white-collar workers outnumber blue-collar ones and in which the professional, scientific, and technical occupations become predominant. For Bell, this latter trend follows from the essential principle underlying the new type of society: the emergence of "theoretical knowledge" as the basis for innovation and policy making. Post-industrial society is thus a "knowledge society," and it is taken to follow that those occupations that possess theoretical knowledge will—on the principle that knowledge is power—come to exert a controlling influence on society.

Some social theorists have argued that the greatest weakness in Bell's thesis lies in his assumption that there is anything novel about the centrality of knowledge to economic and working life. For example, Tony J. Watson (1987) contends that "the growth of industrialism and the rise of capitalism were both dependent on the increasing application of rational-calculative thinking to social life—thus, the growth of scientific and technical qualifications among the population is all part of the rationalization process that Max Weber saw as characterizing western history over several centuries."

It has also been argued that Bell's thesis underplays the significant role of conflict in society emerging from the rise of a technocratic elite in the post-industrial era.

48. Benders, Jos, Job de Haan, and David Bennett, eds. *The Symbiosis of Work and Technology*. London: Taylor and Francis, 1995.

Keywords: work design, sociotechnical, anthropocentric, case study, comparative

"Symbiotic approaches" to work design is the subject of these workshop papers. The term encompasses the approaches usually referred to as sociotechnical, human-centered or anthropocentric. The term symbiotic is preferred by the editors because, unlike the others, it does not imply that social or human aspects are more important than the technical aspects. The articles seek to gather information on various symbiotic approaches from around the world in order to answer questions such as: "Why have previous symbiotic methods not realized their promising potential? What actions need to be undertaken to create more favorable conditions for the implementation of contemporary symbiotic approaches? What are the basic differences and similarities between the different methods? Is there anything new, or are these approaches basically the same?" The contributions cover various symbiotic approaches and issues such as the new paradigm of *Leitbild* for the design of production systems, modern sociotechnolgy, the history of the Swedish sociotechnical approach, the comparison of Swedish and Japanese management systems, German experiences with *Technikgestaltung* (shaping of technology), managing sociotechnical change, a case study on the "smart manufacturing techniques" project, the American perspective and a British application of human-centered design techniques for computer-aided design for control engineers.

49. Bengtsson, Jarl. "Human Resource Development." *Futures*, December 1991: 1085-106.

Keywords: technology, human resources

In addressing the complex issues of the relationship between new technologies and human resources, different methodological approaches can be applied. A rich source of studies exists at the micro level, i.e., enterprises and/or sectors that focus, in particular, on the qualitative changes taking place. Fewer studies exist on the macro level for this subject, given its complexity and lack of adequate data. This article addresses the issues from both perspectives, but findings from the micro perspective predominate. It is structured around developments and changes on the demand and supply side and their interaction. The final section identifies some principal policy issues for governments as they relate both to demand and supply measures, as well as the need to strengthen the database for a better understanding of the issues involved. It draws heavily on recent and ongoing work on the subject carried out with OECD/Center for Educational Research and Innovation (CERI).

50. Berberoglu, Berch, ed. *Labor and Capital in the Age of Globalization: The Labor Process and the Changing Nature of Work in the Global Economy*. Lanham, MD: Rowman & Littlefield, 2002.

Keywords: labor, United States, labor movement, working class, capitalism, globalization, economic aspects, social conflict, Marxian economics

Globalization has become an ever increasing factor in everyday life, and this in turn has had an effect on the nature and dynamics of work in the global economy. The essays provided in this book illustrate the varied forms of labor control and exploitation by the transnational corporations of the dominant imperialist states by providing insights on the labor process and modes of work, and the impact of globalization on the labor movement, on the role of women and minorities in the labor force, and on the terms of class conflict.

51. Berger, Peter L., ed. *The Human Shape of Work: Studies in the Sociology of Occupations*. Chicago: Henry Regnery, 1964.

Keywords: division of labor, case study, stress, work design, sociology, psychology

This collection of essays by sociologists seeks to understand the social relations involved in various occupations from a firsthand view. The writers explore the impact of the social surroundings on the worker as well as how the worker influences his or her environment. Five chapters on five occupations—the apartment building janitor, the assembly-line worker, the engineering technician, the advertising man and the business executive—and a final chapter entitled "Some General Observations on the Problem of Work" make up this book. This concluding chapter addresses deskilling, job dissatisfaction, the extreme division of labor and the meaning of work to the individual.

The chapter on the assembly-line worker is of particular interest. Ely Chinoy outlines the history of the division of labor, standardized parts and conveyor belts. By working on the assembly line, the author learned that the inability to determine one's own pace of work was the principal complaint, although meaninglessness, limited opportunity for socialization, repetitiveness and the absence of interest or challenge are also major problems. Two other finds were that not a single person interviewed in the plant was willing to trade their job for a line job, and that no line workers had anything positive to say about their jobs (except for repair men and fill-in workers who performed a variety of tasks). The paper goes on to look deeper into the effects of assembly-line jobs on the worker. The extremely saddening accounts of job stress, the mad rush to the punch clock at the end of the shift, the need to tranquilize oneself with alcohol and the inability to function at home at the end of the day are told through the words of workers and their families. Although written back in 1964, the author recommends job modification through shortening the line, providing opportunity to change one's pace of work, rearranging the line to allow more interfunctional dependence, group incentives and job enlargement. The main thrust of this classic chapter is that assembly-line work can be separated from other manual labor and treated as a special category on its own because it has distinct problems.

52. Berggren, Christian. "The Evolution and Transplantation of Toyotism." 22-55 in *Alternatives to Lean Production: Work Organization in the Swedish Auto Industry*, edited by Christian Berggren. Ithaca, NY: ILR Press, 1992.

Keywords: lean production, Toyotism, skill, teams

This chapter summarizes the main features of the successful Japanese auto manufacturing production philosophy named "the Toyota system" as developed during the 1950s and 1960s. It includes a description of the basis for its small-batch, flexible, mass production system. "Toyotism" and Taylorism are compared and related in terms of work process, labor deployment, managerial structure and employment relations. Later in the chapter the focus shifts to Japanese plants in North America and the United Kingdom and the conditions necessary for successful operation of these factories, as well as examining the nature of work in these plants. The author concentrates on issues of work in the Western world that include skill development, multiskilling or reskilling, JIT control and worker autonomy, teamwork and the problem of physical strains and work hazards.

53. Bernstein, Paul. *American Work Values: Their Origin and Development.* SUNY Series in the Sociology of Work. Albany: State University of New York Press, 1997.

Keywords: work ethic, United States, history, industrialization, public welfare

The Lutheran-Calvinist emphasis on work for the glory of God is used as a starting point, after which the book shifts to the change in work values that occurred from early industrialization in America to the end of the Great Depression, a period characterized by both opportunity and alienation. This was followed by modern trends that led to the empowerment of employees even as that empowerment tested the values of such participation in a time where downsizing was common. Also touched upon are the debates related to work and welfare during these transformations. The author concludes with a more recent focus on self-fulfilling employment in the context of industrial downsizing.

54. Bertil, Gardell. "Worker Participation and Autonomy: A Multilevel Approach to Democracy at the Workplace." *International Journal of Health Services* 12, no. 4 (1982): 527-33.

Keywords: health, democracy, participation, stress, productivity, case study

The article describes a process toward democracy in the workplace in a Swedish middle-sized manufacturing company producing for the export market. The change process was initiated and engineered by the trade union local in close cooperation with management. Within an overall strategy for increased worker control, the democratized work organization combines codetermination for the local trade union board in strategic management decisions with a system of autonomous production groups, where supervisors have been replaced by "contact people" elected by and responsible to the groups. Through the autonomous groups, all workers participate in decisions about production. The groups decide on all matters related to work performance and take collective responsibility for production results. As an introduction to the case, the paper puts this trade union model for democracy at the workplace in the perspective of a fifty-year development of productivity and worker participation in Scandinavia. The case report deals both with the change process (why and how it came about) and with the outcome of the new work organization for the workers, the union, and the company. It is shown that the new work organization has meant richer job content, increased dignity for workers, increased solidarity among workers, increased trade union activity and strength, as well as a more effective use of productive resources in the company. Despite local peculiarities, it is concluded that the experiences gained from this case can be transferred to other workplaces where workers are interested in having more say, more security, and a more meaningful work situation.

55. Bessant, John, and Sam Cole. *Stacking the Chips: Information Technology and the Distribution of Income*. London: Frances Porter, 1985.

Keywords: technology, human resources, unemployment, comparative, information technology, productivity

The authors examine the potential within the information technology revolution for radical change in the structure of society in terms of the pattern of employment, education, power and wealth. In particular, the impact of information technology on unemployment and on the "pecking order of nations" is considered. The book includes empirical reviews of information technology (with data reflecting a global perspective) and projected effects using computer modeling and analysis. Some of the research questions addressed include the following: "What will be the effect on labor and capital productivity; will the technology create or destroy jobs, where and what kind?"; "What is the relative importance of the indirect versus the direct effect of the technology? How important are intersectoral and international processes?"; "Will the new technology create wealth but destroy jobs? What will be the impact on the distribution of income between capital and labor, or between different kinds of labor?"; "Can domestic and international social policy foster the potential gains and alleviate the potential inequities arising from the new technology?"; and "How can the technology be used to confront the development needs of low income countries?"

See especially chapter 2 "Who Holds the Cards," chapter 3 "The Game So Far: Experiences with Applications of Information Technology," and chapter 4 "Probable, Plausible, and Possible Alternatives: Weighing the Odds."

56. Besser, Terry L. *Team Toyota: Transplanting the Toyota Culture to the Camry Plant in Kentucky*. SUNY Series in the Sociology of Work. Albany: State University of New York Press, 1996.

Keywords: automobile industry workers, employees, industrial sociology, case study, automobile industry and trade, management, corporations, Japan

Toyota's Camry assembly plant in Georgetown, Kentucky, is the focus of an in-depth study in this book. Based on employee interviews, newspaper accounts, analyses of company publications, attendance at company events, and interaction with company employees over a five-year period, both the management and non-management perspectives were documented on how Toyota is replicating its style of management and its team culture in the United States. By using the term "team" as an organizing metaphor, the author is able to demonstrate how Toyota is able to penetrate the small work group, thus increasing employee commitment and recruit support for organizational goal achievement. This metaphor is also used to demonstrate how Toyota coordinates all levels the plant into a "we're all in this together" ethos. Also provided is the team concept that is used to delve further into the issue of work disabilities, as well as an overview of the position of female employees and wives of Japanese executives.

57. Beyerlein, Michael M., Douglas Johnson, and Susan T. Beyerlein, eds. *Team Performance Management*. Advances in Interdisciplinary Studies of Work Teams 6. Stamford, CT: Jai Press, 2000.

Keywords: teams in the workplace

The chapters in this book provide in-depth coverage by addressing the hows and whys that underlie team effectiveness, including such issues as learning, compensation, and empowerment. This topic is growing in interest due to a growth in work teams being tried in many settings, including research and development, government, support services, manufacturing, sales and education, just to name a few. The author finds that high performance levels are not guaranteed by the use of teams; they require flow from the proper design and the continued support of the teams via skill building, empowerment, reward system changes, and information access.

58. Biggs, Lindy. *The Rational Factory: Architecture, Technology and Work in America's Age of Mass Production*. Studies in Industry and Society. Baltimore: Johns Hopkins University Press, 1996.

Keywords: history, rational factory, mass production, efficiency, plant design, work design, case study

This is basically a work of industrial history that combines three elements into its analysis: industrialization itself, industrial architecture, and the transformation of work brought about through industrialization. It examines, as the title indicates, the idea of the thoroughly rational factory, and the engineers who made use of the notion to build the factories of the nineteenth and early twentieth centuries. The author notes that the idea of the rational factory "guided development in large-scale industries whose success depended on control of production." The book is not, however, a history of engineers and their work but, rather, "an exploration of the quest for the perfect factory and what it meant for the people who worked within the system as well as those who designed it."

Biggs examines the manner in which the owners and engineers of industrial plants translated the ideal of the "perfect factory" into a physical design embodying the principles of efficiency, order and control.

The two fundamental stages in the development of the rational factory are analyzed in detail: first, the mechanization of distinct individual operations to facilitate increased production and control; and second, the standardization and regulation of the entire production process through redesign and mechanization of materials handling.

Separate chapters consider such topics as the role of industrial engineers, factory welfare work, rationalization of production methods, and the modernization of factories in both the nineteenth and twentieth centuries. This book provides a good historical overview of the conditions and ideals through which modern work regimes evolved. Two extensive case studies are also presented.

59. Bills, Daniel B., ed. *The New Modern Times: Factors Reshaping the World of Work*. SUNY Series in the Sociology of Work. Albany: State University of New York Press, 1995.

Keywords: human resources, technology, sociology, social change, social aspects, industrial sociology, technological innovations, labor supply

The authors in this volume are concerned with analyzing how technological developments, institutional transformations and demographic changes are altering the nature and pace of work, and how these factors are in turn being transformed by emerging work arrangements. One of the strengths of the book is its recognition of the fact that work and employment are embedded in larger structural/institutional/cultural contexts.

The text is based on strong empirical data and well-documented research—resisting the common tendency in this field of study to make exaggerated claims and speculative projections about future work trends.

Part 1 of the book focuses on "Historical Perspectives" of work, skill, technological change and education. An overview of the industrialization process is presented, touching on major developments in the division of labor, work reorganization, mechanization, etc.

Part 2 discusses "Current Transformations and the Future of Work." Topics examined include the following: working class culture, workplace democracy, collective action, organizational behavior, and technology and work. In addition, a research program is presented that investigates how new organizational structures affect the people who work in them.

All contributors to this book share a common perspective that an understanding of the workplace is basic to an understanding of where our society has been, where it is presently, and where it will be in the future. The assessments, in the American world of work, are made from historical, contemporary, and projected trend points of view. There is also focus on many of the broad causes and consequences of trends in the demographic, institutional, and technological spheres of American society that are continuing to influence both the working and non-working lives of the American public. In doing so, many issues such as the social consequences of new technologies, the fundamental changes in terms of employment, the changing skill levels, and the emerging economic role of women are addressed.

60. Bjerkness, Gro, Pelle Ehn, and Marten Kyng, eds. *Computers and Democracy*. Aldershot, UK: Avebury, 1987.

Keywords: computers, democracy, sociotechnical systems, skill, automation, work design

This volume is "an interdisciplinary collection of articles on design and use of computer-based systems and tools in the context of democratization of work." The first part of the book, "Systems Design and Industrial Democracy," presents different approaches to the question of computers and democracy. These include the following: "the trade union-based Scandinavian tradition," the sociotechnical systems perspective, and "an American contribution advocating a form of enlightened management."

The second part of the text "Skills and Automation" contains a number of articles "ranging from analysis of the impact of computers on skills and work, to cases in which criteria such as the preservation and development of skills have been used as guidelines in design."

The third part of the book, "Not Only Waged Men," discusses "the importance of developing strategies that provide unwaged groups, consumers, and clients with opportunities to influence technology."

The fourth and final section examines "Future Perspectives." Topics discussed include "The Perspective Concept in Information," "Systems Development and Use," and "Safe Expert Systems."

61. Blackburn, Phil, Rob Coombs, and Kenneth Green. "New Technology & Neo-Fordism." 88-107 in *Technology, Economic Growth and the Labor Process*. London: Macmillan Press, 1985.

Keywords: automation, labor process, Fordism, organizational design

This fifth chapter offers a consideration of neo-Fordism within the theme of the book: a comprehensive historical treatment of the relationship between mechanization and the labor process. After raising the point that Fordism can no longer significantly improve productivity, the authors consider how the barriers to successful mass production could be overcome. That is, they are searching for neo-Fordism. The importance of work organization and technological change is emphasized.

After a brief critique of Braverman's theory, the results of Kelly's studies are summarized in detail. The authors settle on a definition of neo-Fordism that involves the following: "*technological* developments in control mechanization that weaken the link between mechanization and scale. This 'flexible' form of mechanization permits increased variability in products and processes to be accommodated at higher levels of mechanization," "*organizational* changes that tend to favor the adoption of work roles, rather than individual repetitive tasks organized on an hierarchical basis," and "*informational* infrastructures that integrate different productive sub-units (semi-autonomous groups, machining centers or different interdependent, geographically-separated production units) with control of materials flow, stock control, and production planning."

62. Blackler, Frank, and David Oborne, eds. *Information Technology and People: Designing for the Future*. Leicester, UK: British Psychological Society, 1987.

Keywords: computers, information technology, anthropocentric

This volume offers a psychological perspective on the issues of technological design and management in relation to information technology (IT). The contributors argue that ineffective application and implementation of IT all too often result in wasted resources, time and effort. "Unless the new technologies are designed and introduced with an appreciation of the needs and reactions of those who will use and be affected by them, the chances that they will operate effectively are slight."

The basic premise of the book is that when it comes to the introduction of information-based technologies, "the application of knowledge about human behavior, actions, thoughts, feelings, education etc. have often been insufficient or missing." In other words, this is a human-centered approach to the subject.

Part 1 deals with "Information Technology and Organizations," part 2 looks at "Information Technology in Health and Education," and part 3 examines "Society and the New Technologies." Sample chapter titles from the book include "Managing Factory Automation," "Ergonomics and the New Technologies," "Expert Systems in the Health Field," "The Computer in the Classroom—Attitudes to Information Technology," and "Information Technology in the Home."

63. Blackwell, Gerry. "Productivity: The Great Leap . . . Sideways." *Canadian Business*, 1992: 78-82.

Keywords: computers, productivity, case study

This article questions the widespread belief that the billions of dollars invested in information technology by companies have resulted in significant productivity gains. It is suggested that many business enterprises have been so busy spending money on all the latest computer and automation equipment that the value of these investments has not been questioned enough.

The case of London Life Insurance Company of London, Ontario, is examined. This particular company held back on the purchase of laptop computers for its sales force (when its competitors rushed out to do so) in order to experiment with a small pilot program designed to determine the effectiveness of sales force automation.

Statistics are cited in the article that show "a discouraging trend in productivity growth in Canada." Meanwhile, spending on information technology has increased dramatically, "making it one of the economy's fastest-growing capital expenditure items." A research and consulting firm quoted in the article contends that "the service sector . . . is now spending 50 percent to 60 percent of its capital investments on information technology. . . . However, the increase in productivity that comes from an increase in expenditures on information technology seems to be—zero." Statistics are also cited from the manufacturing sector—"many companies are overinvesting in information technology—for each additional investment of $1, they are getting only $0.80 back."

The article concludes with some insights on how to better assess the actual benefits of introducing information technology, and how to properly prepare people and companies for the new technology, so as to maximize productivity by paying closer attention to human factors.

64. Blanpain, R., ed. *The Harmonization of Working Life and Family Life*. The Hague: Kluver Law International, 1995.

Keywords: work and family, women, policy, comparative, labor relations, QWL

This volume presents a cross-cultural perspective of issues related to the harmonization of working and family life. Contributions, in the form of regional reports, are from France, Belgium, Italy, Japan, Sweden, Britain, and the United States. Topics discussed include the following: time flexibility; reduction of working hours; parental leave; child benefits and child care facilities; and maternity leave with the right to a guaranteed job upon return to the workplace.

Emphasis is given to the role of government policy and legislation in improving the quality of work and family life, with special attention paid to government policy as it affects working women. The diverse approaches taken by trade unions and employer organizations are also included in the reports.

The editor notes that "in many cases, measures such as working time flexibility and part-time work have been passed without the specific intention of facilitating working and family life but nonetheless this has been a beneficial result. Other countries have made the harmonization of work and family life the hallmark of their labor relations systems."

65. Blauner, Robert. *Alienation and Freedom: The Factory Worker and His Industry*. Chicago: University of Chicago Press, 1964.

Keywords: alienation, sociology, general, case study, assembly line

This is one of the most influential books in modern industrial sociology and the sociology of work and occupations. Blauner reformulates Marx's classic theory of alienation and applies it to workers in four different industrial settings—the print shop, the textile mill, the automobile assembly line, and the automated chemical plant. These four types of industry are chosen to highlight the experience of work in the context of four distinct types of technology: craft, machine-tending, assembly line and "process" technology.

The overall concept of alienation is used to bring together the factors influencing job satisfaction. These "dimensions of alienation," as he calls them, include the following: powerlessness, meaninglessness, isolation and self-estrangement.

Essentially, the work is "a sociological study of the relationships between technology, social structure, and personal experience." The author tries to show that "the worker's relation to organization of the factory determines whether or not he characteristically experiences in that work a sense of control rather than domination; a sense of meaningful purpose rather than futility."

To sum up Blauner's research results, he found that alienation was relatively low in the craft printing industry and the process chemical industry, higher in the machine-tending textile setting and highest on the car assembly line. Since the early 1970s, specialists in industrial sociology and the sociology of work have found serious problems with Blauner's thesis. Some have argued that he trivializes Marx's notion of alienation by conceptualizing it in subjective terms. Others have questioned his inferences from attitude survey data and the representativeness of his sample areas.

The most problematic aspect of his study is probably its failure to consider political context of technology. Blauner suggests that as technology becomes more automated in the future, so will the opportunity for employees to experience increased control, purpose, meaning and self-realization at work. Of course, this completely overlooks the fact that the deskilling of work and greater control exercised over workers are major potential consequences of the introduction of new technology.

Despite the weaknesses in Blauner's classic study, its contribution to sociological theory and a host of research fields that examine the relationship between work organization and health is profound.

66. Bluestone, Barry, and Irving Bluestone. *Negotiating the Future: A Labor Perspective in American Business*. New York: Basic Books, 1992.

Keywords: unions, industrial relations, participation, teams

This comprehensive volume by two leading industrial relations specialists in modern labor-management relations analyzes some of the changes required if American business and industry are to be successful in increasing their productivity, improving the quality of their products and stepping up their rate of innovation. The authors argue that significant change in the workplace is essential for economic survival in an age of fierce international competition.

The book is introduced with a discussion of traditional labor-management practices characterized by "adversarialism" and "authoritarianism." These outdated features of the workplace, which proved to be unworkable in challenging the economic climate of the 1980s and 1990s, are then contrasted with some of the new characteristics of labor-management relations: "teamwork, cooperation, and mutual trust."

Various work reorganization experiments by firms and unions, including "employee involvement," "quality circles," "problem-solving teams," "autonomous work groups" and "participative management," are assessed, both for their strengths and for their limitations.

"Management rights" and "union demands" are also examined in the context of the tension between management's long-standing desire for total control and labor's struggle for the rights of workers and improved working conditions.

In relation to possible applications for preventive work strategies and healthy workplace design, see especially chapter 6 "Employee Involvement in Action" and chapter 7 "Does Participation Work?"

67. Blumberg, Melvin, and Donald Gerwin. "Coping with Advanced Manufacturing Technology." *Journal of Occupational Behavior* 5 (1984): 113-30.

Keywords: computers, automation, comparative, case study, sociotechnical systems

Computer aided manufacturing equipment is supposed to revolutionize batch production by increasing control over this highly uncertain mode of manufacturing. However, as computerized equipment becomes more complex, it becomes less compatible with the sociotechnical system of most firms. The ensuing problems, with which management, staff specialists and workers have great difficulty in coping, lead to the new technology being only partially under control. It is difficult to evaluate whether to purchase a computerized manufacturing system, and there are problems in evaluating their efficiency once they are implemented. Evidence is presented from case studies of five firms in three nations that have purchased computerized production systems. Policy recommendations and research suggestions are provided for dealing with the situation.

68. Blyton, Paul, John Hassard, Stephen Hill, and Ken Starkey. *Time, Work, and Organization*. London: Routledge, 1989.

Keywords: labor relations, psychology, sociology, time discipline

In our industrial society, work is the primary shaper of the concept of time. The economic orientation to time dominates. Time is rationalized and commodified. Thus, managers constantly search for the most efficient use of time. Time-discipline and job routinization are forced upon workers. Recognizing that an interdisciplinary approach would be valuable, the topic of time, work and organization is broached from the perspectives of industrial sociology, psychology, economics and labor relations.

In chapter 2, it is argued that time does not receive adequate attention in the study of industrial sociology. A social-anthropological perspective with a focus on the metaphors of time as a line and as a cycle is recommended. It is revealed that the notion of time as a line prevails in industrialism, ignoring human-paced work and concentrating on machine-paced work.

Chapter 3 draws on cognitive and social psychology to gain a better understanding of the experience of work. Occupational stress, time of work and the occupational group are also examined.

The economic perspective is taken in chapter 4 to analyze working time. The traditional theory that presumes leisure time and income from work generate satisfaction equally is critiqued. Time allocation studies are also considered.

How does time organize our lives? Chapter 5 illustrates how important time is in organizing socialization and, of course, work. The author argues that organizations exist because collectives need to solve three main time problems: the reduction of temporal uncertainty, interunit conflicts of interest over temporal matters, and the inevitable scarcity of time.

Finally, in chapter 6, the relationship between time and industrial relations is contemplated. The duration of working-time, overtime, shiftwork, holidays, early retirement and flexible working-time are some of the issues explored. The difficulty in matching flexible human time to technological/machine time is noted.

69. Boguslaw, Janet. *Social Partnership and Social Relations: New Strategies in Workforce and Economic Development*. New York: Routledge, 2002.

Keywords: industrial sociology, textile workers, work and family, New Bedford (Massachusetts), social conditions

The effect that social relations have on social partnerships and how the partnerships themselves affect change in regional social relations are examined. The author shows how social relations can be understood not as a descriptive characteristic of social partnerships but as part of what makes social partnerships effective problem-solving initiatives.

70. Bosma, Hans, et al. "Low Job Control and Risk of Coronary Heart Disease in Whitehall II (prospective cohort) Study." *British Medical Journal* 314 (22 February 1997): 558-65.

Keywords: stress, health, work design, case study

This large research study examines "the association between adverse psychological characteristics at work and risk of coronary heart disease among male and female civil servants in London, England." Results of the research reaffirm conclusions made by R. A. Karasek and other social scientists with regard to the relationship between low control in the work setting and employee ill-health. The findings of the study are as follows: (1) "Low job control in the work environment contributes to the development of coronary heart disease." (2) "The risk of heart disease is associated with both objective low job control and perceived low job control." (3) "Increase in job control over time decreases the risk of coronary heart disease." The authors also suggest that "policies giving people a stronger say in decisions about their work or providing them with more variety in work tasks may contribute to better cardiovascular health."

Implications for preventive strategies in the workplace, the reorganization and planning of work design and public health are very strong in this research paper.

71. Bourbounais, Renée, et al. "Job Strain and Psychological Distress in White-Collar Workers." *Scandinavian Journal of Work, Environment and Health* 22 (2 April 1996): 139-45.

Keywords: stress, psychology, case study, support

The objective of this study was "to determine whether workers submitted to high job strain, a combination of high psychological demand and low decision latitude, develop more psychological distress than workers not submitted to high job strain. A second objective was to determine whether social support at work modifies the association between job strain and psychological distress." The design of the study was cross-sectional and included white-collar workers in the Quebec City area. "A self-administered 26-item questionnaire (the Job Content Questionnaire) measured psychological demand, decision latitude, and social support at work. Psychological distress was measured by the Psychiatric Symptom Index, a 14-item self-administered instrument." The study results offer "support for an association between job strain and psychological distress among white-collar workers. This association tended to be stronger when there was a combination of high psychological demand and low decision latitude. However, exposure to one or the other of these constraints was also associated with an elevated level of psychological distress. It is notable that the association between job strain and psychological distress remained important even after adjustment for variables often pointed out to explain mental health problems at the discharge of work conditions: age, gender, employment status, occupation, social support at work and nonwork social support, cynicism, hostility, domestic load, and stressful life events during the last 12 months. . . . Social support at work, although associated with psychological distress, did not modify the association between job strain and psychological distress." Moreover, this study showed that more women than men declared a high level of symptoms of distress. Less educated subjects, those with an annual family income of less than Can$ 40,000 and clerical workers also showed more severe symptoms.

72. Bowers, John M. "The Janus Faces of Design: Some Critical Questions for CSCW." 333-350 in *Studies in Computer Supported Cooperative Work*, edited

by J. M. Bowers and S. D. Benford. Amsterdam: Elsevier Science Publishers B.V. (North-Holland), 1991.

Keywords: democracy, skill, participation, work design

The author attempts to make explicit the thesis that most technology-led work has implicit sociological and political themes embedded in it. He examines this by looking at the design process through which production eventually takes place. He addresses questions such as: What aims are embodied in the final products—is it an enhancement of workplace democracy or of managerial control? Does it lead to deskilling and the routinization of work or does it heighten pre-existing skills? Is computer supported cooperative work possible? and if so, under what conditions?

73. Boyce, James K. *The Political Economy of the Environment*. Amherst: University of Massachusetts, 2002.

Keywords: environmental economics

The natural environment is often profoundly affected by how we distribute wealth among ourselves, since some claim more of its resources than others. When disparities are great between those with economic power and those without, those at the top of the political economic ladder can more easily pollute the air and water and waste the natural resources for those at the bottom.

Some even believe that the ethical basis of policy should supercede human needs and pertain solely to the well-being of nature, since the environment accounts for so much of our daily needs and living. Those who base their reasoning more on self-interest typically do so from the advantageous perspective of market exchange and income.

Both sides of the environmental debate juxtapose nature with humans, the preservationists arguing that nature cannot renew itself if the negative impacts of human exploitation go uncontrolled, while the proponents of market rationality believe human ingenuity will overcome environmental constraints. In both cases, the poor are maligned.

Starting with the idea that humans are not apart from nature but a part of it, the book discusses how inequality is a cause of environmental degradation, power distribution and public health, the globalization of market failure, and democratizing environmental ownership.

74. Boyett, Joseph H., and Henry P. Conn. *Workplace 2000: The Revolution Reshaping American Business*. New York: Dutton, 1991.

Keywords: case study, teams, participation, organizational change

The authors present a large empirically-grounded body of research related to the organization and structure of the rapidly changing business/industrial work environment. Particular attention is given to those aspects of work organization that must undergo significant adaptation "if Americans are to survive in the workplace of tomorrow." Numerous and varied case studies are included along with considerable academic research, as well as material from the popular press.

A wide range of predictions are made by the authors concerning the future of work and the role expected of workers. The following examples represent some of the most important of these forecasts: "Companies . . . will be flatter, leaner and more aggressive. . . . Downsizing . . . and the trend toward flattening the organization will continue." "Flexibility and creativity will be more important for success than endurance and loyalty." "The sharing of information will be of critical importance to sustain performance. . . . The most valued individuals will be those who can work effectively with other employees in a team effort." "Much more than basic literacy will be required for success in the new organization. Americans will need to know how to solve problems, think creatively, and work effectively in a group."

For case study material on "employee involvement" strategies and "team" systems, see especially chapter 7 "Experiments in Workplace 2000" and chapter 8 "Employees Take Charge." Although this volume goes some distance in outlining the likely organizational realities of the future workplace, it gives far less attention to the psychosocial effects on workers and society at large.

75. Boyle, Daniel C. "The 100 Club." *Harvard Business Review*, March-April 1987: 26-7.

Keywords: productivity, labor relations

This brief article gives a description of a program developed by one of four plants, the Palmer factory, run by Diamond International Corporation, that rewards employees for work well done, good attendance and good behavior. The program is called "The 100 Club" and was designed to reward employees but not to act as the sole incentive for improvement. It is a simple system whereby employees accumulate points for various qualities such as good behavior, attendance and work, that add up to modest gifts, such as jackets (upon reaching 100 points) and others from a list. The program has continuously raised productivity, company earnings and worker morale. Since then, it has been expanded to encourage group efforts (where points for reaching certain group goals can be attained).

76. Bradley, Gunilla. *Computers and the Psychosocial Work Environment*. London: Taylor and Francis, 1989.

Keywords: computers, information technology, stress, psychology, QWL, technology, rationalization

This book represents the results of a ten-year research project on "The Effects of Rationalization on the Work Environment" (known as the RAM project) carried out in Stockholm, Sweden. The aim of the project, and the book as well, is "to make a detailed analysis of the psychosocial work environment and its link with rationalization, primarily with changes brought about by advances in electronic data processing (EDP) technology."

The first chapter discusses the opportunities and risks inherent in computer technology. Chapter 2 contains a brief review of the development of computer technology and considers future developments in telecommunications technology. Chapters 4, 5, and 6 offer case study material on the implementation of computer systems in three different companies. Chapter 7 examines stress and mental strain, and chapter 8 discusses "the significance of the psychosocial work environment in terms of the benefits we derive from our leisure time and family lives and in terms of the individual's health." Chapter 9 deals with more general issues in the sphere of computerization and the work environment, and chapter 10 looks at "Future Research" into the "Quality of Working Life and New Technologies."

77. Bradley, Gunilla E., and Hal W. Hendrick, eds. *Fourth International Symposium on Human Factors in Organizational Design and Management*. Stockholm: Elsevier Science, 1994.

Keywords: QWL, stress, health

This book contains a massive collection of professional papers that were presented at a Human Factors Symposium, held in Sweden in 1994. The objective of the symposium was to "provide an interactional forum for the dissemination and exchange of scientific information on organizational design and management (ODAM)."

An extremely broad range of papers are offered, providing a wealth of recent data on the subject of work organization, design and human health. Included are papers "on theory, methodology, research findings, reviews, and case studies from leading scientists . . . throughout the world." Particular attention is given to "the development, introduction, and use of new technologies."

The text is broken down into five major themes: (1) organizational and psychosocial work environments, (2) human resource development and human competence, (3) labor markets and society in change, (4) front line technologies, and (5) well-being and health. The latter is of special interest in the context of preventive strategies in the workplace. Topics discussed in this part include the following: "Preventive Strategies in Automated Offices, Employee Participation, and Preventing Occupational Diseases Caused by New Technologies"; "A Systems Approach to Reducing Physical and Psychological Stress"; "Prevention through Worker Participation Intervention"; and many others.

78. Bradshaw, David J., and Suzanne Ozment, eds. *The Voice of Toil: Nineteenth-Century British Writings about Work.* Athens: Ohio University Press, 2000.

Keywords: working class, nineteenth century, working class in Great Britain, working class in literature, work as oppression

Work had been one of the most controversial subjects of the nineteenth-century, when many thinkers associated work with the honest pursuit of doing good, or comprising a commitment to serve others and promote a better future for all. This soon changed when the satisfaction of what work could do for individuals had its counterbalance in the anger and dismay expressed at the conditions of those whom Robert Owen, in 1817, first called the "working class." Working class people were confronted, both at the labor site and at their lodgings, with oppression, and the misery of their lives became the subject of sentimental poetry, government reports, popular fiction, and journalistic accounts. The separation of the spheres for men and women was also a topic that was heatedly discussed and thus found its way into public discourse and literature as well. *The Voice of Toil* uses a collection of stories, poems, essays, and a play in order to reflect four prominent ways in which the subject of work was addressed.

79. Bramwell, Ros, and Cary L. Cooper. "VDUs in the Workplace: Psychological and Health Implications." 213-27 in *International Review of Industrial and Organizational Psychology 1995*, edited by Cary L. Cooper and Ivan T. Robertson. Chichester, UK: John Wiley and Sons, 1995.

Keywords: computers, stress, work design, psychology, health

The article provides an overview of the research findings of health effects of video display units (VDUs). First, the VDU is defined and the cathode ray tube explained. Five groups of health hazards associated with VDUs are studied: musculoskeletal, visual, skin and reproductive health problems and stress.

The considerable number of musculoskeletal damage complaints suggests that VDU use could be a cause. But job design, not only workplace design, seems to play a role. While visual strain and headaches are very common symptoms related to VDUs, permanent eye damage and sight deterioration are not generally accepted as results of VDU use. The same conclusion is drawn regarding skin problems. The impact on occupational stress is difficult to study, it is noted, because of the vast differences among job characteristics of VDU users. The link between VDUs and miscarriages, difficulty in becoming pregnant, and fetal health problems are explored. The authors conclude that no clear cause-effect relationships are discernible but are possible for subgroups such as very heavy users. The radiation, ergonomic and psychosocial stress effects of VDUs on pregnancy are also discussed.

80. Braverman, Harry. *Labor and Monopoly Capital: The Degradation of Work in the Twentieth Century*. New York: Monthly Review Press, 1974.

Keywords: general, Taylorism, skill, labor process, division of labor, case study

This exceptional and groundbreaking social science text still stands out as one of the most comprehensive analyses of the labor process as a whole and Taylorism in particular. The author draws on an enormous range of Marxist and more traditional labor and management literature, combining it with his own considerable work experience.

Braverman is best known for the contribution his book has made to the labor process debate engaged in by sociologists, industrial relations specialists and organizational theorists. His basic thesis is that the pursuit of capitalist interests has led to a general trend toward deskilling and mechanization of jobs across the employment spectrum, from manufacturing to retailing and from design to clerical work.

Braverman further argues that the working class will become increasingly homogenous through the process of deskilling and work degradation, that all employees (blue collar, white collar, technical and manual) will find themselves in a more and more similar position.

The greatest criticism of Braverman's thesis is not directed against the claims of trends toward deskilling but against his views on increasing homogenization.

This volume contains detailed discussions on a wide range of labor topics, including: the division of labor; the history of scientific management; the scientific-technical revolution and the worker; surplus value and surplus labor; the modern corporation; the roles of the state; and the structure of the working class.

81. Bridger, R. S. *Introduction to Ergonomics*. New York: McGraw-Hill, 1995.

Keywords: ergonomics, human factors, sociotechnical systems, workplaces, work design

This is a broadly-based introductory text on the ergonomic approach to the analysis of work systems. As noted in the introduction, "Ergonomics aims to ensure that human needs for safe and efficient working are met in the design of work systems."

The first chapter of the book discusses the ergonomic approach to design in the work environment using simple models. The history of the discipline, its present state and future trends are also described. Topics include the following: the human components of a work system; human-machine systems; the physical environment and work organization; classification of design issues; sociotechnical implications, etc.

Chapter 2 examines anatomy, posture and body mechanics. Chapter 3 looks at anthropometric principles in workspace and equipment design. Chapter 4 considers workspace design for standing and seated workers. Chapter 5 analyzes the upper body at work. Chapter 6 discusses the design of manual handling tasks. Chapter 7 is concerned with physiology, workload and work capacity. Chapter 8 looks at the industrial implications of physiology. Chapter 9 considers heat, cold and the design of the physical environment. Chapter 10 examines vision, light and lighting. Chapter 11 considers hearing, sound and noise. This is a good introductory treatment of ergonomics from the perspective of theory and practice. Implications for healthy workplace design are substantial.

82. Brief, Arthur P., Randall S. Schuler, and Mary Van Sell. *Managing Job Stress*. Boston: Little, Brown and Company, 1981.

Keywords: stress, coping, women, management, organizational behavior

This is a very readable and fairly comprehensive (in spite of its brevity) treatment of the subject of job stress. The authors draw on the research findings of doctors, sociologists, and psychologists and summarize them for a wide audience. Although the book is primarily directed toward "courses in management, organizational behavior, and personnel administration," it serves as a good general introduction to the field. Contents include sections on job stress and the quality of life, major sources of work stress, personal mechanisms for coping with job stress, management strategies for stress reduction, and working women and stress.

83. Brinkerhoff, Merlin B., ed. *Work, Organizations and Society: Comparative Convergences*. Westport, CT: Greenwood Press, 1984.

Keywords: comparative, sociology, participation, family, women, organizations

The contributions to this volume focus broad attention on family, work, organizations, and societies using a comparative sociological perspective. The authors express a holistic view of social life, resisting the common academic tendency toward specialization.

The introductory chapter, a "preview at the macro-level" looks at the major units of analysis—work, organizations, and society—and related concepts, for example occupations, technology, and interdependent systems and institutions. The author explores how these elements fit together into a meaningful whole, and how comparative studies facilitate a holistic approach.

Chapter 2 sets out a model for analysis using concepts from organizational theory that deals with workers' control, participatory management, and workers' councils.

The author of Chapter 3 considers which organizational features impede participation in the workplace, proposing a workers' control model in contrast to traditional "oligarchical control."

Chapter 4 explores the relationship between modernization and "the socio-cultural-personality system" and effects on female labor participation.

Chapter 5 reports on a survey of organizational characteristics in fifty Japanese factories in order to determine "whether organizational size or production technology is more important in shaping organizational structure."

Chapter 6 contains an extensive annotated bibliography on "Work, Organizations, and Society in Comparative Perspective."

84. Brodkin Sacks, Karen, and Dorothy Remy, eds. *My Troubles Are Going to Have Trouble with Me: Everyday Trials and Triumphs of Women Workers*. New Brunswick, NJ: Rutgers University Press, 1984.

Keywords: women, family, skill

Eighty percent of working women in the United States were employed in the clerical, sales, service and manufacturing sectors in the late 1970s, when the research for this book was being done. The articles aim to encourage and publicize research to help women improve their working conditions and to gain economic independence. Part 1 "Working Families and the Domestic Code" investigates the relationship between family and work life. Part 2 "Technology and the Changing Shape of Women's Work" questions corporations' claims that jobs are being upgraded and require more skill. On the contrary, it seems that the use of new technologies in clerical, service and even some professional jobs are resulting in deskilling and routinization. Women in the manufacturing sector, especially the textile and clothing industry, are the focus of the final section, entitled "Work and Resistance in the Global Factory." Here, women's skills are clearly a necessity, even in a highly mechanized process. However, they are treated and paid as if they are in entry level, unskilled jobs. The essays collectively show that women do have a sense of their skill and do rebel against oppression at work. Two themes tie the fifteen contributions together: an exploration into capitalism's effect on women's work; and how women work together to resist oppression and help each other.

85. Brödner, Peter. *The Shape of Future Technology: The Anthropocentric Alternative*. London: Springer-Verlag, 1990.

Keywords: Fordism, Taylorism, anthropocentric, sociotechnical, skill, automation, tacit knowledge

Written by a renowned specialist in German advanced manufacturing technology, this work examines an alternative form of industrial production utilizing "anthropocentric systems." The author argues the case for this human-centered type of production rather than the conventional American Fordist, Taylorist form. He contends that "technology should be perceived as part of culture" and that "there should be different forms of technology . . . which reflect the cultural, educational, political, and ideological realities of the countries in which the technology is to be implemented."

In anthropocentric systems, "the worker deals with the qualitative subjective judgements and the machine merely deals with the quantitative elements. At the production planning and scheduling level, the object is to render processes highly transparent." Moreover, "the deep tacit knowledge of the skilled worker is accepted as valid scientific knowledge."

In the text, political, sociotechnical and ideological considerations are taken into account, as well as the types of organizational forms that reinforce control and power relationships. The author "reveals on the one hand the inefficiencies of Taylorist forms of production and on the other, provides statistical and economic evidence to support his searing critique of the existing forms of manufacturing technology."

Mass production techniques are contrasted with those of workshop production, and the impact of automation on intellectual work and knowledge-based systems is analyzed.

Most importantly, the book offers sound technological proposals of interest to industrial sociologists, engineers, systems designers and trade unionists.

As noted by Mike Cooley in the introduction, "this book will provide one of the intellectual and political building blocks necessary in the process of constructing a form of technology that enhances human skill and our environment rather than diminishing it."

86. Brödner, Peter, and Waldemar Karwowski, eds. *International Conference on Human Aspects of Advanced Manufacturing and Hybrid Automation*. Gelsenkirchen, Germany: Elsevier Science Publishers, 1992.

Keywords: automation, work design, anthropocentric, skill, safety, expertise

Contemporary models for the development and implementation of advanced manufacturing systems reflect a growing awareness of the importance of social design (as opposed to a preoccupation with the use of technology). The papers presented in this volume examine the new design perspective that, in Europe, has often been referred to as the anthropocentric systems model. At the core of the new or emerging paradigm is "a holistic approach to work design which considers the mutual dependencies of people's needs, organization, and technology."

The authors in this collection share the belief that in today's highly competitive manufacturing environment "the development and comprehensive use of human abilities, skills, and expertise have become the most crucial factors for economic success."

The book contains 75 papers from engineers, computer scientists, and sociologists and is organized into six sections. The first part "Design of Advanced Manufacturing Systems" considers issues of design of advanced manufacturing systems as "a unity of people, organization, and technology." See especially "Advanced Manufacturing and Anthropocentric Production Systems in the European Community" by W. Wobbe. Also see "Designing Organizations for Factory 2000" by J. Bessant et al. and "Human Issues in Manufacturing Technology" by C. N. Day et al.

Part 4 on human resources management, part 5 on skill formation and training, and part 6 on safety have the greatest relevance for preventive and healthy work strategies. In particular, see "A Training Method to Promote the Integration of Preventive Maintenance Tasks at the Shop-Floor Level" by D. Gude and "Skill and Technology" by M. Florin et al. in part 5. In part 6, see especially "Worker Safety in Computer-Integrated Manufacturing Systems: Needs for Research" by W. Karwowski.

87. Bullinger, H. J., and E. D. Ammer. "Work Structuring Provides Basis for Improving Organization of Production Systems." *Industrial Engineering*, October 1984: 74-82.

Keywords: workplace design, work design

Two industrial engineers outline a planning process that restructures work organization through cooperative teamwork among various departments of a production system. They include a brief case study of work restructuring at the Daimler-Benz factory.

88. Burbidge, J. L. "Change to Group Technology: Process Organization is Obsolete." *International Journal of Production Research* 30, no. 5 (1992): 1209-19.

Keywords: work design, teams

The traditional type of organization for manufacturing is process organization, in which organizational units each specialize in a particular process. This is gradually being replaced by product organization in the form of either continuous line flow (CLF) or group technology (GT). Group technology (GT) is a method of organization for manufacturing in which the organizational units (groups) complete all the parts they make at their particular processing stage and are equipped with all the machines and other facilities they need to complete these functions. CLF is the preferred type of organization for process industries and for a few cases of mass production in other types of industry. GT is the preferred type of organization for batch and jobbing production. This paper finds that if "production flow analysis" (PFA) is used to plan the division into groups of machines and associated families of parts, then it is always possible in batch and jobbing production to find a total division into groups, with very few exceptions and with no back-flow or cross-flow between groups. It bases this finding on 33 listed examples from practice, and on the observation that because most routing data is very flexible, it would be very surprising if one ever found a case where GT was impossible. As GT is always possible where it is appropriate and can always lead to major increases in efficiency, it follows that process organization is obsolete.

89. Burnes, Bernard. *New Technology in Context: The Selection, Introduction and Use of Computer Numerically Controlled Machine Tools*. Aldershot, UK: Avebury, Gower Publishing, 1989.

Keywords: work design, Taylorism, labor process, CNC, technology, case study, skill

This book examines the impact of new technology on work organization and job design. Part 1 provides a general overview of the impact of new technology on society. The first chapter reviews the literature while the second one provides an historical perspective of work organization and job design. The useful third chapter critiques the following four approaches: scientific management, job design (work humanization), contingency theory, and labor process theory. The history, description and criticisms of each approach are outlined. It is concluded that factors such as organizational culture, ideology, economic and social climate, organizational goals and managerial strategy affect the choice of approach and need to be studied.

Part 2 of the book presents nine longitudinal case studies of organizations that adopted computer numerically controlled (CNC) machine tools. The companies are studied in the categories of small, medium and large organizations. A comparison and discussion of the case studies is also undertaken. The author calls for a greater involvement by all and special care by managers when planning change. Throughout the book, deskilling and work centralization/decentralization receive attention.

90. Butera, Frederico, Vittorio Di Martino, and Eberhard Köhler, eds. *Technological Development and the Improvement of Living and Working Conditions: Options for the Future*. Luxembourg: European Foundation for the Improvement of Living and Working Conditions, 1990.

Keywords: QWL, technology, Taylorism, participation

What will be the effect of technological development on work? Technological Taylorism, freedom from monotonous and tedious work, or no significant change? All of these outcomes are possible, argue the contributors. How best to plan for the outcome with the most healthy working conditions is the challenge addressed by the European Foundation for the Improvement of Living and Working Conditions, for whom this book was prepared. Chapter 2 shows that technology is only one factor that affects the organization of work. Chapter 3 argues that the consumer benefits when computers are introduced in banking, insurance, hospital, government, supermarket, and home entertainment services. Worker participation in the decision making process regarding new technologies is advocated in the next chapter. An especially important chapter is chapter 5, which presents a model to explain how new technologies bring about physical and psychological stress. Here, Mogens Agervold contends that the entire context of the work environment—especially control over one's work, work quality and participation, not just technology—must be considered in order to evaluate the causes of stress. In chapter 6, the possibilities of new technologies improving shift work are considered. The final chapter summarizes the conclusions reached.

91. Button, Graham, ed. *Technology in Working Order: Studies of Work, Interaction and Technology*. London: Routledge, 1993.

Keywords: computers, sociology, ergonomics, work design, human factors

This is a collection of sociological studies that investigate the way in which computer systems technology is ordered and produced and the interactional work of participants in its design, construction, implementation, and use. Although aimed primarily at sociologists, the book is also of considerable relevance for specialists in the disciplines associated with computer systems development such as computer science, software engineering, human-computer interaction, psychology, ergonomics and design.

See especially part 3 "Work Practices in the Use of Technology," which addresses technology use in work settings that are organized around technology and how technology is built into the interactions of those who use and consume it. Also see part 5 "Human-Computer Interaction" for case study material dealing with this theme and especially chapter 3 "The Use of 'Intelligent' Machines for Electrocardiograph Interpretation."

92. Campbell, David N., R. L. Fleming, and Richard C. Grote. "Discipline without Punishment—At Last." *Harvard Business Review*, July-August 1985: 162-78.

Keywords: labor relations, case study

This article presents a new way for companies to deal with problems arising with workers: the "nonpunitive approach to discipline." When company supervisors began to realize that punishing employees did not rehabilitate them but only caused anger, resentment, and an overall negative attitude about their work environment, other options began to be discussed. This new approach takes most of the onus off the supervisors and places it on the employees. When disciplinary problems occur, the employees are "reminded," instead of warned, of their responsibilities to the company. On the first occasion, the event is not recorded in their personnel file. On the second occasion, a "written reminder" is issued. In both cases, the employee is encouraged to take steps to better their behavior on their own, with the help of an action plan laid out in the meeting with the manager. When this fails, the employee is put on a one-day paid "decision-making leave." The pay shows the company's desire to see the employee remain a member of the team, yet it forces the employee to make a choice between improving his/her behavior or risking dismissal. The entire system was designed to create a more positive atmosphere to allow employees to maintain a positive outlook toward the company, themselves, and their working environment. It has been found that this new system also benefits the business aspect of the company in terms of reducing paid sick leave, turnover and the number of disciplinary incidents and grievances, thus cutting down on lost revenue.

93. Campbell, John P., and Richard J. Campbell and Associates. *Productivity in Organizations: New Perspectives from Industrial and Organizational Psychology*. Jossey-Bass Management Series, Jossey-Bass Social and Behavioral Sciences Series. San Francisco: Jossey-Bass Publishers, 1988.

Keywords: QWL, quality circles, productivity, autonomous work groups, participation, self-management, policy, psychology

Industrial and organizational perspectives are used to examine the relationship between performance/productivity and various job redesign/employee involvement strategies such as Quality Circles (QCs), job enrichment, self-managing teams, QWL, autonomous work groups, etc. The role of new technologies is given considerable attention in this relationship, as is the role of company management. Both qualitative and quantitative methods are used in the research to assess the effectiveness of the strategies noted above. In addition, summary data from a large number of empirical studies is reported and analyzed to provide an overview of findings in the literature. Chapter 9 "Job Enrichment and Performance Improvement," chapter 10 "The Quality Circle and Its Variations," and chapter 11 "Groups and Productivity: Analyzing the Effectiveness of Self-Managing Teams" are especially noteworthy.

The following is a selective sample of some of the conclusions reached in the research: In general, "job characteristics are correlated with improved performance" (although the strength of the relationship varies with such factors as motivation and worker resistance, effectiveness of structural and design changes, etc.); "The evidence available so far suggests that QCs do not have very powerful effects on attitudinals such as job satisfaction and commitment. Negative effects of QCs have less commonly been reported than neutral or positive effects"; and while "self-managing groups do change organizational effectiveness outcomes . . . the effects are greater on . . . quality of life indicators than on business criteria such as productivity."

The research in this volume offers some rather surprising and unexpected conclusions regarding the relationship between job performance and various job characteristics. These could have significant implications for future policy decisions.

94. Capelli, Peter, et al. *Change at Work*. Oxford: Oxford University Press, 1997.

Keywords: organizational change, downsizing, labor relations

This study of work organization and change was sponsored by the National Planning Association in the United States, a private-sector group whose aim is to "promote a more competitive US economy and to focus on both macroeconomic strategies and ways to use human resources more effectively." The book is "a major attempt to gather and use systematic data on the changing nature of employment and to develop a better understanding of emerging employment relationships." Although the original focus of the work was to study work organization and assess "high-performance systems," it gradually broadened to include other issues such as employment security, training and labor market outcomes.

The implications of organizational restructuring for employment are detailed in chapter 1. Chapter 2 documents trends in downsizing and in the use of contingent workforces. Chapter 3 discusses the changes within work organizations. Chapter 4 describes arrangements for employer-provided training and employee work incentives. Chapter 5 examines the changing skill requirements in high-technology workplaces. Chapter 6 considers the consequences of the changing employee relationships for employees.

In the context of healthy work programs and preventive strategies, chapters 3 and 6 are the most relevant, although the implications for these areas of concern are often not well drawn out.

95. Carlsson, Chris, ed. *Bad Attitude: The Processed World Anthology*. London: Verso, 1990.

Keywords: computers, alienation, unions, health, safety, expert systems

This volume offers a collection of writings and graphics from *Processed World* magazine. The book combines satire and critical analysis to expose the alienation and exploitation of information workers in the computer age. It contains firsthand accounts of corporate computer culture from the perspective of those at the bottom of the ladder in big banks, defense contractors, computer manufacturers and food processing factories. The contributors—through articles, letters, poems, art and autobiographical stories—provide an insightful picture of the underside of the so-called information age. They document their day-to-day experiences "handling information" as workers at all levels of the modern computerized office. The book deflates much of the hype surrounding excessive claims about the potential of the new service economy and the high-tech jobs that will liberate the masses of unemployed workers. Many of the hazards of office computer work are highlighted, along with a discussion of the role of trade unions in improving the quality of working life for information workers. See especially "Work's Diminishing Connections" for a look at the psycho-social effects of work in the electronics industry. Also see "Mind Games" for a discussion of artificial intelligence and expert systems, and their implications for information workers. And see "Computer Education = Processed Kids?" for a scathing critique of computer-based education and our culture's steadfast devotion to instrumental rationality.

96. Carre, Francoise, Marianne A. Feber, Lonnie Golden, and Stephen A. Herzenberg, eds. *Nonstandard Work: The Nature and Challenges of Changing Employment Arrangements*. Industrial Relations Research Association Series. Champaign, IL: Industrial Relations Research Association, 2000.

Keywords: employment, full-time/part-time, workforce, unions, nonstandard employment

During the 1980s and 1990s, the workforce saw a downward trend in standard employment job security. With the increasing number of nonstandard employment options available, the job market has seen long-term mutual attachments as well as structured labor markets declining in place of more "flexible," often short term, employment. As the epidemic of newly emerging employment arrangements sweeps through the ranks of the workforce, affecting not only blue-collar workers but managers and professionals, it has attracted an increasing amount of attention.

Due to the complex nature of the nonstandard workforce, comprised of people of all manner of gender, race, and age, the problem of understanding its nature is a complex one. Key questions arise around the differences between perceived concepts of "standard" and "nonstandard" work. Of no less importance is determining to what extent these jobs meet the needs of the company and employer, and what can be done to improve arrangements that may be inadequate in this respect.

While few definitive answers are given on this controversial issue, the various analytical approaches provided by the authors seek to identify and recommend solutions to undesirable outcomes of nonstandard work arrangements.

This volume also examines the economic consequences of the development of a nonstandard workforce. These consequences include the following: market mediated employment, part-time and self-employment, differences in work regarding race and gender, companies' profitability and productivity, contemporary responses, historical perspectives, the structure of postindustrial labor markets, and transforming contract work into union jobs. Several case studies are also provided.

97. Cavendish, Ruth. *Women on the Line*. London: Routledge and Kegan Paul, 1982.

Keywords: women, assembly line, case study, stress, unions, work design

This is a personal account of women's experience of assembly-line work in a large British factory. Central issues discussed include the following: social, psychological and health effects of repetitive, exhausting work; consequences of a rigid sexual and racial division of labor; and the role of labor and union movements.

A very compelling, firsthand analysis and a solid example of participatory field work, with many insights into the stressful world of the assembly line. This book has implications for the area of work redesign, although these are not explicitly spelled out.

98. Chatterjee, Piya. *A Time for Tea: Women, Labor, and Post-Colonial Politics on an Indian Plantation*. Durham, NC: Duke University Press, 2001.

Keywords: tea plantation workers, India, history, twentieth century, tea trade, women

Using a historical critique of the labor practices on an Indian plantation, the production, consumption and circulation of tea are examined. This reveals how the female tea-pluckers seen in advertisements—picturesque in mist-shrouded fields—came to represent what colonialism in India was all about. The reality behind these made-up images is exposed to show the truth: terrible working conditions, low wages, and coercive labor practices enforced by the patronage system. By exposing the reality of the situation, the author tells the story of the women workers and then concludes by reflecting on the cultures of hierarchy, power and difference in the plantation's villages. In turn, the overlapping processes by which gender, caste and ethnicity constitute the patronage system of villages and their fields of labor are explored.

99. Chew, W. B. "The Case of the Machinist's Mutiny." *Harvard Business Review*, November-December 1990: 14-30.

Keywords: labor relations, case study, technology

This case study is based on a real situation (using fictitious names) in which there is a clash between management eager to implement new technology and long-time workers resisting the change. The workers see no need for the technology, are comfortable with and extremely knowledgeable about the existing machinery, and are somewhat scared of the computer programming skills that must be learned. The detailed description of the situation is followed by responses by four business professionals. They have been asked what they would do to handle the problem. Two of them stress the importance of considering the emotions and concerns of the employees and the social context of the shopfloor. The two other commentators focus on the importance of change and new technology in order to remain competitive.

100. Ciulla, Joanne B. *The Working Life: The Promise and Betrayal of Modern Work.* New York: Three Rivers Press, 2000.

Keywords: work ethic, psychological aspects, work and life

Ciulla examines why so many people today have let their jobs take over their lives. Technology was meant to free us from work, however, we work longer hours and are often tethered to the office at home by cell phones and e-mail. People still seek self-fulfillment, community and identity from their work, but these things may be increasingly difficult to find in today's workplace. The social contract in which employees and employers shared a sense of mutual loyalty is all but gone, yet many of us still sacrifice personal time for jobs that we could lose at the drop of a stock price. By tracing the evolution of the meaning of work from Aesop to Dilbert and critically examining the past 100 years of management practices, the author asks questions that we often fail to ask at our own peril. Some examples of these questions include the following: "When you are on your deathbed, will you wish you had spent more time at the office?" "Why do we define ourselves by our jobs rather than by other activities we do outside of work?" and "What can employers and employees promise each other in today's business environment?"

101. Clegg, Chris, and Martin Corbett. "Research and Development into 'Humanizing' Advanced Manufacturing Technology." 173-95 in *The Human Side of Advanced Manufacturing Technology*, edited by T. D. Wall, C. W. Clegg, and N. J. Kemp. Chichester: John Wiley and Sons, 1987.

Keywords: automation, technology, skill

This chapter discusses the lack of investment in the research and development of the human side of advanced manufacturing technology (AMT). The first part justifies the claim that the human side of AMT has been neglected and outlines five benefits of humanizing AMT. One such benefit is that such a system would pay attention to people's need for more complex jobs rather than deskilled, simplified ones and thus would promote a good quality of working life. Other benefits include improvements in performance and competitiveness. The second part of the chapter explains the reasons why the human side of AMT has been neglected in the past, and whether these reasons are still relevant today in light of highly automated manufacturing processes. A research and development strategy for the humanizing of AMT is outlined in the third section. Incorporated in the discussion is the improvement in the health of workers due to an optimal allocation of functions for the worker and a more humanized interface.

102. Clement, Andrew, P. Kolm, and I. Wagner, eds. *IFIP WG9.1 Working Conference on NetWORKing*. Vienna: Elsevier Science, 1993.

Keywords: computers, networks, participation, control, women, teams, privacy

At its most general level, the conference on which this volume is based was focused on the implications of computerization for working people. More specifically, this book concentrates on "responding to, and hopefully influencing, the development and implementation of various forms of computer based networks, both within and between workplaces." It addresses the technical challenges involved as well as consequences for work, organization, and social practices. The book also gives considerable attention to the political and power dimensions of computing work—issues that are often not well covered in computer-related texts. For example, in part 2 of this book, "Participation and Power," the essay on "Networking: Participation and Power Aspects" by Tone Brattetieg provides a good overview of the major issues involved. See also "Social Control and Social Contract in Networking: Total Quality Management and the Control of Knowledge Work" by Heinz Klein and "Computer-Mediated Communication as Employee Voice" by Libby Bishop and David Levine. Part 3 "Reaching Over Distances" deals with electronic networks and mediated collaborative research including the social effects on everyday work life. Part 4 explores networking, computers and privacy issues. See "Working in the Electronic Fishbowl? Privacy Aspects of Multi-Media Communications" by Andrew Clement and "Networking: Transparency versus Privacy" by Jörg Flecher. Part 5 explores "Information Policy" concerns. See especially "The Politics of Networking in Health Care" by Ole Hanseth and Langdon Winner. The final part 6 looks at how "Networking Changes Organizations and Their Management." See especially "Integrated Gender Perspectives on Human-Centered Approaches to Developing Computerized Office Systems" by Eileen Green and "Empowering Team Work with Coordination Technologies: An Organizational Learning Perspective" by Timo Käkölä for particularly insightful discussions.

103. Coates, Joseph F., Jennifer Jarratt, and John B. Mahaffie. *Future Work: Seven Critical Forces Reshaping Work and the Work Force in North America*. San Francisco: Jossey-Bass, 1990.

Keywords: policy, sociology, family, human resources

This well-organized book is a combination of documented past trends and specific interpretations and conjectures about long-term implications regarding work. It is a good description of conventional work-related problems and an excellent source for demographic, economic and sociological information. The seven themes of the book are: (1) increasing diversity in the workforce, (2) reintegration of work and family responsibilities, (3) globalization of business and the workforce, (4) restructuring of the workforce and human resource planning, (5) shifting to a knowledge-based workforce, (6) rising employee expectations, and (7) expanding corporate social responsibility.

104. Cockburn, C. *Machinery of Dominance: Women, Men and Technical Know-How.* London: Pluto Press, 1985.

Keywords: women, skill, case study, technology, policy

This ethnographic treatment of what happens to women's work when new technology is introduced in various workplaces concentrates on experiences and relations between men and women in light of new technology. It suggests that it is important to develop policies that enable women to transcend their historically disadvantaged relationship to technology (in a broad sense) and develop mastery over it. One of the strengths of the book is its exploration of how technology shapes identity. Comparative case studies of workplaces using traditional techniques and using new technologies are presented in the following areas: the clothing industry where the computer has changed many cutting and pattern processes; mail order firms where goods handling has been mechanized and computerized in the warehouse; and computed tomography scanning that is fast gaining importance in the radiology departments of hospitals.

105. Cohen, Marcy, and Margaret White. *Playing with Our Health: Hazards in the Automated Office.* Vancouver: Press Gang Printers and Publishers, 1986.

Keywords: computers, health, video display terminal, automation, stress, family, radiation, safety

This book is designed as an educational and resource guide for clerical workers, union officials, students, and teachers interested in the health and safety problems associated with video display terminals (VDTs). There are specific suggestions for workshops and educational exercises, as well as a resource list of books referenced in each section. There is also a general resource section outlining health and safety organizations, newsletters, books, films, etc. Section 1 of the text deals with "Work Stress"—how it affects our health, why clerical work with computers is so stressful, and ways to reduce harmful stress. Specific topics discussed here include the following: electronic monitoring, radiation-induced stress, dual responsibilities of work and family life, shift work and related health and safety problems, job redesign, the control of electronic monitoring, relaxation techniques, and limits on VDT use. Section 2 looks at radiation hazards, especially for pregnant women. Existing scientific research is considered, current standards are examined and inadequacies noted, and details are provided on how to protect VDT operators from radiation. Section 3 focuses on "Taking Action on Health and Safety." Topics explored here include the following: employees rights under the law, employers' obligations, joint union-management committees, forming a union health and safety committee, union gains for VDT workers, investigating the workplace, and compensation/legislation issues. Also see the resource section, the appendices, and the excellent survey questionnaires at the end of the text.

106. Cohen-Rosenthal, Edward. "Sociotechnical Systems and Unions: Nicety or Necessity." *Human Relations* 50, no. 5 (May 1997).

Keywords: sociotechnical systems, unions, organizational change, labor relations

The author of this article argues that "sociotechnical systems (STS) theorists have largely ignored the role of unions both in their theoretical framework and in STS implementation. This oversight weakens the potential application and dissemination of STS theory and practice. STS democracy is frequently seen by its proponents as preferable to union democracy except when they come to the same conclusion. Unions have historically played a key role in the development and success of seminal STS initiatives but are not seen as a critical specification for success. Many practitioners have noted the instrumental importance of unions in unionized settings without acknowledging class, conflict, or union values. As such, many unions have dismissed or resisted STS innovations. Despite these serious shortcomings, the labor process argument has failed to produce a credible alternative to STS principles. In some cases, the union role has been central to STS reforms and examples like these have prompted some national union movements to promote work reform with an STS base. Recently, the labor movement in the United States has endorsed work reform approaches akin to STS approaches. STS changes are seen not just as ways to change managerial practices but also to alter union structures and functioning. As such, a union-rooted STS approach provides greater societal and workplace impact benefiting employees, employers, trade unions, and the society." In order for STS to have the breadth of impact it should, the author maintains that "true union engagement is a necessity."

107. Cole, Robert E. *Strategies for Learning: Small-Group Activities in American, Japanese and Swedish Industry*. Berkeley: University of California Press, 1989.

Keywords: comparative, quality circles, teams, organizational behavior

Robert Cole, a leading figure in industrial relations research and organizational behavior, provides a detailed comparative study of "small-group activities" in American, Japanese and Swedish industrial settings. The author defines small group activities as "workshop- or office-based groups that are given a greater opportunity to exercise direct control over everyday work decisions and the solving of workshop problems." In the United States such groups are commonly referred to as quality circles or employee-involvement groups. Cole sets out to examine the reasons why "American firms moved more slowly and less effectively in adopting small-group activities than Swedish and, especially, Japanese ones." Management behavior, rather than workers' behavior, is the central concern of the study, although the implications for the self-esteem, well-being and performance of the employees are fully acknowledged.

Various theories that attempt to explain the emergence of small-group activities are advanced. Some cite "the role of new technologies of flexible manufacturing, combined with growing global competition" in encouraging increased teamwork and employee participation. Others propose that small-group activities are "a strong democratizing force that finally brings the benefits of political democracy into the workplace." Still others, such as the neo-Marxist perspective, subscribe to the belief that these activities "are just one more management technique to control workers."

Finally, theories of human growth and development "with their stress on self-actualization" speak about participation and greater employee involvement in terms of the "humanization of work."

In sum, Cole attributes much of the success among Japanese firms in quickly and efficiently deploying small-group activities for competitive advantage to the creation of an effective national infrastructure. See chapter 14 "Summing Up" for a succinct summary of the study results.

108. Confer, Robert G. *Workplace Health Protection: Industrial Hygiene Program Guide*. Boca Raton, FL: CRC Press, 1994.

Keywords: health, safety

The author has compiled a reference book for evaluating industrial hygiene programs. He presents 50 criteria in nine categories: management, technical aspects, support activities, personal protective equipment, special materials, special operations, emergency preparedness, and medical surveillance. This checklist begins the book. Then the criteria are described and established based on industry practice, consensus standards, technical literature, trade association publications, and other procedures that have proved to be effective. The author developed this reference document in order to provide a practical tool for consistently evaluating the applicability and/or effectiveness of workplace health protection programs. The criteria can be used for implementing a program from scratch or for evaluating and modifying an existing program. They are applicable worldwide and the author hopes that they can be used to improve working conditions in overseas operations.

109. Cook, Peter. *The Industrial Craftsworker: Skill, Managerial Strategies and Workplace Relationships*. London: Mansell, 1996.

Keywords: craftswork, unions, labor relations, knowledge embedded in experience, skill

Craftsworkers have their own worldview and consider themselves different from other industrial workers. Their view that craftswork has its own moral value arose from the time when work, particularly craftsworking, was considered the most honorable of secular activities. Chapters 1 and 2 trace the history of craftsworking as a cultural force and what it means to be a craftsworker. They also investigate what skill is and compare real, socially constructed, and tacit skill. Because of the uniqueness of craftsworkers, tension exists between them and other industrial workers as well as between them and managers. These two relationships are probed through two case studies. The first one is presented in chapters 3 through 6 and deals with toolmakers and tool and die makers in American car factories and the second (chapters 7 through 9) in the British context. The conclusion is that the behavior of "industrial craftsworkers" can, during the development of unionization and of collective bargaining, be roughly characterized as both aristocratic and militantly vanguardist. Which of the two characterizations applies most can be to some extent explained by key contextual factors, including the historical development of particular national labor movements, the nature of the state, the predominant management style, and differences in employment conditions between craft and production workers. Important also is the presence or absence of a legacy of earlier successful workplace control struggles that, combined with the factors above, have created a very different industrial climate in Britain—even for the quintessential American activity of "volume car-making." More importantly, the case studies analyze the fate of knowledge embedded in experience in the age of advanced manufacturing technology.

110. Cooley, Mike, ed. *Architect or Bee? The Human Price of Technology*. London: Hogarth Press, 1987.

Keywords: computers, automation, tacit knowledge, skill, human factors, knowledge embedded in experience, knowledge separated from experience

This book offers both a critique of contemporary technologies (especially computer automated systems) and a constructive attempt to redesign them to better respond to human needs. The author suggests that we must look closely at those forms of technology that meet our particular historical and cultural requirements, and develop more appropriate forms of technology to meet our long-term aspirations.

Cooley questions the widespread belief that automation, computerization, and robotic devices "will free human beings from soul-destroying, routine, backbreaking tasks and leave them free to engage in more creative work." He also doubts that computer innovations will automatically lead to a shorter working week and more leisure time. The book questions these assumptions and shows that "we are beginning to repeat in the field of intellectual work most of the mistakes already made in the field of skilled manual work at an earlier historical stage." The author looks critically at technological change as a whole "in order to provide a framework for questioning the way computers are used today."

Topics discussed in the book include the following: common sense and tacit knowledge, skill acquisition in the context of human and computer "intelligence," the changing nature of work, human-machine interaction, CAD-CAM systems, competence, skill and "training," intellectual and manual work and the political implications of new technology.

111. Cooley, M. J. E. "Problems of Automation." 199-207 in *Proceedings of the First International Conference on Human Factors in Manufacturing*, edited by T. Lupton. Bedford: IFS and North-Holland, 1984.

Keywords: Taylorism, division of labor, alienation, skill

This brief paper begins with Cooley declaring the importance of questioning our underlying assumptions of science and technology and our failure to examine the full range of technological choices open to us. This failure amounts to "closing of technological options and alternative forms of human organization."

Cooley then recounts a brief history of the Tayloristic division of labor, the Western scientific methodology, and the myriad of problems it created when dealing with complex systems. His discussion also covers computer pacing and related mental stress, intellectual workers (white-collar), CAD and deskilling, alienation, and routinization of creative design.

112. Cooper, Cary L., and Roy Payne, eds. *Current Concerns in Occupational Stress*. Wiley Series on Studies in Occupational Stress. New York: John Wiley and Sons, 1980.

Keywords: stress, health, psychology

At first glance, this is a rather dated volume of essays by psychologists and behavioral scientists in the field of occupational stress and health. Nevertheless, the editors of this book are two of the leading researchers on stress in the workplace (at least in the 1980s) who have put together a solid and diverse collection that remains relevant today.

Part 1 focuses on jobs at particular risk of stress-related problems. Part 2 discusses various aspects of work life that contribute to stress, such as job transfer, two-career couples, Type A behavior and Western society's work values. Part 3, on coping with stress, provides the best material in the text in terms of preventive strategies for stress reduction. Issues explored include techniques for reducing managerial stress and organizational stress among employees, social support of stress, and various coping mechanisms. Little emphasis, however, is given to technological and structural factors. Still, the overall result is an insightful volume with some classic material.

113. Cooper, Cary L., and Roy Payne, eds. *Causes, Coping and Consequences of Stress at Work.* Wiley Series on Studies in Occupational Stress. Chichester: John Wiley and Sons, 1988.

Keywords: stress, work design, white-collar work, coping

This volume is an extensive update of the authors' classic work *Stress at Work,* published in 1978. The previous book focused on blue-collar and managerial stress; this one examines in greater detail "stress in the office, the impact of new technology, the pressures of industrial relations difficulties, and the continuing problems of repetitive manual work." Moreover, this edition includes a comprehensive section on "health promotion in the workplace" and "interventions for stress reduction and prevention."

Part 1 of the book concentrates on "The Epidemiology of Occupational Stress," revealing the extent to which the medical and psychological fields are merging in this area of research. Part 2 looks at "Factors in the Person's Environment" by considering managerial and professional stress in large organizations, new technology and operator stress, the nonwork factors in stress at work, and the psychological stressors associated with industrial relations. Part 3 explores "Factors in the Person" including "hardiness, locus of control, trait anxiety, and a range of personality characteristics." In addition, "the significance of coping, both as a determinant and consequence of stress" is examined.

Part 4 "The Person in the Work Environment" has a strong preventive component, with emphasis given to health promotion, job redesign, stress management, and other approaches to stress reduction. The final section of the book, part 5, examines methodological issues and future directions for research. This is an outstanding and comprehensive volume with an extensive bibliography.

114. Cooper, Cary L., and Ivan T. Robertson, eds. *International Review of Industrial and Organizational Psychology 1996.* Chichester: John Wiley and Sons, 1996.

Keywords: psychology, division of labor, Taylorism

The first two chapters are the most relevant to healthy work. Chapter 1 "Self-Esteem and Work" demonstrates that self-esteem is a profound psychological need. The next section reviews various theories of self-esteem. The theories of Freud, White, Ellis, Deci and Rand and the social approval theory are outlined and critically assessed. Next, the differences between self-esteem, self-efficacy, locus of control, and self-concept are explained. The various methods of measuring self-esteem and the corresponding problems are noted next. The nonwork correlates of self-esteem—physical attractiveness, gender, ethnic group and social class—are discussed. As well, the workplace correlates (causes and/or consequences) of self-esteem found in the literature are probed. These correlates include thinking, decision making, job search, occupational choice, job choice, goal choice, persistence, performance, job characteristics, job satisfaction, stress and plasticity.

The historical and contemporary theories of job design are the focus of chapter 2. The work of division of labor proponents Babbage and Smith, Taylor's scientific management and Herzberg's Motivation-Hygiene Theory are briefly introduced. Then, three contemporary approaches are reviewed and analyzed. These are the Job Characteristics Theory, Campion's Integrated Framework, and design of work for teams. The chapter concludes with suggested avenues for future inquiry such as the effects of workers comparing their jobs to others' jobs, the physical work environment, the process of changing jobs and the nonwork outcomes of job design.

115. Cooper, Cary L., and Michael J. Smith, eds. *Job Stress and Blue Collar Work*. Wiley Series on Studies in Occupational Stress. Chichester: John Wiley and Sons, 1985.

Keywords: stress, alienation, blue-collar work, coping

This collection of essays, written by industrial engineers and organizational psychologists, provides a comprehensive analysis of the unique occupational stress problems faced by blue-collar workers. Insights into the stressful working conditions of this group are offered, along with "alternative strategies or courses of action to help alleviate, minimize or cope with them."

Chapter 1 explores trends in blue-collar worker attitudes and worker alienation. Chapter 2 gives a historical review of these workers' attitudes and perceptions from the early 1970s to the mid-1980s. Chapter 3 discusses "one of the underlying reasons that blue-collar work is so stressful, lack of control." Part 2 of the book examines "a variety of stressful working conditions and situations. Topics considered include machine-paced work, stress and repetitive work, the impact of new technology, and alternative work schedules and their potential implications for health. Part 3 provides "an overview of various approaches and techniques for controlling worker stress, including Employee Assistance Programs (EAPs), union efforts to relieve stress, social support, and individual coping." The final section of the book further explores the "application of individual coping strategies, their usefulness in symptom reduction, and examples of successful use."

In the context of healthy work promotion and preventive strategies, chapter 8 "Alternative Work Schedules: Flextime and the Compressed Work Week" and chapter 13 "Social Support and Stress Reduction" are especially relevant.

116. Corbett, J. M. "Technically Embedded Constraints on Job Design and How to Overcome Them." 67-71 in *IFAC/IFIP/IMACS Symposium on Skill Based Automated Production*, edited by Peter Kopacek and Robert Genser. Vienna: Pergamon Press (for IFAC), 1989.

Keywords: work design, organizational behavior, automation, technology

Many consider the effect of technological systems on job design to be negligible compared to the effect of organizational systems. Corbett contends that advanced manufacturing technology is not neutral and significantly constrains an organization's choice of shopfloor design. The first section of the article critically examines the case for technological neutrality in job design and exposes its weaknesses. The case for "soft" technological determinism is put forth in the next section. In order to account for the constraining effects of the technology, an alternative to the traditional sequential decision-making process—in which first the technology and then the organizational and human factors are considered—is necessary. Such an alternative process is outlined in the third section. Finally, several multidisciplinary design methods that aim to overcome the constraints imposed by production technology choices are evaluated.

117. Corbett, J. Martin, Lauge Baumgaard Rasmussen, and Felix Rauner, eds. *Crossing the Border: The Social and Engineering Design of Computer Integrated Manufacturing Systems*. Springer Series on Artificial Intelligence and Society. London: Springer Verlag, 1991.

Keywords: sociotechnical systems, anthropocentric, computers, advanced manufacturing technology, work design

"This book discusses and develops concepts and methods of interdisciplinary collaboration between engineers, social scientists, and users in the process of developing 'human centered' production technology." The title *Crossing the Border* refers to the disciplinary border that the authors attempt to cross in the course of their research—particularly between social science and engineering design, as well as between "conventional social science research (which takes a reactive stance to the world of technology and work) and applied research . . . of a more proactive kind."

The authors speak of a "bifunction of the technical and social realms of working life," which this text attempts to break through by "opening up the black box . . . which so often constitutes advanced manufacturing technology in most social science research and by exploring . . . methods with which social scientists, engineers, and users may work together to design human-centered technology and humane computer-aided work systems."

See chapter 1 for a discussion of the existing paradigm crisis in the field of technology and work. Three different perspectives are identified and assessed—the technique-oriented, the sociotechnical and the human-centered approaches—and a work-oriented approach is outlined. Chapters 2 and 3 focus on the interdisciplinary collaboration developed in human-centered CIM systems. Various project results are documented and assessed. Chapter 4 deals with the problem of design method generalizability and considers how greater collaboration in the design and development of human computer-aided work systems can be fostered. The final chapter offers a number of meta-rules to guide interdisciplinary collaboration in the design of work and technologies.

118. Corlett, E. N., and J. Richardson, eds. *Stress, Work Design and Productivity*. New York: John Wiley and Sons, 1981.

Keywords: work design, anthropocentric, stress, psychology, ergonomics

The design of a machine or a process usually emphasizes the importance of technical efficiency but rarely sees the influence on the efficiency of the people in the system. What people do arises almost by accident from what the machinery does not do. Moreover, not only is the content of a person's job often decided by convention or in other implicit ways, but the workplace in which s/he does it may also owe more to the convenience of the machinery than the operator.

If we accept that physical adaptation takes a matter of centuries, and social adaptation takes decades, it follows that to take full advantage of the potential of technology we must use its flexibility to design primarily for humans, not for itself.

Part 2 concentrates on an ergonomic and industrial psychology approach. Part 3 concentrates on methods of assessing psychosocial and mental stress in industry. Part 4 focuses on job design and stress.

119. Cornfield, Daniel B., Karen E. Campbell, and Holly J. McCammon, eds. *Working in Restructured Workplaces: Challenges and New Directions for the Sociology of Work*. Thousand Oaks, CA: Sage Publications, 2001.

Keywords: reconfiguring workplace status hierarchies, casualization of employment relationships, restructuring and worker marginalization, comparative labor responses to global restructuring

By bringing together works based on the fundamental changes in the nature of work in the global economy, the editors hope to answer such questions as: What are the current trends in workplace restructuring and the impact of these trends on workers' lives? and Around what concepts will work be organized and groups and individuals motivated in the changing nature of today's work environments? To do so, they use works that present a new theoretical framework for thinking about "workplace restructuring." Also, new research and a policy agenda were charted for examining the nature, prevalence, and consequences of workplace restructuring. In doing so, both the human consequences of workplace restructuring as well as cross-national variations in a wide range of global worker responses to the changing nature of work were examined.

120. Courchene, Thomas J. *A State of Minds: Toward a Human Capital Future for Canadians*. Montreal: Institute for Research on Public Policy (IRPP), 2001.

Keywords: human capital, Canada, manpower policy, globalization, information society, information technology, social aspects

This book examines the political structures that link local, provincial, and federal governments and challenges many longstanding beliefs about how society should be organized and financed. The author, while focusing on Canadian competitiveness in a global economy, shows us how an open federal state like Canada can achieve both social justice and economic prosperity.

121. Crandall, Rick, and Pamela L. Perrewé, eds. *Occupational Stress: A Handbook*. Washington, DC: Taylor and Francis, 1995.

Keywords: stress, coping, psychology, organizational behavior

A number of well-known scholars contribute to this comprehensive attempt at examining occupational stress. The five sections of the book balance theoretical perspectives with empirical findings, thus enhancing its value. Section 1 critically appraises the strength of the transactional approach in psychology to the study of stress and compares it to other theoretical perspectives.

Section 2 is devoted to the organization of the theoretical perspectives developed in section 1 through various models and their testing. The models range from ones that focus on individual and organizational characteristics, stress as an intervening variable, and organizational effectiveness and health outcomes, to others that test the moderating influence of social support, mastery, active coping, as well as the differences between problem-focused versus emotion-focused coping styles.

The next section is devoted to an explicit analysis of various modes of coping with stress and naturally segues to section 4 where the failure of coping styles, namely "burnout," and its consequences are examined.

The final section of this book provides a critical evaluation of various interventions aimed at reducing job stress—from counseling at work to exercise as a possible buffer to job strain.

122. Crompton, Rosemary, Duncan Gallie, and Kate Purcell, eds. *Changing Forms of Employment: Organizations, Skills and Gender*. London: Routledge, 1996.

Keywords: technology, skills, women, multinational, human resources

Separating underlying trends from short-term economic fluctuations can be difficult. But the editors have identified three recent trends in employment patterns. The first pattern discussed concerns changes in the organization of production and productive activity. This, of course, is the shift from Fordism to post-Fordism. Chapter 2 argues for the rebuilding of labor market institutions while chapters 3, 4, and 5 are concerned with deregulation and the resulting broadening of boundaries. Multinational corporations, international contract services and the shipping industry are studied. The second trend commented upon in this collection is the large role that changes in technology, particularly information technology, now plays. The implications for the recomposition of skills and employment are investigated by the contributors to this second part. The third trend is that the "male breadwinner" model of employment is no longer applicable; thus the third section explores the change in gender relations. The relationship between national, institutional, cultural and sectoral factors that obstruct these changes are examined.

123. Daniels, Cynthia R., ed. *Lost Fathers: The Politics of Fatherlessness in America*. New York: St. Martin's Press, 1998.

Keywords: fatherless family, paternal deprivation, African American fathers, absentee fathers

This collection of articles by scholars from diverse backgrounds provides the reader with a culturally and politically charged concept of fatherlessness that illustrates the divisions that constitute public debate on this issue. Debates arise over the proper or desirable place of fathers in the lives of children and revive old areas of controversy and initiate new ones. Tied into the issue of fatherlessness are questions regarding the nature of mothering and fathering, the biological roots of sexuality and parenting, the relationship between family structure and poverty, and the efficacy and desirability of alternative family structures.

124. Dankbaar, Ben. "Lean Production: Denial, Confirmation or Extension of Sociotechnical Systems Design." *Human Relations* 50, no. 5 (May 1997).

Keywords: sociotechnical systems, lean production, teams, Fordism, innovation

This article offers "a comparison between the basic elements of lean production and sociotechnical systems design (STSD) and compares them both with the characteristics of the traditional Fordist system of mass production. It argues that lean production can hardly be considered as an alternative to mass production, as its proponents suggest, but is on the contrary extending the life of mass production methods. However, lean production does appear to contain some building blocks for the innovative production systems that are expected to prevail in the 21st century." Dankbaar argues that STSD, which has always presented itself as an alternative and possible successor to Fordist methods, "will need to link its traditional concerns for quality of work and flexibility of work organizations with the new issues of continuous improvement, learning, and innovation." The author adds that "the fact that lean production appears to prevail in car manufacturing can hardly be accepted as proof that it represents the production system of the 21st century." Finally, Dankbaar suggests that "STSD may satisfy itself that it can match LP in terms of creating flexible organizations (with a higher quality of work), but it can still learn quite a bit about the design of innovative organizations. If it wants to remain a relevant tradition, it had better learn those lessons. If it does, because of its attention to the quality of work, it may show itself to be far more capable of creating high-motivation high-innovation organizations than lean production ever will."

125. Darrah, Charles N. "Workplace Skills in Context." *Human Organization* 51, no. 3 (1992): 264-73.

Keywords: work design, computers, automation

The contents of this chapter are most accurately summarized in the words of the author himself: "Concerns about people who are ill-prepared to perform in workplaces of the future have resulted in various policy reports identifying 'basic skills' and postulating appropriate educational responses. Much of the supporting data are thin, and yield descriptions that characterize work through a limited and biased sample of possible observations. Work is made to appear unambiguous, instrumental, rational, and subject to universal categorization. Fieldwork in a manufacturing plant presents a richer picture of work that counters these distortions by demonstrating the importance of alternative styles of work, strategies for managing ambiguity, and the importance of local knowledge. The conventional focus on skills in isolation is replaced by one in which both skills and our ability to describe them is constrained by the technological and organizational contexts of workplaces. Incentives, opportunities, the expressive function of skilled performance, and feedback about results all influence skills. Finally, the role of factors mediating the effects of macroscopic economic forces is explored. I argue that the restricted focus on skill of individual workers is misplaced, and that educational reforms must address the social nature of work, including the capacity to understand and modify technology and organization."

126. Davenport, Thomas H. "Saving IT's Soul: Human Centered Information Management." *Harvard Business Review*, March-April 1994: 119-31.

Keywords: information technology, management, anthropocentric, technocentric, computers

This article offers a detailed analysis of a relatively new approach to information handling in organizations known as Human-Centered Information Management. The author argues that many managers today who promote information technology (IT) as the key catalyst of business change "become prisoners of their own fascination, constructing elaborate technology architectures, and enterprise information models to guide systems development." It is further argued that "such technocratic solutions often specify the minutiae of machinery while disregarding how people in organizations actually go about acquiring, sharing, and making use of information. In short, they glorify information technology and ignore human psychology." The author notes that technocrats are often insensitive to the unpredictable aspects of human nature; "[they] are constantly caught off guard by the 'irrational behavior of end users.'" For the author, only one thing is certain for the many diverse information users in large organizations: "Effective information management must begin by thinking about how people use information—not with how people use machines." The following three observations made by the author exemplify how a human-centered approach to information management contrasts with the standard IT view:

(1) "Information evolves in many directions, taking on multiple meanings . . . rather than forcing employees to simplify information so that it will fit into a computer, a human-centered approach to information calls for preserving the rich complexity we prefer in our information diets."

(2) "People don't share information easily. Assuming that different departments, professionals, or line workers will want to use technology to share information is one of the biggest mistakes executives make. Yet it is one of the fundamental assumptions made in planning any IT system. That is, if you build it, people will use it."

(3) "Changing an IT system won't change a company's information culture. The presence of technology, in and of itself, cannot wholly transform a corporation. . . . Changing the technology only reinforces the behaviors that already exist. . . . Too many managers still believe that once the right technology is in place, appropriate information storing will follow."

The author goes on to suggest that most good managers do not rely on computer-based information to make decisions.

See also "The Information Facts of Life" on page 122 and the chart on page 123 that contrasts traditional information architectures with human-centered approaches to information management.

127. Davidson, Marilyn J., and Cary L. Cooper, eds. *Women and Information Technology*. Wiley Series in Psychology and Productivity at Work. Chichester: John Wiley and Sons, 1987.

Keywords: women, computers, health, video display units, information technology, automation

This particular volume in the Wiley Series in Psychology and Productivity at Work (edited by David Oborne) presents "a comprehensive overview of the impact of new information technology on women in terms of both employment and human and organizational issues—present and future."

The book is divided into four main sections. The first section presents a cross-cultural perspective of the effects of information technology on girls and women. The second section concentrates on how new information technology has affected women working in different industries in the United Kingdom. The third section provides chapters investigating the psychosocial and health effects of IT on women workers (see especially "Visual Display Units—Psychosocial Factors in Health" by Raija Kalimo and Anneli Leppänen). The fourth and final section looks at the future—new trends and initiatives related to women and IT—that includes homeworkers, union involvement and new training initiatives.

The book offers broad coverage of information technologies with a focus on policy and health and is of particular value to psychologists, occupational health specialists, and women's organizations. The contributors also make a number of important recommendations to improve the long-term prospects of women in information technology.

128. Davidson, Marilyn J., and Jill Earnshaw, eds. *Vulnerable Workers: Psychosocial and Legal Issues*. Wiley Series on Studies in Occupational Stress. Chichester: John Wiley and Sons, 1991.

Keywords: women, vulnerable workers, part-time work, abuse harassment

This book is one of the more recent additions to the excellent Wiley Series on Studies in Occupational Stress. This particular volume "attempts to explore the psychosocial and legal issues involved in the employment of certain groups of workers who are more disadvantaged than others at work." Some of the vulnerable groups examined include women workers, disabled workers, part-time workers, black and ethnic minority workers, homosexual workers, HIV-positive workers, and workers with AIDS.

Part 1 of the text presents a cross-cultural perspective of vulnerable workers in the European Community and the United States. Topics of concern here include equal treatment of men and women, independence for people with disabilities, social protection and social security, combating poverty, reducing unemployment and alternative employment measures. Part 2 concentrates on the psychosocial and legal issues relevant to two groups of workers who are particularly vulnerable in terms of physical and health disabilities, namely the disabled and sufferers of HIV and AIDS. Part 3 deals with three types of workers who are susceptible to physical or verbal abuse or victimization generally, i.e., victims of violence at work, victims of sexual harassment at work, and homosexuals and transsexuals at work. The final part of the book covers two groups of vulnerable workers whose numbers do not justify their commonly-assigned "minority" label (i.e., part-time workers and job sharers, and black and ethnic workers).

129. Davis, Ed, and Russell Lansbury, eds. *Democracy and Control in the Workplace*. Melbourne: Longman Cheshire, 1986.

Keywords: democracy, comparative, case study, participation

This volume examines developments in the industrial democracy movement, primarily in Australia, but also in Britain, West Germany, Sweden, Yugoslavia, Japan, and the United States. Detailed case studies of various employee involvement schemes are provided, along with analyses of innovations in occupational health and safety. Particular emphasis is given to the role of labor unions in fostering worker participation strategies. The authors identify three basic criteria for the assessment of industrial democracy programs: "the extent of workers' influence on decision-making, the scope of decision-making, and proportion of the workforce involved."

See especially chapter 3 "Industrial Democracy and the Question of Control," chapter 6 "Worker Participation in Occupational Health and Safety: 'Applied' Industrial Democracy?," chapter 14 "Industrial Democracy and the Control Issue in Sweden," chapter 16 "Employee Participation in Japan," and chapter 17 "Workers' Participation in the United States."

130. Davis, Jim, Thomas Hirschl, and Michael Stack, eds. *Cutting Edge: Technology, Information, Capitalism and Social Revolution*. London: Verso, 1997.

Keywords: technology, alienation, capitalism, knowledge, automation, computers

This volume brings together contributions from workers employed in the new electronics and information industries with leftist theorists in economics, politics, and science to provide an extensive and current analysis of the complex relations between technology and work. Individual essays look at topics including "the cyclical nature of a technologically driven economy, the privatization of knowledge that new information industries demand, the convergence of different economic sectors under the impact of digitalization, and the strategies that trade unionists and governments might deploy to protect jobs and living standards." The authors begin their analysis by noting that the explosion in the development of computer- and robotic-based manufacturing is seeing the rapid expansion of laborless production systems. Such systems, it is argued, create enormous instability, both for the overall world economy where money previously paid in wages is now invested in labor-saving technology and therefore cannot be spent on goods, and for workers whose jobs are being deskilled or are simply disappearing. The editors maintain that "technology has the potential to end material scarcity and lay the foundations for higher forms of human fulfillment. But under existing power structures, it is more likely to exacerbate the poverty and misery under which most people live."

See especially "Robots and Capitalism" by Tessa Morris-Suzuki, "Capitalism in the Computer Age and Afterward" (by the same author), "Value Creation in the Late Twentieth Century: The Rise of the Knowledge Worker" by Martin Kenney, "The Information Commodity" by Dan Schiller, "The Digital Advantage" by Jim Davis, "Structural Unemployment and the Qualitative Transformation of Capitalism" by Thomas Hirschl, and "A Note on Alienation and Automation" by Ramin Ramtin.

131. Davis, Louis E., and James C. Taylor, eds. *Design of Jobs*. Santa Monica: Goodyear Publishing Co., 1979.

Keywords: work design, assembly line, technology, QWL, sociotechnical systems, history, psychology

This classic compendium of essays focuses on the history and methods of job design. Chapters 4 and 5 explore the history and methods of work concepts and provide a historical overview of various job design strategies. Traditional and novel assembly-line techniques are the subject of chapter 11, and chapter 12 discusses the relationship between new technologies and organizational restructuring. Chapter 13 further examines the interactions between technical and social systems by looking at the characteristics and psychological effects of the new technology, as well as the implications for workers' skills. Chapter 14 considers job enlargement from a theoretical and methodological perspective, and chapter 15 offers an assessment of "Job Satisfaction and Quality of Working Life." Chapter 16 explores orthodox job enrichment and chapter 17 looks at "New Leads in Job Design—The Phillips Case." Also see part 5 of the text on "Work Systems Studies." Essays in this section include the following: "Improving the Quality of Working Life: Sociotechnical Case Studies"; "A Sociotechnical Approach to Problems of Process Control"; "A Measure of Work Group Autonomy"; and "An Experiment in Work Satisfaction." At the time of the publication, this text represented one of the best collections in the field by well-known specialists in the area of job design.

132. De Keyser, Véronique, Thoralf Qvale, Bernhard Wilpert, and S. Antonio Ruiz Quintanilla. *The Meaning of Work and Technological Options*. New Technologies and Work. Chichester: John Wiley and Sons, 1988.

Keywords: information technology, history, comparative, skill, sociotechnical systems

This book, one of a series on new technologies and work, is produced by an international interdisciplinary study group. It presents a "problem focused volume of texts concentrating on . . . some of the most important perspectives on the meaning of work in the context of new information technologies."

The introductory chapter offers a historical perspective on traditional work ethics and a discussion of the meaning of work as a scientific construct, which can be linked to technology-related changes in work settings. This is followed in the next chapter by an overview of recent trends in work life (related to technological developments) "that are likely to have an impact on how work is experienced and valued by working persons." The third chapter evaluates the foregoing issues in the context of modern market economies. Chapter 4 applies an international comparative perspective to reflect on the question of a universal technical imperative (i.e., whether one exists or not). Chapter 5 considers the possibilities for implementing modern job design criteria with respect to new information technologies. Case studies are used in chapters 6, 7, and 8 to examine "how different choices in the use of new information technologies impact on working conditions, organizational structure, social relations, skill requirements, skill use." The remaining sections of the book consider the relationship between the sociotechnical systems approach and the perceived quality of work life as well as various methodologies for furthering our understanding of the ties linking technological development to the meaning of work.

133. Dean Jr., J. W., and S. A. Snell. "Integrated Manufacturing and Job Design: Moderating Effects of Organizational Inertia." *Academy of Management Journal* 34, no. 4 (1991): 776-99.

Keywords: manufacturing, industrial relations, total quality management, work design

The article is summarized in the abstract as follows: "This study investigated the difference between integrated manufacturing, a new manufacturing paradigm comprising advanced technology, just-in-time inventory control, and total quality management, and job characteristics (task uncertainty and interdependance). We hypothesized that performance, size, and external control would moderate this relationship. Data from plants and personal managers and nonmanagerial employees in 123 companies showed no main effects of integrated manufacturing on job design among employees in operations, quality control and assurance, and production control. Rather, the relationships were contingent on organizational context. We discuss organizational inertia and resource availability as alternative theoretical perspectives on the impact of organizational context."

134. Dean Jr., James W., and Gerald I. Susman. "Organizing for Manufacturable Design." *Harvard Business Review*, January-February 1989: 28-36.

Keywords: manufacturing, organizational design, industrial relations

One large obstacle to creating well-designed, high quality, low production cost, and efficient products is the lack of communication and collaboration between designers and manufacturers. Four approaches to organizing for manufacturable design are outlined in this article. The first is for companies to invest in software for the designers that helps to guide designs to be more manufacturable. The second approach is to use an integrator, someone who works with both the design and manufacturing groups and who serves as a liaison between the two. This position is a difficult one, as the person must have a reasonable knowledge of both aspects of the product's creation. The third approach uses cross-functional teams that collaborate together from the start of a project. In the least, this team consists of a designer and a manufacturing engineer who work together throughout the project and are often in the same office. This allows for each side to become familiar with the work of the other as well as allow manufacturing to begin its work soon after the design team begins and for them to finish within relatively the same timeframe. The last approach consists of the creation of a single department, which is the largest change of the four. It entails having a single manager for both teams or subunits, one for design and the other for manufacture. However, this demands that the people possess the skills to overlap into the other aspect of the product's creation. These approaches are not cast in stone, and should be customized for individual organizational use.

135. Deem, Rosemary, and Graeme Salaman. *Work, Culture and Society*. Milton Keynes, UK: Open University Press, 1985.

Keywords: sociology, labor process, industrial relations, skill, Taylorism, work design

This text offers a good introduction to many of the current debates in sociology and industrial relations on the nature of work and culture in modern societies. A wide range of issues is covered including the organization of contemporary manufacturing, the labor process debate, labor market segmentation, work outside of formal employment, leisure and unemployment, and "the design of work in capitalist and socialist societies." Conceptual concerns and their practical implications are dealt with in a clear, straightforward manner. See chapter 4 "Work Organization" by Stephen Wood for a good discussion of the deskilling thesis, Taylor's scientific management, technology and the labor process, and work humanization.

136. DeMatteo, Bob. *Terminal Shock: The Health Hazards of Video Display Terminals*. Toronto: New Canada Publications, 1986.

Keywords: video display terminal, health, radiation, stress, ergonomics, policy

This volume, written by a specialist in occupational health and safety, is an excellent source of practical information on video display terminals (VDTs) "for employers and employees, parents and teachers, doctors and public health professionals." The well-researched text is also "a hard-hitting detailed indictment of the social forces that have permitted the unregulated and untested introduction of automaton-like factory-like conditions into the modern workplace." The author lays out the health problems related to VDTs in a very straightforward, readable manner, and offers many suggestions for properly setting up VDT-based work environments.

The book includes "clear, illustrated explanations of what radiation is, and the types of radiation emitted by VDTs," advice on "how to shield your terminal," "descriptions of the ergonomic and stress hazards of VDTs and how they can be mitigated," a review of Canadian and American legislation, "sample health questionnaires and recommended opthamalogical examinations," and an "international overview of proposed technical and workplace standards for VDT operators."

This volume is of special importance for policy makers and design experts interested in creating a healthier interface between machines and human operators. Since its publication, many of its suggestions have been incorporated into policies and today's VDTs are as a consequence much safer. Some other safety concerns, however, are still present.

137. Dembe, Allard E. *Occupation and Disease: How Social Factors Affect the Conception of Work-Related Disorders*. New Haven, CT: Yale University Press, 1996.

Keywords: occupational disease, health, sociology

This rather unique sociological approach to the subject of occupational health examines the process by which certain medical disorders come to be regarded by physicians as work-related. The author's thesis is that "this process is not merely a matter of gathering and interpreting empirical evidence but rather a complex social phenomenon. The determination that a disorder is caused by a patient's job occurs in a rich social context colored by the unequal power relationships that generally prevail between employees and management in the work environment and between patients and physicians in the health care setting. The intense social dynamics that permeate these two contexts help determine whether a particular disorder eventually becomes known as an occupational disease."

The author contends that the question of how disorders come to be regarded as occupationally related is a crucial one, not only because of the direct costs to society associated with occupational illness and injuries, but also because there are substantial effects on worker health, job satisfaction and labor regulations. Moreover, public health and safety officials always strive to anticipate and control significant workplace hazards. Rather than concentrating on the narrow issue of causality, Dembe examines "how the issue of causality is embedded in a particular social and political context" and shows "how that context molds and influences the way in which the causality question is formulated." The author's principal objective is to identify key social factors that affect the initial emergence and recognition of occupational disorders.

See chapter 1 "The Social Context of Occupational Disease" (historical case studies, a pluralistic model of occupational disease, etc.), chapter 2 "Cumulative Trauma Disorders of the Hands and Wrists" (the history of carpal tunnel syndrome, repetitive strain injuries, etc.), chapter 3 "Back Pain" (history of and medical reporting of), and chapter 4 "Noise-Induced Hearing Loss" (control methods, community response to noise exposure, etc.). See especially chapter 5 "Conclusion" (new technologies, labor activism, environmental concerns, economic costs, implications for policy making).

138. Derber, Charles. *Corporation Nation: How Corporations Are Taking Over Our Lives and What We Can Do about It.* New York: St. Martin's Press, 1998.

Keywords: corporations, political aspects, sociological aspects, social responsibility of business, business and politics, industrial policy, moral and ethical aspects, labor policy, international trade, democracy, sovereignty

Our social landscape is changing. The emerging twenty-first century is dominated by corporations that are bigger and more powerful than most countries. Many corporations already manage huge domains of the public sector and they are threatening to further invade traditionally public sectors such as medicine, education, social services, and law enforcement. Large movie, computer, and bank corporations are not only influencing but controlling our lives and identities, and the lives of children. As well as discussing the above issues, this book offers a new vision and suggestions for programmatic reform that address the political and spiritual problems of corporate ascendancy. Also discussed are personal and political changes that are necessary to put them into practice.

139. Dertouzos, Michael L., Richard K. Lester, Robert M. Solow, and MIT Commission on Industrial Productivity. *Made in America: Regaining the Productive Edge.* Cambridge, MA: MIT Press, 1989.

Keywords: general, productivity, case study

The authors of this classic volume, in conjunction with the MIT Commission on Industrial Productivity, provide a comprehensive study of America's industrial performance. They examine weaknesses in U.S. industrial practice and possible causes, as well as changes in the international economic system and "how these changes might alter the requirements for successful industrial performance in the future."

The researchers involved in the study are an interdisciplinary team made up of technologists, economists, political scientists and management and organizational specialists. The main focus of the study is "the nation's production system: the organizations, the plant, the equipment, and the people from factory workers to senior executives that combine to conceive, design, develop, produce, market, and deliver goods and services to the customer."

The authors start "by examining specific firms and industries and work up to more general conclusions and recommendations." Eight sectors of the economy are chosen for detailed study: automobiles, chemicals, commercial aircraft, computers, semiconductors and copiers, consumer electronics, machine tools, and steel. See especially chapter 5 "Technological Weaknesses in Development and Production," chapter 6 "Neglect of Human Resources," chapter 9 "Emerging Patterns of Best Industrial Practice," and chapter 10 "Imperatives for a More Productive America."

140. Dohse, K., Ulrich Jurgens, and Thomas Malsch. "From 'Fordism' to 'Toyotism'? The Social Organization of the Labor Process in the Japanese Automobile Industry." *Politics and Society* 14, no. 2 (1985): 115-46.

Keywords: Fordism, Toyotism, labor process, knowledge embedded in experience, knowledge separated from experience, labor relations

A detailed examination of post-Fordist labor process techniques in Japan by a team of German researchers interested in the automotive industry is presented here. The article does not argue for any particular thesis and remains an excellent description of the changes that were required in labor relations, the knowledge base of the workers, their skills, as well as management styles, before Toyotism could become firmly entrenched in the automotive industry of Japan. This is one of the most succinct introductions to the labor process in Japan; it gives due consideration to the wider cultural and political contexts that helped to bring this process into being.

141. Donkin, Richard. *Blood, Sweat and Tears: The Evolution of Work.* New York: Texere, 2001.

Keywords: work, history of work

The fall of manual labor was regarded as a liberation as society was progressing and industrializing. However, this was followed by a more troubling realization that the new forms of work were dominating people's lives. The question that begs to be asked is, How did it get like this? The concept of work lags several decades behind the current reality. Our outdated concept is founded on an agricultural and industrial past and thus has been "reinforced by a centuries-old theological and cultural sanctification of a manner of work that is no longer even performed by most of us." To delve into this issue further, the author studies the first forms of work performed by our ancestors many generations ago, the growth of the modern job, both the positive and negative results of industrialization, serfdom, slavery, the exploitation of child labor, and finally the modern computer age.

142. Dore, Ronald. *British Factory, Japanese Factory: The Origins of National Diversity in Industrial Relations*. London: George Allen and Unwin, 1973.

Keywords: comparative, technology, labor relations, organizational structure, sociology

This classic work in industrial sociology examines, through a detailed study of a British and a Japanese factory, "the various ways in which two methods of organizing industry differ from each other." The author explains the fundamental differences between the two systems by analyzing the contrasting ways they order social relations and organizational structures.

The book also explains differences in the British and Japanese industrial methods in the context of the "convergence thesis"—a grand-level theory that suggests that the same technology is likely to produce the same sort of institutions (since human nature is basically the same everywhere). The author provides a critique of the generally accepted version of convergence and then, based on his research of the two factories in the study, offers his own alternative version of the thesis. The distinct cultural traditions of the two nations, says the author, ultimately "allows for a good deal of idiosyncratic national variation."

Part 1 of the volume explores in detailed fashion the factory relations themselves, the workers (who they are, how they are recruited and trained), wage structure, union membership and organization, industrial relations, etc. Part 2 provides an extensive discussion of the convergence thesis, and part 3 focuses on the origins of the Japanese employment system and its implications for Western industrial practices.

143. Dosi, Giovanni, David J. Teece, and Josef Chytry, eds. *Technology, Organization, and Competitiveness: Perspectives on Industrial and Corporate Change*. New York: Oxford University Press, 1998.

Keywords: economics, organization studies, business history, corporate strategy

There is a growing consensus that one perspective of a single discipline is unable to explain the complexities and dynamics of firm behavior, organizational structure, and corporate strategy. This work, however, overlaps the ideas of economics, business history, organizational studies, innovation, and corporate strategy in order to interplay ideas of competition, organization, and technology.

144. Driskell, James E., and Eduardo Salas, eds. *Stress and Human Performance*. Series in Applied Psychology. Mahwah, NJ: Lawrence Erlbaum Associates, 1996.

Keywords: stress, human performance, human factors, psychology

This book examines human performance under stress. "It attempts to balance two concerns. The first is theoretical—the desire to understand how human performance is impacted by stress. Accordingly, this volume highlights current research on topics such as stress and decision making, stress and team performance, and factors that moderate stress effects. The second concern is more applied—to examine how stress impacts performance in real-world settings . . . and how we may intervene through selection, training, and system design to avoid future stress-related errors and accidents." This book does not discuss stress-related disorders, clinical interventions, or coping. "Most books on stress invariably devote a considerable amount of pages to disordered behavior, illness, and treatment, and yet there are typically precious few pagers devoted to performance and effectiveness under stress. This work is meant to fill that gap." The authors make the point that "as technology expands, as airplanes become faster and airways more crowded, as naval battleships become more lethal, as decisions to launch or not launch a space shuttle become more complex, the demands imposed by these systems increase. Those who work in these settings face an environment in which they must perform under more pressure and under greater task load, in which stress is more prevalent, and in which the consequences of poor performance are more critical than ever before." The volume is intended as a resource tool for researchers in the areas of applied psychology, human factors, training, and industrial/organizational psychology.

145. Drori, Israel. *The Seam Line: Arab Workers and Jewish Managers in the Israeli Textile Industry*. Stanford: Stanford University Press, 2000.

Keywords: textile workers, Israel, Palestinian Arabs, employment

There are many Arab communities in Israel's Galilee region that are home to export-oriented textile factories, owned by multinational corporations, whose Jewish managers employ local Arab and Druse women as low-level work supervisors and seamstresses. How these managers and workers integrate work culture with the norms and values of the region in order for work arrangements to succeed is explored. The introduction of industrial corporations into developing areas of the world has created tension between social roles, family life and the demands of industrial working life. This has been further accentuated by the tension already present due to the political dynamics of Arab-Jewish conflict, as well as the restricted role of women in Arab society. In order for the business to meet its goals and obligations, it must cooperate with the community and accept its social restrictions.

146. Drucker, Peter F. *Post-Capitalist Society.* Oxford: Butterworth-Heinemann, 1993.

Keywords: capitalism, knowledge, organizational change, information society, general, corporate ethics

This book examines the social transformation of modern society in terms of its basic values, political structure, and key institutions. In the "post-capitalist" era, the author maintains that the free market continues to be "the proven mechanism of economic integration" but "the center of gravity, in the post-capitalist society—its structure, its social and economic dynamics, its social classes, and its social problems" is fundamentally different. Drucker argues that the basic economic resource "is and will be knowledge."

The text discusses the "productivity of the new workforce" in chapter 4 (topics include team work, concentration, restructuring organizations, outsourcing, and averting a new class conflict). Chapter 5 "The Responsibility-Based Organization" considers corporate ethics—social responsibility, power and organizations, and power and information. See also part 2 of the text, on knowledge. Topics discussed here include the economics of knowledge, the productivity of knowledge, management requirements, new performance demands, and the changing role of education and training.

147. Dubin, Robert, ed. *Handbook of Work, Organization and Society.* Chicago: Rand McNally College Publishing Co., 1976.

Keywords: general, leisure, work design, technology, industrial relations, sociotechnical systems, democracy

Though compiled more than twenty-five years ago, this collection of essays contains excellent sociological research on the subject of work behavior, work organization, and the broader societal implications of work. This volume is rather unconventional in its approach, especially for a large volume written in the 1970s. It adopts a holistic perspective by attempting to integrate all the components in the working life of an individual, in order to obtain a "whole picture" of the work experience.

A broad range of topics is included: work and leisure, socialization to work, working behavior, management practices, work and political behavior, and industrial relations in Japan. See especially part 4 on "Work Organizations" for information on technology and job structure, the sociotechnical approach to industrial democracy, and job enrichment and "reinforcement theory."

148. Dubofsky, Melvyn. *Hard Work: The Making of Labor History*. The Working Class in American History, edited by David Brody, Alice Kessler-Harris, David Montgomery, and Sean Wilentz. Chicago: University of Illinois Press, 2000.

Keywords: labor, United States, history, working class, trade unions

The central overriding theme of this work is the study of labor history and how its has metamorphosed over time. This work uses themes on labor history such as Western working class radicalism, United States labor history in transitional and comparative settings, as well as the impact of technological change on U.S. workers' movements. In presenting his ideas, the author gives a firsthand account of the perspective on the academic and political climate of the 1960s and early 1970s and on the development of labor history as a discipline over the past four decades.

149. Dunlop, Charles, and Rob Kling, eds. *Computerization and Controversy: Value Conflicts and Social Choices*. Boston: Academic Press, 1991.

Keywords: computers

This comprehensive anthology introduces some of the major social controversies about the computerization of society, highlighting many of the key value conflicts and social choices relating to computerization. The contributors focus primarily on the present and near future because they believe "computerization presents many important social choices to be made now, and some of them will restrict our social options in the 21st century." The authors present different sides of key debates and examine the social processes that drive and shape developments in computer technology.

"Each of the seven sections opens with an extensive essay that identifies major controversies and puts the articles in the context of key questions. . . . These essays also point the reader to a large body of additional literature about the topics."

Part 1 of the text looks at "The Dreams of Technological Utopianism," and part 2 considers the "Economics and Organizational Dimensions of Computerization." Part 3 explores "Computerization and the Transformation of Work," while part 4 discusses "Social Relationships in Electronic Communities." Part 5 is on "Social Control and Privacy," part 6 examines "Security and Reliability," and part 7 examines "Ethical Perspectives and Professional Responsibilities." This is a first-rate overview of the subject with excellent articles by Wendell Berry, Rob Kling, Joseph Weizenbaum, Terry Winograd and many other specialists. See also the 1996 edition, under Kling, Rob.

150. Eckenrode, John, and Susan Gore. *Stress between Work and Family*. New York: Plenum Press, 1990.

Keywords: stress, family, coping, unemployment

This volume of social science studies presents research on stress that stems from interactions between the environments of work, family, and community. The contributors to the book emphasize the importance of the context in which stress occurs, the reaction to various stressors, and the complex relationships involved. The fluidity of the boundaries between work and family life (known as "spill-over") is another aspect of stress that is dealt with throughout the text. The authors examine, for example, the stress resulting from the inability of working mothers to keep family responsibilities from impinging upon their workday. Also considered are the effects in high stress occupations of not being able to dissipate the tensions that accumulate over the workday.

Chapter 1 focuses on "Stress and Coping at the Boundary of Work and Family" and chapter 2 looks at the multiple effects of "Bringing Work Stress Home." Chapter 4 explores "Stress, Support, and Coping among Women Professionals with Preschool Children." Chapter 6 considers the stresses associated with "Single Parenthood and Employment." Chapter 7 examines "Stress and Blue-Collar Working Wives" and chapter 8 explores "The Individual and Family Effects of Unemployment."

151. Eder, Klaus. "Culture of Crisis: Making Sense of the Crisis of the Work Society." In *Theory of Culture*, edited by Richard Münch and Neil J. Smelser. Berkeley: University of California Press, 1992.

Keywords: alienation, work ethic, skill, deskilling, leisure

In this article, the author examines the "theory of the crisis of the work society." Eder begins his analysis by noting that whether or not the crisis actually exists, "there is a strong cultural pessimism in intellectual and everyday life that fuels the discourse. But there is no consensus as to its extent or its character, nor even a consensus as to what is meant by a crisis." It is further noted that "this lack of consensus makes it difficult to transcend cultural pessimism and to turn to social analysis, to an 'objectifying' account of the supposed crisis." The author maintains that there are two contradictory aspects of the theory of a crisis of the work society, the structuralist and the culturalist, which are in themselves insufficient to explain the crisis. "The structural part claims that the labor market has become significantly more competitive (if unevenly so), that (educational) status no longer guarantees work, and that work is being de-coupled from status. It even claims that work has become scarce and the object of intensifying struggles between status groups. The cultural part says that there is a de-coupling of work from self-realization and that people are retreating from work. Thus the crisis of the work society is seen to result from work's increasing importance on the structural level and from its decreasing importance on the cultural level." The author insists that such a contradictory relationship cannot be reduced to a structural and a cultural crisis. He argues that the crisis of the work society consists precisely in this contradictory relationship, "a relationship that could not be understood if we did not account for the specific contributions of structure and culture." In developing his argument, Eder looks at "the developmental processes in the social organization of work that are held to be responsible for changes in the work ethic." Eder considers "how changes in the modern work ethic open new possibilities for social actors to invent and defend specific versions and adaptations. The emergence of antagonistic groups defined in terms of structural location and cultural orientation points to a social crisis that will have far-reaching effects upon the course and intensity of structural and cultural changes that accompany the transformation of advanced modern societies into postindustrial societies."

152. Edvardsson, Rúnar. "Skill, Gender and Technical Change in a Nordic Environment: Typesetting in Iceland and Sweden." *New Technology, Work and Employment* 9 (1994): 30-42.

Keywords: gender, deskilling

The printing industry is an archetypal industry for studying technical change and workers' skill levels. The author rejects the deskilling argument for technicized typesetting based on his study of Icelandic and Swedish printing houses. He shows that workers' skills depend on firm size, country, labor legislation, gender and original skill level and that deskilling has occurred in some cases but not in others. Detailed descriptions of the various printing houses and tasks are included along with a history of the printing industry.

153. Edwards, Richard. *Rights at Work: Employment Relations in the Post-Union Era*. Washington, DC: Brookings Institution, 1993.

Keywords: employee rights, unions, enterprise rights

In this work, common ground between employers and their workers is sought on which to shape the future of employment relations and of workers' rights in particular. If this common ground were to be found, the federal government should be obligated to play a central role in moving us toward it. However, policy makers must be able to articulate a clear vision of where we are going or their efforts will be interpreted within the polarities of traditional liberal-versus-conservative discourse.

154. Ehn, Pelle. *Work-Oriented Design of Computer Artifacts*. Stockholm: Arbetslivscentrum, 1988.

Keywords: computers, democracy, participation, philosophy, skill, knowledge embedded in experience, design

This is "an inquiry into the human activity of designing computer artifacts that are useful to people in their daily activity at work." The author is committed to two design ideas. The first is "industrial democracy . . . the attempt to extend political democracy by also democratizing the workplace—the social life of production." The second is "quality of work and product . . . the attempt to design skill-enhancing tools for skilled workers to produce highly useful quality products and services." The author's reflections on these design ideals and their realization are referred to as "work-oriented design of computer artifacts."

The book places considerable emphasis on involving end-users in the design process, emphasizing their qualifications and participation as resources for democratic control. The role of skill and participation in design as creative and communicative process is also given special attention.

The author does not argue "for a reinvention of the wheel: the instrumental power of systems thinking for purposive rational action is beyond doubt, and many of the computer applications that function well today could not have been designed without rationalistic design methods." Instead, he suggests "a reinterpretation of design methods to take us beyond the so strongly embedded Cartesian mind-body dualism and the limits of formalization, toward an understanding that hopefully can support more creative design ways of thinking and doing design as co-operative work, involving the skills of both users and designers."

In its consistent emphasis on the importance of uniting knowing and doing and designing and using, this work has considerable preventive potential.

155. Elger, Tony, and Chris Smith. *Global Japanization? The Transnational Transformation of the Labor Process*. Critical Perspectives on Work and Organization. London: Routledge, 1994.

Keywords: labor, management, comparative, just-in-time, quality circles, case study

This volume offers an extensive analysis of "the current debate about the global role of Japanese corporations, firstly by reassessing how far such corporations are pioneering new social relations in their own workplaces at home and abroad and secondly by analyzing the wider influence of their innovations in non-Japanese firms."

The chapters in part 1 address the debate about the character of the Japanese management model in Japan. There is systematic case analysis of the distinctive features of work organization in a large Japanese car assembly plant as well as a discussion of the impact of restructuring on the employment status and job security of employees in a large manufacturing firm. Implications for the organization of the Japanese labor market and employment patterns are also considered.

Part 2 of the book examines the transplantation of Japanese production management techniques overseas. A firsthand account of work in a Japanese auto transplant in the United States is given, along with critical commentary and assessment of such techniques as "continuous improvement," JIT production, and the team concept of working. This part of the book also includes a case study report on worker's responses to new management techniques (such as QCCs) at a Canadian General Motors–Suzuki joint venture.

Part 3 of the volume focuses on the influence of the Japanese production model on the procedures and employment practices of non-Japanese companies. Case study material is presented on the Swedish model of work organization, Total Quality in Italy and the "Joint Process" model in the United States.

156. Elliott, Glen R. *Stress and Human Health: Analysis and Implications of Research*. New York: Springer Publishing Co., 1982.

Keywords: stress, health, case study

This volume offers the results of a comprehensive study carried out by the Institute of Medicine and National Academy of Sciences in the United States. It is a broadly integrative inquiry that intends to promote interdisciplinary research into complex health problems, including that of environmental stress. Research areas include the following: "Stress and Life Events"; "Stress in Organizational Settings"; "Work Stress Related to Social Structures"; "Psychosocial Assets and Modifiers of Stress"; and "Biological Substrates of Stress and Stress and Illness."

157. Ellwood, David T., Rebecca M. Blank, Joseph Blasi, Douglas Kruse, William A. Niskanen, and Karen Lynn-Dyson. *A Working Nation: Workers, Work, and Government in the New Economy*. New York: Russell Sage Foundation, 2000.

Keywords: labor, United States, industrial relations, labor policy

New inequalities and new opportunities are being created in the workplace as the United States economy changes. One of the main questions confronted is, How could per capita national income have steadily risen while the wages of most male workers froze? It is found that basically none of the growth in the economy between 1973 and 1996 went to middle and working class male workers, whose wages were in the bottom two-thirds of income distribution. Instead, almost half of the new income in the economy was paid to women, which only means that women have been catching up to the pay rate of men. It is then suggested that the connections that workers and employers share have weakened, and as a result, the number of workers with long-term employment with one firm has declined. Thus, the impact and prevalence of a variety of what might be labeled "high-performance workplace strategies"—from quality circles to training to self-managed work teams—are examined. The final two parts of the book examine whether we should be troubled by the trends in inequality and what, if anything, should be done about them.

158. Ennals, Richard. *Artificial Intelligence and Human Institutions*. Springer Series on Artificial Intelligence and Society. London: Springer-Verlag, 1991.

Keywords: computers, artificial intelligence, tacit knowledge, case study, skill, management, technology

This volume argues that truly successful applications of artificial intelligence (AI) are possible only with an understanding of human institutions, social considerations and the limitations of technology. The book has a strong practical component and explains how insights from AI can be used to deal with real-world problems. A number of case studies are presented from the fields of education, training, business, engineering, health, and community work. Suggestions for future directions in research are also offered.

See especially chapter 4, entitled "Work." Topics discussed include the following: the strategic significance of skills; transferring skills; tacit knowledge; knowledge-based systems and work-based learning; understanding the individual and technology; the politics of skills; and work, skills and management.

Throughout the text, a human-centered approach is evident, with concern for the limitations of technological capability in the workplace also apparent. Questions of responsibility, proper management training, and adequate understanding of complex technological systems are given considerable attention.

Above all, the author contends that AI must be seen "as a tool for social, or collaborative, problem-solving rather than for individual procedural problem-solving of the conventional kind."

159. Epstein, Cynthia Fuchs, Carroll Seron, Bonnie Oglensky, and Robert Saute. *The Part-Time Paradox: Time Norms, Professional Lives, Family, and Gender.* New York: Routledge, 1999.

Keywords: part-time lawyers, practice of law, division of labor in the family

Due to time constraints, most professionals must ask themselves if it is possible to build a career and a family at the same time. It is this conflict between escalating time demands of career and family life and the consequences of part-time work as a solution that are explored. Drawing on interviews with full- and part-time attorneys, the authors delve into the multiple dimensions of the part-time work solution, considering issues of job security, the consequences of new technology, the economics and stigmatization of part-time work, and the division of labor in the family.

160. Erikson, Kai, and Steven Peter Vallas, eds. *The Nature of Work: Sociological Perspectives*. New Haven, CT: Yale University Press, 1990.

Keywords: work, industrial sociology, unemployment

The collection of works all agree that the nature of work in America is being transformed in important ways. In the United States, work is shifting toward the use of complex technologies, the processing of information, and the provision of services. All the while, blue-collar factory jobs in industries such as steel and automobiles are being exported to countries where lower wages are the rule. This is also putting the familiar patterns of the working world at risk with the shift in values and expectations of those who work.

161. Eriksson, I. V., B. A. Kitchenham, and K. G. Tijdens, eds. *International Conference on Women, Work and Computerization*. Helsinki: North Holland/Elsevier, 1991.

Keywords: women, computers, automation, participation

This volume is the result of the International Conference on Women, Work and Computerization held in Helsinki, Finland, in 1991. Seven major themes are reflected in the papers: improving the quality of women's work, labor markets within firms, division of labor and computerization in different countries, female orientation in systems design, training and education, women in EDP jobs, and gender, symbols and technology.

The basic premise of this book is that "the written history of technological development is the history of resourceful and ingenious men. Men made the inventions and were responsible for their adaptation to use. . . . Women have started to lay claims for a better footing for women in this new era of technological development where computers are taking the main role. Women want to give their insights into the development of computer systems and their adaptations to working life."

The book also gives special attention to participatory system design approaches and interdisciplinary cooperation in the implementation of computer technologies.

162. Ermann, M. David, ed. *Computers, Ethics, and Society*. 2nd ed. New York: Oxford University Press, 1997.

Keywords: computers, deskilling, comparative, democracy, unemployment

This is an excellent collection of articles on the ethics of various computer uses and their impact on society. Four of the articles deal with "Work in the Computerized Society." In the article "Computers Transform the Work Setting," Ian G. Barbour surveys the many ways computers may impact our lives. He asks whether they will increase unemployment (likely), deskill workers (unlikely), or democratize our work lives (mixed).

In chapter 18, "The authors examine how computer technologies affect lesser-developed countries (LDCs). As electronic data transmission rapidly improves, many companies in industrial nations are relocating their data processing facilities to LDCs. These relocations have created jobs in countries such as Ireland, Malaysia, and Brazil. The jobs, however, are heavily skewed toward low-skilled occupations. The authors warn that work environments in LDCs are inflexible, that many occupational health hazards are present, and that pay scales are below those of industrialized nations."

The article "Computing in Small, Energetic Countries" highlights "several small countries that have positioned themselves in the global economy of information technologies. Ireland, Israel, New Zealand, and the city-states Hong Kong and Singapore have all found niches—whether in hardware production, software production, or the exportation of information infrastructures." The authors conclude that "small countries with active government support, good educational systems, and geographical advantages are most likely to prosper in the Information Age."

Finally, Tom Forester's article "'Whatever Happened to the Information Revolution in the Workplace?" argues that computers have caused neither profound workplace changes nor the profound societal changes that were predicted. Computers, he argues, have not caused serious changes in leisure time, unemployment, the use of paper records, the tendency to work at home, and so forth. Forester also explains why he thinks predictions fell so wide of the mark.

163. Esland, Geoff, and Graeme Salaman, eds. *The Politics of Work and Occupations*. Toronto: University of Toronto Press, 1980.

Keywords: sociology, management, unions, psychology

The contributors to this book all share the belief that "in order to understand work experience one must analyze the relationship between the nature, design, and organization of work on the one hand and the form of society within which it occurs on the other." In particular, they seek to analyze the impact of the political nature of work arrangements on employees. Each article has a specific focus, namely occupational development, occupational placement, the meaning of work, dirty work, professions and professionalism, control and resistance at work, humanized management, trade unions and power. One conclusion that seems evident from these writings, prepared for a third-year Open University course, is that workplaces reflect the power structures, relationships and injustices that exist in the larger society.

Alan Fox's classic chapter on "The Meaning of Work" deserves a closer look. He first makes a distinction between personal meanings and social meanings of work and asserts that they must both be studied. However, the relationships and interactions between the two must also be considered. He begins an in-depth analysis of these meanings and interactions by asking questions such as, "How many people in our society can be said to enjoy even an approximation to a free choice of the work meanings they live by? What are the constraints, influences, and organizational pressures that cause an individual to live by one set of meanings that they live by, and what are the consequences for the social groupings or classes of which they are members? Are any structural regularities observable in our answers to these questions? How is the situation changing, and what are the possibilities for the future?"

He posits that sharp differences in work experience exist between the deprived majority and privileged minority. This privileged group has the power to shape the design and organization of work. But they are driven to maintain the "instrumental" approach to work. By instrumental, Fox means the dominant attitude that is consistent with scientific management and based on minimizing immediate costs and maximizing immediate productivity. The privileged minority will, Fox declares, most likely resist changes to the meaning of work to include worker self-actualization if this interferes with immediate economic goals. Thus a major challenge to current power structures in the workplace as well as in the larger society is necessary for the majority of workers to be able to attach a richer meaning to work.

164. Evans, Gary W., Gunn Johansson, and Sybil Carrere. "Psychosocial Factors and the Physical Environment: Inter-Relations in the Workplace." *International Review of Industrial and Organizational Psychology* 9 (1994).

Keywords: psychology, stress, health, management

How might "physical and psychosocial elements of the work environment interrelate to affect human health?" This is the question posed in this chapter. Psychosocial characteristics under the headings of structural, organizational, interpersonal, and task parameters and physical characteristics, categorized into ambient, layout and arrangement of space, architectural design, and ergonomic factors are listed. Then, two conceptual models of how the work environment affects human models are presented. "Moderation occurs when the relation between one work environment characteristic and health is altered by the level of another work environment variable. . . . The moderator variable qualifies the work environment-health relation uncovered, specifying when or under what conditions the association between the initial environmental characteristic and health holds. Mediation occurs when the relation between one work environment factor and health can be explained by or accounted for by some underlying process. . . . A mediating variable is a mechanism or an explanatory process that helps explain how the work environment is linked to health."

For the moderator model, physical and psychosocial interactions, physical and physical interactions, and psychosocial and psychosocial interactions are explored. Physical antecedents and psychosocial mediators, psychosocial antecedents and physical mediators, psychosocial antecedents and psychosocial mediators, and physical antecedents and physical mediators are considered for the mediator model. Numerous studies and their results are cited in these sections to summarize what possible relations exist. Further conceptual implications are discussed for both models.

165. Ezorsky, Gertrude, ed. *Moral Rights in the Workplace*. Albany: State University of New York Press, 1987.

Keywords: QWL, freedom, health, whistleblowing, management, industrial relations

The contributors to this volume focus on "moral problems that arise for people who labor in ordinary workplaces—factories, schools, mines, stores, and farms." The book examines "problems of freedom and coercion that develop on the job, issues of the right to meaningful work, occupational health and safety, whistle-blowing, the right to union organization, unemployment, and the flight of factories, the rights of health care workers, and workers' self-management." Other important concerns, such as employment discrimination, comparable worth, seniority, affirmative action, and worksharing, are also discussed.

Published under the sponsorship of the National Society for Philosophy and Public Affairs, the book considers three moral values that predominate in debates over workplace policy: freedom, fairness, and the general good.

The editor notes that the first value, freedom, is endorsed both by those who criticize and those who defend this capitalist organization of the workplace. In chapter 3, for example, Kurt Nutting claims that the employer's right to determine working conditions is inherently coercive; in chapter 2, Tibor Machan argues that the establishment of working conditions by management is the outcome of a free exchange in the marketplace between employers and workers. The second value, fairness, is invoked in the controversy over affirmative action for minority persons and women (see the essays in chapter 7). The third value discussed by writers in this book is the general good. In R. M. Hare's essay, for example, a utilitarian philosophy is proposed that suggests that "usefulness in promoting the general good should be the only moral standard for adopting a policy in the workplace."

166. Fan, I. S., and Robert Gassmann. "A Study of the Practicalities of Human-Centered Implementation in a British Manufacturing Company." 586-9 in *Advances in Agile Manufacturing*, edited by P. T. Kidd and W. Karwowski. Amsterdam: IOS Press, 1994.

Keywords: anthropocentric, case study, work design

Three cells in a British vehicle braking systems manufacturing company were compared to gain insight into how to introduce human-centered cells. Cells X, Y and Z differed in terms of the age of the cell and the degree of human-centerdness. Cell, X, the youngest cell, most resembled the traditional techno-centered cell. On the other hand, cell Z, the eldest cell, had adopted the most participative management strategies and the most human-centered approach. Cell Y was the intermediate cell. As predicted by the demand-control model, members of cell Y were more confident and motivated than those of cell X. However, the expected improvement for cell Z did not result because of a dramatic decrease in demand for this cell's components.

167. Fassel, Diane. *Working Ourselves to Death: The High Cost of Workaholism, The Rewards of Recovery*. New York: Harper Collins Publishers, 1990.

Keywords: job stress, workaholics, psychology

There is a pervasive modern addiction to work, and this book reveals the difference between healthy productivity and obsessiveness, all the while offering empowering methods for recovery. With the use of case histories and examples, the author demonstrates how the compulsion to work excessive amounts damages personal relationships, work performance, and physical well-being.

168. Feldman, Steven P. "The Idealization of Technology: Power Relations in an Engineering Department." *Human Relations* 42, no. 7 (1989): 575-91.

Keywords: psychology, sociology, engineering, organizational culture

The author summarizes the article as follows: "The management of technological development involves a dilemma; the manager must strive to understand the diverse specializations required to develop new technology, but he must focus on integrating these specializations. The former requires knowledge, the latter power. It is my contention, however, that in technologically-oriented work groups, there is a tendency for the importance of technology to be exaggerated while power issues are ignored. This process is referred to as the idealization of technology. The result is an inattention to organizational goals and cooperative processes. In this essay, the interpretive concept of culture and the psychoanalytic theory of idealization is used to investigate this problem. The framework is applied to an engineering department whose primary work is the development of advanced technological products. The process of idealization distorts organizational reality in such a way that continual distortions are needed, is a cultural mechanism that is used to mediate the conflict between the exercise of power and the fear power, integrates the individual into the organizational culture while simultaneously undermining cooperative relations, and encourages conformity while undermining power relations."

169. Fincham, Robin, and Peter S. Rhodes. *The Individual, Work and Organization*. Totowa, NJ: Rowman & Littlefield, 1988.

Keywords: sociology, psychology, stress, work design, skill, deskilling, alienation, sociotechnical systems, technology, rationalization

Written by an industrial sociologist, this volume of essays on behavioral studies is primarily designed as an introductory textbook for management and business students. Unlike many other versions of behavioral studies that are based on organizational theory or the subdiscipline of occupational psychology, this approach is drawn from the two major disciplines of sociology and psychology. The authors use this critical discipline-based approach to examine, among other topics, work-related stress, attentive job design, and current debates on the labor process and new technology. There is also an emphasis throughout the text on "practical problems of the workplace, such as the development of occupational skills, the control of effort, and motivation and organizational goals." Both the qualitative and quantitative dimensions of behavioral studies are reviewed.

Chapters 2, 8, 9, and 13 are especially relevant to the subject of healthy workplace design, although their consideration of preventive strategies and health effects is rather minimal. Particular topics explored in these chapters include the following: types of stress at work; the sociotechnical systems approach; autonomous work groups; constraints on work redesign; alienated labor; Weber and rationalization; technology and the labor process; the deskilling debate; new technology and management; and the effects of new technologies on employment. This volume offers a solid, comprehensive treatment of many central issues in the sociology and psychology of work, from a behavioral perspective, with good insights into major theoretical and methodological concerns.

170. Fineman, Stephen, ed. *Unemployment: Personal and Social Consequences.* London: Tavistock Publications, 1987.

Keywords: unemployment, poverty, crime, women

This collection of articles by social researchers examines "what unemployment does to people: how it affects individuals, how it penetrates families, and its implications for communities and societies." Various themes explored include the following: "the tangle between unemployment, poverty and crime; the particular problems for women in the job market; and the disappointments for those leaving education with little prospect of employment. The book also highlights implications for change—in forms of support, in definitions of work, and in the very nature of work itself." See especially part 2 "Families and Communities," part 3 "Social Responses and Structures," and chapter 13 "Alternative Routes to Work."

171. Finlayson, Ann. *Naming Rumpelstiltskin: Who Will Profit and Who Will Lose in the Workplace of the 21st Century.* Toronto: Key Porter Books, 1996.

Keywords: technology, unemployment, unions, workplace change, forecasting

The author of this book originally set out to examine the current transformation of work in the context of rapid technological change, with a particular emphasis on the implications of these changes for young Canadians. As the author engaged herself more deeply in the debate on jobs and workplace change, she began to question the motives of some of those participating in the debate and also wondered whether much of the debate was really about the future of work.

Several important questions arose that shaped the eventual context of the book. For example, "Why was no one addressing such questions as the appropriate role of employers in reconciling profits with the interests of their employees and of the society in which they do business? . . . Why did everyone assume that unions had become historical artifacts, and that the search for a creative working relationship between employers and unions was passé? Why didn't concerns for equity or for the environment seem to matter anymore?"

This volume fully accepts that "technology *is* changing the way we work and that global competition *is* forcing corporations to re-examine the way they do business." However, the author seriously questions whether the "grim determinism that has characterized the debate about jobs and joblessness" is serving us well. She also suggests that this "determinism" has paralyzed us with fear, "causing us to abandon efforts to find better ways to work" and making us believe that there are no real decisions to be made.

The author rejects the rigid determinism of self-interested proponents of workplace change and offers both a critique of their methods and philosophy and positive suggestions for alternative change in work environments.

For material relevant to healthy work concepts and preventive programs for change, see especially chapter 8 "The Value of Work" and chapter 9 "Working Better."

This is a well-written, insightful account of contemporary workplace trends that uses the metaphor of modern-day Rumpelstiltskins to dramatize its central theme.

172. Fishman, Daniel B., and Cary Cherniss, eds. *The Human Side of Corporate Competitiveness*. Newbury Park, CA: Sage Publishing, 1990.

Keywords: psychology, family, health, human resources

Written from an applied psychology perspective, this book presents findings that are of practical use in promoting the health of workers, their families and their communities while also facilitating organizational competitiveness. The authors maintain that a psychologically healthy work environment is the key to improving organizational effectiveness.

See especially chapter 4 "New Attitudes and Motivations in Workers: Growing Interdependencies among the Work, Personal, Family, and Educational Spheres of Life." It focuses in a phenomenological manner upon the personal values and perspectives of contemporary workers with an emphasis on some of their expectations regarding day care, maternity leave, comparable pay for women, wellness programs, facilities for the disabled, etc.

Also see chapter 8 "Strategies for Integrating the Family Needs of Workers into Human Resource Planning." It includes a discussion of flexible work arrangements, health benefits and employee assistance strategies.

The summary of the book discusses "Emerging Managerial Themes for the 1990s: Interdependencies and Synergies among the Individual, Organizational, and Societal Well-Being." Topics considered here include: managing clashes in corporate culture and transnational cultural conflict (for example, the issue of American industry adopting Japanese management practices).

173. Fletcher, Ben. *Work, Stress, Disease and Life Expectancy.* Wiley Series on Studies in Occupational Stress. Chichester: John Wiley and Sons, 1991.

Keywords: stress, health, disease

This is another volume in a series of works on occupational stress. Chapter 1 "Models of Stress and Disease" in particular is of special relevance to the subject of healthy work and preventive strategies in the workplace. A number of influential general models of occupational stress are outlined in order to closely examine the link between work and health. The final section then develops a new "configural model" based on the strengths of earlier ones. As the name suggests, this model incorporates the common findings verified in the other models.

The author also describes the distinction between stress, stressors, and strain, and then analyzes the multiple effects of "decision latitude" as formulated by Karasek and Theorell.

As well as providing an overview of how work factors (intrinsic and extrinsic) in the work environment can affect mental and physical health, the author considers the personal differences between people that must be taken into account when studying occupational stress.

The latter part of the chapter offers details on the testable assumptions and predictions that can be made from applying the "configural model." By integrating many of the best aspects of other general models of occupational stress, the author is able to come up with a comprehensive and encompassing construct that includes many more environmental and personal variables of interest to those examining the relationship between work and stress.

See also chapter 2 "Life Events and Disease," chapter 3 "Stress and the Immune System," chapter 6 "Transmitting Occupational Stress," and chapter 7 "The Epidemiology of Work Stress."

174. Florida, Richard. "The New Industrial Revolution." *Futures*, July-August 1991: 559-76.

Keywords: work design, industrial relations, technology

This article outlines a new framework for understanding the current period of global restructuring, focusing on the relationship between technological change and organizational change. After reviewing the major approaches in the debate over future pathways to industrialization, a new perspective for understanding the "new industrial revolution" is presented. At the core of this revolution is the emergence of a series of powerful new industrial technologies that are giving rise to new forces of production and a concomitant transformation in production organization. A new shop floor is emerging, in which innovation and production, intellectual and manual labor are increasingly integrated. As this process of industrial restructuring evolves, success will depend on organizational forms that effectively harness and mobilize collective intelligence.

175. Floyd, Michael, Margery Povall, and Graham Watson, eds. *Mental Health at Work*. London: Jessica Kingsley Publishers, 1994.

Keywords: mental health, rehabilitation, coping

About 3.7 million people in Britain suffer from severe mental illness and 71 million working days are lost to mental illness each year. Thus, preventing, detecting, and dealing with mental illness are important for an employer. The book, based on the conference and workshop Mental Health at Work explores issues such as vocational rehabilitation and training, occupational health services and overcoming barriers to employment for the workers suffering from mental illness. The only chapter that is significant for healthy work is the chapter entitled "Creating a Healthy Workplace" that studies the relationship between work characteristics and worker well-being. Dr. Michael Banks presents a framework and model based on research on unemployment, job design, clinical studies of stress, job transitions and shiftwork. First, the concepts of affective well-being, competence, aspiration, autonomy and integrated functioning are defined and their importance to workplace health noted. Second, Dr. Banks identifies nine influential characteristics of the work environment: (1) opportunity for control, (2) opportunity for skill use, (3) externally generated goals, (4) variety, (5) environmental clarity, (6) availability of money, (7) physical security, (8) opportunity for interpersonal contact, and (9) valued social position. The third section of this brief chapter discusses possible interventions such as the development of personal coping strategies, flexible work arrangements and keep-fit programs, with little emphasis on preventive measures.

176. Forester, Tom, ed. *The Information Technology Revolution*. Cambridge, MA: MIT Press, 1986.

Keywords: computers, automation, general

This well-known volume of essays covers the key technological developments in a relatively early period of the information revolution—1980 to 1985. It also tracks many of the major social changes that began to emerge during this time, especially those initiated by computerization and automation.

The book aims to bridge the gap between the "two cultures" of scientists and liberal arts students. The pattern of each chapter is designed to be useful for teaching purposes: an introductory article is usually followed by either case studies or pieces that explore some of the issues in greater depth. Comprehensive guides to further reading are included at the end of each chapter (and at the end of the book); these are well organized and very helpful for research purposes.

Directly relevant to healthy work is part 3, which includes three comprehensive articles on how computers have changed the way we work now; the increase in the amount of work expected from workers; the changing skill requirements at the workplace; and the altered relationship between management and labor. Part 2 also has articles that impinge on work, though it is a little uneven from the perspective of healthy work. See especially chapter 6 "Factory Automation," chapter 7 "Office of the Future," and chapter 8 "Banks, Shops, Hospitals."

177. Forester, Tom. "The Myth of the Electronic Cottage." *Futures* 20, no. 3 (June 1988).

Keywords: home-based work, electronic cottage, social decentralization

This article examines the truth of claims made over the last twenty years by futurists that we will see a significant increase in computer-based home activities and the consumption of information technology-based services—amounting to a revolutionary change in lifestyles. The author reviews the evidence on use of "home informatics" gadgetry and participation across a range of home-based activities and discusses why home working, home banking, home shopping, and home information services have not taken off as predicted. Forester draws on case study material and personal experiences to argue that "1) writers have consistently underestimated the psychological problems of working at home and 2) consumers have by and large not found new information technology-based services to be cheaper, usable or useful—nor do they fulfill their psychological needs." In short, the article offers a sustained critique of the notion of the "electronic cottage." The author concludes that "while 'home informatics' may be of interest for various reasons, developments on this front are unlikely to lead to a substantial increase in economic activity in the home or an increase in the consumption of information technology based services in the home of a sufficient volume to amount to the revolutionary change in lifestyles depicted in the electronic cottage scenario." It is further argued that the process of technology transfer into the home is a slow and complex business. "The mistake of some home informatics enthusiasts has been to assume that IT will transfer swiftly and smoothly into homes with inevitable social changes following on." After reviewing the relevant evidence, Forester contends that the electronic cottage is largely a myth.

178. Fox, Matthew. *The Reinvention of Work: A New Vision of Livelihood for Our Time*. San Francisco: HarperCollins, 1994.

Keywords: alienation, secularization, spiritual work, reenchantment

This book is an extended essay on the spiritual dimensions of work. The author suggests that "during the Newtonian era, in a nonsacred, secularized society . . . the desocialization of work . . . [that took place] . . . lies at the heart of our alienation." It is further argued that "when it comes to the pressing issue of work and jobs in an era of postindustrialization, we can learn much from the wisdom of our mystical traditions." The book draws from the wisdom not only of Western mystics such as Hildegard, Eckhart, Aquinas, Rilke, and others, but from mystics of Eastern and Middle Eastern traditions as well. In addition, the author calls on the thoughts of contemporary scientists such as Gregory Bateson, Thomas Berry, Fritjof Capra, and Erich Jantsch. In the first part of the book, "The Great Work and the Inner Work: Revisioning Work," Fox deals with work as non-action, "the inner work of our species that has been so long neglected in our industrial work world." (See especially "Work as Lamentation," "Feminist Perspectives," "Work as Addiction," and "Work as Healthy Nothingness.") In the second part, "The Great Work and the Outer Work: Reinventing Work," the author applies the principles from part 1 on "non-action" to "outer work." Examples are given of "contemporary persons and movements that are beginning to reenchant our work by transforming various work worlds and professions." Examples are also offered of this transformation (or reenchantment) of work worlds ranging from the environment, farming, and politics (chapter 5) to education, youth, and sexuality (chapter 6) to health care, psychology, and art (chapter 7) to economics, business, and science (chapter 8).

The third part of the text, "Ritual: Where the Great Work of the Universe and the Work of the People Come Together," promotes the notion of ritual as an effective means of reinventing work in our time. Emphasis is given here to "the need for a cultural shift toward inner work on persons and communities alike"—what E. F. Schumacher calls "putting our inner house in order."

179. Francis, Arthur, and Peter Grootings, eds. *New Technologies and Work: Capitalist and Socialist Perspectives*. London: Routledge, 1989.

Keywords: case study, work design, CNC, industrial relations, policy, comparative

Production developments of manufacturing companies in ten different companies are examined. The focus is on how societal conditions have an impact on the social/organizational consequences of the introduction of new technology at work. All the case study researchers focused on the relationship between new technology (e.g., CNC machines) and the national education system, industrial relations, social and political policy, and industrial structure within their respective countries, and upon the consequences of technological introduction for work organization, work content and load, qualification, work culture, and intra-organizational industrial relations. Case studies include Czechoslovakia, Hungary, GDR, USSR, Poland, Belgium, FDR, US, Finland and the Netherlands.

180. Frankenhaeuser, Marianne, and Bertil Gardell. "Underload and Overload in Working Life: Outline of a Multidisciplinary Approach." *Journal of Human Stress*, September 1976: 35-46.

Keywords: stress, health, case study, machine-paced work

A research project is outlined in which concepts and methods from social psychology and psychophysiology are integrated in the study of human adaptation to underload and overload related to technically advanced work processes. Attempts are made to identify aversive factors in the work process by studying acute stress reactions, for example catecholamine excretion, in the course of work and relating these to long-term, negative effects on well-being, job satisfaction, and health. Data from a pilot study of sawmill workers support the view that machine-paced work characterized by a short work cycle and lack of control over the work process constitutes a threat to health and well-being.

181. Fraser, Steven, and Joshua B. Freeman, eds. *Audacious Democracy: Labor, Intellectuals, and the Social Reconstruction of America*. New York: Houghton Mifflin Co., 1997.

Keywords: labor movement, United States, working class, intellectuals

The central dilemma that is addressed is: How can a newly revitalized and combative labor movement challenge the corporate domination of American life and help win the fight for economic security, social justice, and a more "audacious democracy"? To answer this, a collaboration is required between American intellectuals and labor movement activists. Also addressed is the possibility of social change over the next decade.

182. Fraser, T. Morris. *The Worker at Work: A Textbook Concerned with Men and Women in the Workplace*. London: Taylor and Francis, 1989.

Keywords: ergonomics, occupational hygiene, health

This book is quite general in its approach to work-oriented issues such as work environment, workers' physiological and psychological health, design of equipment for human use, and chemical agents in the workplace. It covers elements of ergonomics, occupational hygiene, and occupational health. It is geared not only to professionals in the above-mentioned fields, but also to engineers, industrial designers and managers. It is a good introduction to the area of work and workplace problems.

183. Freeman, Chris, and Luc Soete. *Work for All or Mass Unemployment? Computerized Technical Change in the 21st Century*. London: Pinter Publishers, 1994.

Keywords: unemployment, forecasting, computers, automation

This volume is about the employment/unemployment effects of computer and telecommunications technology. The authors underscore the point that mass unemployment caused by technological change is not just economically wasteful but also socially disastrous. It is argued that the process of job creation will only outstrip that of job loss on the necessary scale when appropriate policies are followed. "These policies for a return to full employment must take into account the special features of computer and telecommunications technology and in particular the need for new infrastructural investment in 'Information Highways' and 'Byways' and in the Education and Training Systems."

Chapter 1 outlines the social consequences of high and prolonged unemployment in the 1990s and chapter 2 summarizes the debate among economists about technical change and unemployment. Chapter 3 presents more evidence on the technical and economic characteristics of new information technology. Chapter 4 deals with the new developments in the international division of labor, international trade and international investment flows. Special attention is given to Southeast Asia. Chapter 5 discusses the question of "flexibility" in wages, in work organization and in patterns of employment over the working lives of men and women (part-time, flex-time, and full-time work are examined). Chapter 6 argues that "information technology offers some serious possibilities of ameliorating the threats to the global environment associated with a pattern of economic growth based on energy-intensive and materials-intensive technologies." Finally, chapter 7 considers a range of policies for future employment in the context of the "Information Age."

184. Freeman, Richard B., ed. *Working under Different Rules*. New York: Russell Sage Foundation, 1994.

Keywords: labor, United States, wage inequality

For the majority of the twentieth century, the American workforce enjoyed what was once considered the "American dream." They were at the forefront in wages, productivity, and positive workplace conditions. Also, unions insured free enterprise and high labor standards. However, despite the relatively high standard of living, Americans have fallen behind the majority of their trading partners and competitors when it comes to providing good jobs at good pay, as has been proven by spiraling income inequality and stagnant real earnings. These essays show that the current U.S. labor market is characterized by a high degree of flexibility, with rapid employee turnover, ongoing creation of new jobs, and decentralized wage setting practices. They also reveal that there is more to this story: inadequate job training, frequent layoffs, and increased numbers of workers forced to accept increasingly popular and common low paying jobs. The virtually union-free work environment that is becoming the norm in an increasing amount of private sectors has stripped workers of a strong collective voice. German apprenticeship programs and the Japanese system of "job rotation" are used to demonstrate more effective approaches to preparing workers for the changing demands of lifetime employment.

185. French Jr., John R. P., Robert D. Caplan, and R. Van Harrison. *The Mechanisms of Job Stress and Strain.* Wiley Series on Studies in Occupational Stress. New York: John Wiley and Sons, 1982.

Keywords: stress, coping, psychology

This second volume in a series, reporting on the results of a large study of occupational stress, strain and mental health (among twenty-three occupations), "concentrates on multivariate analyses of the effects of stress on strain" and develops a general theoretical model for guiding future research. Attention is also given to discovering "environmental variables that have a significant effect on health and that could be altered so as to improve the quality of life." Thus, there are significant implications here for isolating the environmental factors that prevent "maladjustment and excessive strain in normal people." See especially chapter 7 "Summary and Implications" for selective material on reducing job stress.

186. Frenkel, Stephen J., Marek Korczynski, Karen A. Shire, and May Tam. *On the Front Line: Organization of Work in the Information Economy*. Ithaca, NY: Cornell University Press, 1999.

Keywords: work, production management, industrial sociology, service industries, workflow systems, case study

This book offers a comprehensive analysis of the organization dynamics of front-line work that is based on a five-year study of over one thousand employees from eight leading companies in the United States, Australia, and Japan. It reveals similarities and differences found in work environments, such as variance in authority relations and division of labor, as well as different management approaches used in the United States and Australia. It also shows how bureaucratic, entrepreneurial, and network forms of organization coexist in the information economy by examining how work differs among service, sales, and knowledge-based settings.

187. Galegher, Jolene, Robert E. Krant, and Carmen Egido, eds. *Intellectual Teamwork: Social and Technological Foundations of Cooperative Work*. Hillsdale, NJ: Lawrence Erlbaum Associates, 1990.

Keywords: computers, cooperation, work groups

This comprehensive volume offers a broad sample of social science research relevant to the design and evaluation of technology (especially computer-based information technology) for cooperative work. The contributors "demonstrate the relevance of high-level theories of social interaction and social organization, the value of empirical analyses of specific instances of intellectual teamwork, the effects of particular information technologies on the experiences and performance of users, and, finally, they give us a hint of technologies that await us in the years ahead. Together, they suggest to us the mutual benefit that could result from better integration of social science and technological perspectives on intellectual teamwork." The basic premise of the book is that creating practical information technology requires not only technical expertise but also an understanding of the social and behavioral processes that the technology is designed to support.

See especially part 3 "Experiences with Technology for Cooperative Work." This section contains five empirical investigations of "experiences with technologies that have been available long enough to provide us with evidence about whether their potential to aid cooperative work has been fulfilled." The technologies examined include electronic mail, computer conferences, voice messaging, and video teleconferences. Chapters 10, 11, and 12 report studies showing the benefits of information technology that allows communication across space and time. On the other hand, chapters 13 and 14 reveal that experience with new technology to supplement or replace real-time meetings has been more problematic.

188. Galkin, A. "The New Technology and the Problem of Unemployment." 35-58 in *Technological Change and Workers' Movements: Explorations in the World Economy*, edited by Melvyn Dubofsky. Thousand Oaks, CA: Sage Publications, 1985.

Keywords: unemployment, computerization, automation, information technology, deskilling, labor

In this chapter, the author stresses how "the new technology of microcomputers and robotization has caused mass unemployment and social crisis in the capitalist world." It is argued that the widespread introduction of these technologies did not become a feasible venture until the late 1970s and early 1980s, when, after significant improvements, they became quite economical. Galkin notes that "the adoption of a new technological base obviously cannot be carried out overnight. . . . It calls for huge capital investments, complex technologies for each industry . . . specially trained manpower, and many other things." It is further suggested that at first the saving of labor was not among the leading factors contributing to mass unemployment in the developed capitalist countries. The author maintains that the mass lay-offs that began during the mid 1970s "were mainly due to the production slump that was taking place in the process of economic recession . . . by the beginning of the 1980s the saving of labor due to the introduction of new technology and machines became a major determinant of the employment dynamics and, consequently, of unemployment." The author also discusses the growing incidence of temporary employment and home employment, as well as some of their social and economic consequences. Finally, Galkin proposes the adoption of alternative employment/production programs, that, "while not being directed against technological progress, could provide the restructuring of the production process on a new technological basis without harm for the mass categories of the working people." The first program (aimed at solving mainly current problems) would be a more equitable distribution of the available amount of work, to be realized largely through the introduction of shorter working hours and reduced overtime. The second program (aimed at a more profound social transformation) "assumes the creation of new spheres of labor application, predominantly in the infrastructure: culture, education, health services, sports, environmental protection, new social infrastructures, and so on."

189. Gallie, Duncan, Micheal White, Yuan Cheng, and Mark Tomlinson. *Restructuring the Employment Relationship*. New York: Oxford University Press, 1998.

Keywords: industrial sociology, Great Britain, labor, industrial surveys, management, employee participation, effect of technological innovations on employees, industrial hygiene, hours of labor, flexible, women, employment

Drawing on the *Employment in Britain* survey (a national survey providing the richest source of evidence to date about people's experience of employment), the book examines the impact of new technologies, the changing forms of employment contracts, the growth of job insecurity, and the emergence of new management policies on people's experience of employment. Focus is placed on the implications of these developments for the ways in which skills and work tasks have been changing, the flexibility demanded at work, the degree of participation in decision making, and the nature of control at work. The authors then question whether there has been a tendency toward either a polarization or convergence of employment experiences between men and women, and between occupational classes. Insight is offered into how the changing quality of work in the past few years has affected employees' involvement in their jobs and organizations, the propensity for absenteeism and staff turnover, as well as the stress they experience at work. Even though the study provides strong evidence of a trend toward upskilling, the authors argue that the restructuring of the employment relationship has reinforced traditional lines of division in the workforce.

190. Gamst, Frederick C., ed. *Meanings of Work: Considerations for the Twenty-First Century*. SUNY Series in the Anthropology of Work. Albany: State University of New York Press, 1995.

Keywords: industrial sociology, industrial relations, work

A basis for understanding the ever-changing patterns of work in a growing global market that is increasingly struggling to overcome problems such as contingent employment and decline of the middle class is examined by using the interconnected cultural, social, and economic dimensions of human work. By focusing on the sociocultural considerations of work, this book discusses the applications, scope, utility, and ideas about the integration of societies through work organizations and their occupational and other social statuses. Issues of discontent and satisfaction generated by work, the exercise of power in work, the decision making process as affected by emotions and values, the cultural meanings and myths of work, the reactions to and processes of retirement from work, and the social expectations of nonwork and work are also issues into which the authors delve.

191. Gandy, John, and Lorne Tepperman. *False Alarm: The Computerization of Eight Social Welfare Organizations*. Waterloo, ON: Wilfrid Laurier University Press, 1990.

Keywords: computers, social work, organizational change, automation

This volume examines the impact of computerized information systems on organizations and staff. The authors chose social welfare organizations in particular as the setting for their research for several reasons. "First, the programs of these agencies are based on values that many believe are put at risk by computerization, privacy, autonomy, discretion, initiative, and professionalism. Second, the clientele of social welfare agencies are highly vulnerable to centralization and changes in the power between the individual and the organization. Third, in social welfare agencies, personal autonomy, and the exercise of ethical choice are more significant issues than in other types of organizations." This book offers an empirical in-depth examination of computer use in social welfare organizations in Canada. The research study was designed to test the predictions of social welfare specialists and others regarding the impact of computerization on these organizations. A brief but important literature review of the field is included. This literature, and the findings of this study as well, suggest that "continuing vigilance is needed to ensure that computer technology will not destroy human dignity and individual autonomy." However, optimism is also expressed "that ways can, and must, be found to use it to improve the computerized delivery of services." Some of the key questions and problems that are addressed here include the following: "Do social welfare organizations have information needs that, with our present level of knowledge, cannot be quantified without undermining the credibility and indignity of the services provided? Does computerization threaten the value base of social work, the delivery of service and/or relations between clients and staff? If so, what can be done to minimize the impact? Does a computerized information system challenge the existing power structure in the organizations? What are the sources and extent of staff resistance to computerization in social welfare organizations?"

192. Gardell, Bertil. "Worker Participation and Autonomy: A Multilevel Approach to Democracy at the Workplace." *International Journal of Health Services* 12, no. 4 (1982).

Keywords: participation, democracy, productivity, stress, health, history

This article is based on a comprehensive case study coordinated and financed by the Swedish Center for Working Life. It describes the implementation of a workplace democracy program in a mid-sized Swedish manufacturing company "initiated and engineered by the trade union local in close cooperation with management."

The introduction to the article provides a fifty-year historical perspective on the worker participation movement in Sweden and details the specific strategies developed to create more humane/productive work environments. The article then examines the methods used to introduce autonomous work groups in this particular company and reports on the outcome of the new work organization for the workers, the union and the firm.

The author concludes that "the new work organization has meant a richer job content, increased dignity for workers, increased solidarity among workers, increased trade union strength, as well as a more effective use of productive resources in the company." In addition, the author expresses the conviction that "the experiences gained from this case can be transferred to other workplaces where workers are interested in having more say, more security, and more meaningful work situations."

193. Gardell, G., ed. *Working Life: A Social Science Contribution to Work Reform*. London: John Wiley and Sons, 1981.

Keywords: stress, mental demands, shift work, biological rhythms

This is one of the first social-science efforts to consider the impact of highly automated work processes on workers in terms of stress, mental demands, and safety issues. It also looks into the relationship between shift work and biological rhythms. Even though most of the insights contained here have been taken up and enlarged upon by later writers, some of the articles are still useful. The essays by M. Frankenhauser are particularly important from the perspective of healthy work.

194. Garson, Barbara. *The Electronic Sweatshop: How Computers Are Transforming the Office of the Future into the Factory of the Past.* New York: Simon & Schuster, 1988.

Keywords: case study, computers, automation

Fifty percent of McDonald's workers quit within two weeks; many walk out within two days. This extremely high turnover rate has resulted in 7 percent of the American labor force having worked at McDonald's at some point in their lives. McDonald's is the subject of the first of Garson's excellent case studies of automated workplaces. In this engaging work, she shares conversations with various employees to give us a feel for what it is like to work in a routinized, automated workplace where computers seem to be the managers. Garson also interviews airline reservation agents who have been trained in standardized conversations. But automation and computers not only affect the workers at the bottom of the organization. The book chronicles how professionals are being turned into clerks by studying how social workers', psychiatrists' and stock brokers' work is becoming rationalized and automated. Even the work of managers and bosses is being controlled by computer surveillance and record keeping. Centralizing control and moving decision making higher up in the organization seems to be the effect of introducing computers into white-collar work everywhere. Garson notes that she was surprised to discover how far the industrialization of office work had gone. She assumed at the outset of her research that efficiency and cost cutting were the motive. However, she concludes that "the old-fashioned capitalist motives of efficiency, profit, and greed were merely the rational covers for a far-crueler philosophy.

"The goal of modern management—to dictate exactly how a worker does his job and to make him accountable for every minute of the working day—is irrational. It can sometimes be defended in terms of efficiency or productivity, but its only consistent objective is control for the sake of control. That's why any large group of workers who can be automated eventually will be.

"As neo-Taylorists turn their eyes higher up the occupational ladder, the irrational quest for control merges with a primitive struggle for survival. 'Automate or be automated' seems to be the motto as managers and executives turn upon themselves."

195. Garson, Barbara. *All the Livelong Day: The Meaning and Demeaning of Routine Work*. Revised and updated ed. New York: Penguin Books, 1994.

Keywords: automation, routine work, monotonous work, clerical work

"Stacking Ping-Pong paddles in piles of fifty. Entering 50,000 keystrokes an hour into a computer. Performing one weld on one seam on 101 cars an hour, eight hours a day. In factories and offices around this country, work is systematically reduced to the most routine and repetitious tasks. How do workers keep working without losing their minds? To find out, Barbara Garson traveled around the country for two years, spying out the mind-games and minute-to-minute devices workers use to restore meaning to jobs drained of meaning in the name of profit. She found resentment, she found humiliation, she even found sabotage; but above all, she found that people passionately want to work. 'The crime of modern industry,' she concludes, 'is not forcing us to work, but denying us real work.'"

All the Livelong Day has become a classic work that reveals the effects of routinized work. It shows, through conversations with workers and supervisors of a Ping-Pong set manufacturer, a fish cannery, a make-up packaging plant, a car assembly line, a lumber mill and other places how people resist attempts to be turned into machines. It becomes apparent that control over one's work is so important that even workers in the most routinized, machine paced jobs manufacture goals for themselves and invent games in order to exercise their control. This revised and updated edition contains an additional section with stories from the electronic office. Garson concludes that the techniques used to industrialize white-collar work are basically the same as those applied to factory work. Garson shares her experiences in a fascinating and accessible fashion.

196. Gattiker, Urs E. *Technology-Mediated Communication*. Berlin: Walter de Gruyter, 1992.

Keywords: communications technology, organizational change

The contributors to this volume come from the fields of industrial sociology, information systems, public administration, and organization studies; all share a common interest in computer-based communication technology. The focus is on how an organization's structure, its functioning and performance, as well as the behavior of groups and individuals within it, ultimately determine why communication technology is applied in certain ways to transform input into output.

Section 1 explores how the organization's grouping of functions, coordination and task allocation are intertwined with communication technology. This section's macro focus is centered on four essential factors: "Communication technology must be

1) available (e.g., computer installed on the firm's mainframe)

2) accessible to the worker (at or near the workspace)
3) appropriate and, equally important,
4) well suited to an organization's structure."

Section 2 shifts from structural macro to micro issues by studying how individuals and groups can use technology-mediated communication channels differently. Chapter 4, for example, reports on a three-year study investigating the use of voice mail, and chapter 5 analyzes videoconferencing technology utilized by groups (and how this mode of interaction influences the quality of outcome).

Section 3 is the only theoretical piece in the book and it discusses some philosophical, conceptual and paradigm development issues applying to both dimensions of communication technology (i.e., hardware and software as well as the processes of communicating).

197. Gattiker, Urs E., ed. *Women and Technology*. Technological Innovation and Human Resources 4. Berlin: Walter de Gruyter, 1994.

Keywords: women, technology

This volume examines women's experience of technology in different types of jobs and occupations in various organizations. A number of important questions are explored. For example, "If women shift into the male-dominated scientific professions and occupations, how might technology (particularly advanced computer technologies) and continuous education affect their work experience? Could it be that an increased use of technology in the workplace further demarcates gender lines and leads to women receiving positions with lower qualifications than men?"

Section 1 explores how women and men perceive technology, technology-mediated work, and change in the job design and work organization as attributed to technology. Chapter 1 addresses how those women working for federal and state agencies feel about technology-mediated work, especially with respect to information technology. Chapter 2 concentrates on the type and extent of use of an electronic mail system by individuals working in one occupation. Chapter 3 focuses on technology-induced organizational change and its effect upon job design and work organization.

Section 2 focuses on telecommuting. Chapter 4 reports on a study of women trying to prevent their professional obsolescence through continuous education efforts. A comparison with men is presented and gender differences are found. Chapter 5 in this section analyzes how technology may affect job segregation further through telecommuting; some have labeled telecommuting the "re-invention of the nineteenth century sweatshop."

See especially section 3: a theoretical essay that discusses some important philosophical, conceptual, and paradigmatic issues relating to information technology and the work environment.

198. Gavriel Salvendy, and Waldemar Karwowski, eds. *Design of Work and Development of Personnel in Advanced Manufacturing*. Wiley Interscience Series. New York: John Wiley and Sons, 1994.

Keywords: computers, organizational change, work design, manufacturing, personnel management

The authors in this collection of articles all share the position that "as manufacturing enterprises of today rapidly move toward computer-based integration, it becomes clear that their economic survival will depend to a great extent on the symbiosis of social, technological, organizational and management, and ecological design efforts."

Job design in modern manufacturing systems is the subject of chapter 1. Topics discussed are as follows: job design principles for group work, job enlargement, job rotation, autonomous work groups, CAD technologies and their influence on job design, and sociotechnical systems. Three case studies of new job design principles are offered along with a summary of their particular characteristics and results. Chapter 4 considers "Technical Choice and Work Design—Alternatives for the Factory of the Future." This chapter looks at new technologies and the organization of labor, the role of technical choice, the role of education and vocational training, and the requirements for the management of innovation. Chapter 5 "The Design of Work and Technology" explores the concept of flexible specialization, sociotechnical design procedures, criteria for human-centered design of work and technology, and integrated group manufacturing. The concluding remarks at the end of each chapter are particularly useful.

Despite the heavy use of technical language at times in this book, there is considerable value here in the context of preventive work strategies.

199. Gee, James Paul, Glynda Hull, and Colin Lankshear. *The New Work Order Behind the Language of the New Capitalism*. Boulder, CO: Westview Press, 1996.

Keywords: capitalism, democracy, management, inequality, knowledge workers, sociology

This is a compelling account of global capitalism and the "new work order" in the information age. In the view of the authors, "this new work order is largely about trying to create new social identities or new kinds of people: new leaders, new workers, new students . . . even new 'private' people who are supposed to dissolve the separation between their lives outside work and their lives inside it." Given that the three authors share an interest in how language, learning and literacy get caught up in social practices to produce and reproduce social identities, with their accompanying interests and values, "the new work order provides a tailor-made focus around which to explore and develop this shared interest."

The book analyzes the "new work order" promoted in the international management literature and uncovers some startling contradictions. On one side are promises of more meaningful and satisfying work, greater respect for diversity and more democratic distribution of knowledge. On the other is escalating inequality in the workplace and between individuals, nations and continents. The authors ask whether the language of management today (e.g., "workplace democracy," "empowerment," "team leaders," "knowledge workers") heralds a brave new workplace or whether it really masks a new form of capitalism. The first three chapters of the book take up the new work order in "theory" and the next three take it up in "practice." See especially chapters 4 and 5, the case study part of the book. They deal in detail, using ethnographic methods, with an electronics assembly factory in the United States that is implementing a major workplace reform, namely self-directed work teams. The authors suggest that such teams represent many of "the major motifs of the new capitalism."

200. Geiss, Gunther R., and Narayan Viswanathan, eds. *The Human Edge: Information Technology and Helping People.* New York: Haworth Press, 1986.

Keywords: information technology, social work, computers, case study, ethics

This volume on the subject of computers in social work contains a collection of papers originally presented at the Information Technology and Social Work Practice Conference, held in Queenstown, Maryland, June 9-12, 1984. The contributors to this comprehensive text examine what is or should be the response of social work to the rapid introduction of information technology into "what some consider the last professional bastion of human values and human concern, social work practice." The editors note in the preface that "there are those who would like to obstruct the intrusion of this technology . . . those who would defend us against what they perceive to be the onslaught of mechanistic thinking, automation, and dehumanization." On the other side, "there are some who propose creative new applications of technology to better fulfill the mission of practice." The editors continue: "If we accept their proposals, how shall we proceed with the construction of a new scheme of practice suited to the needs and resources of a new era? The opportunities offered to us by information technology are quite attractive; yet we know that there are substantial and, often, hidden costs attached." Much of this book concerns itself with defining the appropriate applications of information technology to helping people, especially in social work. Part 1 considers "The Foundations" (intercultural technology transfer, concepts, trends, terms, and impacts). Part 2 examines "Views of Present and Future" (opportunities and threats, applications, and case studies). See part 3 "Issues and Options" for chapters on values and ethics, science and knowledge, management and resource development, blending information technology and social work, and social work education in the new information era.

201. Gelb, Betsy D. "Preventive Medicine and Employee Productivity." *Harvard Business Review*, March-April 1985: 12-6.

Keywords: health, productivity

The link between work performance and preventive medicine is examined. Examples of companies who invested in exercise facilities or programs and improved productivity are given. Although it does not mean that exercise participation *causes* increased productivity, a link does seem to exist. Exercise programs reduce absenteeism and turnover rates. The scarcity of insurance coverage for preventive medicine programs such as exercise, nutrition and smoking cessation programs is demonstrated. Apparently, most organizations cannot justify increased premiums for preventive medicine coverage. Suggestions for how to encourage worker participation in preventive medicine programs are also included in this brief article.

202. Gellerman, Saul W., and William G. Hodgson. "Cyanamid's New Take on Performance Appraisal." *Harvard Business Review*, May-June 1988: 36-41.

Keywords: industrial relations

Critically analyzed in this article are the new approaches that the biotechnology and chemical company Cyanamid is taking toward their performance appraisals for employees. There are several ways to reward good work, as well as to deal with unsatisfactory performance, and these have been disputed for many years. In the past, Cyanamid rated its employees on a scale that included an O (for "outstanding"), an X (for "excellent in several major areas") and an R (for "achieves expected results"). These were distributed following a bell curve where O would account for 20 percent of the workers, and X and R would include 40 percent each of the remaining employees. There was also an N (for "needs improvement") and "+" and "-" for every letter. This system proved to be unsatisfactory for several reasons, so a new one was started. It was simplified, with only three ratings, and it focused, unlike the old system, on each employee's strengths instead of pointing out all their weaknesses. This created a more positive environment for both the employees, who thus felt better about themselves, and the managers, who had to do the employee assessments. The new system was well received, although not without criticism. For example, employees felt G (for "good") was too broad and included too great a range of employee perfomance. Despite this and other minor complaints, the new system was more favorably looked upon than the old one, and was adopted throughout the company.

203. George, Jennifer M., and Gareth R. Jones. "Experiencing Work: Values, Attitudes, and Moods." *Human Relations* 50, no. 4 (April 1997).

Keywords: values, job performance, organizational behavior, work values

The authors introduce this article by noting that there have been hundreds of studies conducted that have examined specific dimensions of the work experience such as job satisfaction or work values, and hundreds more have focused on the relationship between an aspect of the work experience and an outcome such as job performance or turnover. It is further noted that "much of this research is disjointed, however, and the component studies do not fit together in such a way as to give us a rich understanding of the way different factors such as work values, job satisfaction, and performance interact to affect one another." In this paper, the authors discuss a model of the work experience (the Values, Attitudes and Moods, or VAM, model) that integrates three of the most significant dimensions of the work experience, work values, attitudes and moods, into one overarching framework. This model describes how people experience work and the psychological processes through which they define and structure their circumstances and give meaning to them. These three dimensions, according to the authors, "underscore the need for the simultaneous consideration of values, attitudes, and moods for a fuller understanding of the work experience." The VAM model is also used here to examine and reinterpret several ongoing debates in the literature. For example, it is used to suggest reasons why the performance/satisfaction relationship is so low and why social loafing occurs in some work situations and not in others. The goal of the authors is "to show the utility of the model as a way to invigorate research into the work experience and its effects on organizations and their members."

204. Gershuny, J. "Are We Running Out of Time?" *Futures*, January-February 1992: 3-22.

Keywords: leisure

Through analysis of time-use, the proposition that "time is running out" is examined. This view has been based on arguments that the richer a society becomes, the less its members have the opportunity to relax and do as they please. The opposing view is that the "leisure society" continues to emerge in developed countries, and that the experience of the 1980s is somewhat exceptional. Long-term prospects for the leisure society are examined, and the conclusion is reached that the economic development process of the shift of time-use from production consumption is continuing.

This popular image of the future corresponds to arguments from various academic disciplines that suggest that economic development leads to time congestion. These arguments are convincing, at least for the United Kingdom during the 1980s. But do they hold more generally? A new multinational comparative collection of time-use evidence suggests that there may still be some hope for the leisure society.

205. Gibson, John E. "Taylorism and Professional Education." 149-57 in *Manufacturing Systems: Foundations of World-Class Practice*, edited by Joseph A. Heim and W. Dale Compton. Washington, DC: National Academy Press, 1992.

Keywords: engineering education, Taylorism, manufacturing

The manufacturing system needs to be looked at holistically to include relations with subcontractors, suppliers, and customers as well as the interrelationships of the physical manufacturing environment, manager, and worker. This article considers how to educate and train business managers and engineers so that they are a part of this holistic manufacturing system. The author claims that the reasons that American business and engineering schools have not incorporated this restructuring of manufacturing is because they have not yet abandoned Taylorism and they are change-resistant. The author outlines how elements of Taylorism are applied in the workplace and engineering classrooms.

206. Gil, David G., and Eva A. Gil, eds. *The Future of Work*. Cambridge, MA: Schenkman Books, 1987.

Keywords: forecasting, unemployment, poverty, philosophy

This collection of philosophical and normative writings is based on a conference entitled The Future of Work held by the Center for Social Change Practice and Theory at Brandeis University in 1985. The book represents an effort to develop a constructive approach to issues of work and meaningful employment. The contributors begin with the premise that "social and economic justice, or its absence, depend on the way work and the exchange and distribution of its products are arranged and viewed in a society." The authors then ask whether there could be alternative arrangements of work to those currently dominant ones "which would result in greater fulfillment of human potential and social harmony." They also explore the question of "what philosophical and institutional transformations would be necessary toward these ends, considering the available scientific and technological capabilities of humankind and the scope of natural resources?"

All of the authors in this volume share a common belief that "unemployment and poverty, or to use a more analytic phrase, systematic exclusion from sharing in society's collective production and product, are preventable social problems which, directly or indirectly, hurt and diminish everyone."

See especially chapter 2 "Why Work" by Stanley Aronowitz and chapter 6 "Workplace Democracy: Theory and Practice" by Thomas Rice. See also chapter 5 "Women, Work, and Poverty" by Deanne Bonnar.

207. Gill, Colin. *Work, Unemployment and the New Technology*. Cambridge, UK: Polity Press, 1985.

Keywords: technology, unions, unemployment, stress, skill, work design

This concise volume, written from an industrial relations and sociological perspective, explores the implications of advanced technology for work. The microelectronics and telecommunications industries receive particular attention, with additional focus being given to the effects of the "new" technology on employment patterns and trade union involvement.

See especially chapter 2 "The Automated Office" for information on "The Effect of New Office Technology on Skills . . . Job Content and Job Stress, and Health and Safety Aspects of Office Employment." See chapter 3 "On the Shop Floor" for material dealing with "The Quality of Working Life Movement, Group Technology and Quality Circles, Job Redesign, and the Shop Floor Reaction." Chapter 4 focuses on "The Unemployment Threat" and chapter 5 considers "The Trade Union Response." Chapter 6 considers "Alternative Approaches to New Technology: the Scandinavian Experience." Topics discussed here are as follows: "Legislation and New Technology; the Swedish Center for Working Life; the Work Environment Act; and Some Swedish Research Projects." The seventh and final chapter examines "New Technologies and the Future of Work." Topics are as follows: "Future Work Patterns; The Work Ethic; Reduced Working Hours?; Redistributing Work; New Focus of Job Design; and The Politics of Design."

208. Gill, Karamjit S., ed. *Information Society: New Media, Ethics and Postmodernism*. Berlin: Springer-Verlag, 1996.

Keywords: information technology, general, computers

This excellent interdisciplinary volume brings together three critical debates of post-industrial society on culture and technology, information society, and postmodernism. The contributors discuss some of the dilemmas and paradoxes arising from the convergence of information and communication technologies, and examine these issues within the context of an interdependent world of working, living and learning. The book provides theoretical and methodological underpinnings for the analysis and design of information, communication and new media technologies. Based on contributions from major researchers in the field, this volume brings together themes of knowledge and development, ethics and technology, telematics and social innovation, postmodernism and representation, and creativity, cooperation and innovation, and examines the implications for the traditional ways of working, living and learning in post-industrial society. The book will be of particular interest to researchers and practitioners who are concerned with the wider policy, social, cultural, philosophical and ethical problems of an information society. See especially the opening address by Mike Cooley on "Visions and Problems of the Post-Industrial Society," "Knowledge and the Post-Industrial Society" by Karamjit Gill (chapter 1), and "The Keyboard Blues: Modern Technology and the Rights and Risks of People at Work" by Patricia Shipley (chapter 4). This chapter focuses on health and safety concerns in the computerized workplace by using several good case studies. See also "Information System Design: Human Centered Approaches" by Jim Thorpe (chapter 7).

In the second section of the text, entitled "Information Society: Working and Learning Dimensions," see "Technological Change, Social Innovation, and Employment" by Peter van den Besselaar (chapter 8), "Empowerment and Enslavement: The Transformation of Work" by Matthew Jones (chapter 9), and "Information Communication Technology and Society: A Community-Based Approach" by Peter Day (chapter 12).

The final section looks at the postmodernism debate in the information society. See especially "Electronic Mail, IT Productivity, and Workplace Culture" by C. W. Boyne (chapter 19).

This is an outstanding multidisciplinary volume of relevance to the healthy work field of research.

209. Gill, Tom. *Men of Uncertainty: The Social Organization of Day Laborers in Contemporary Japan*. SUNY Series in Japan in Transition. Albany: State University of New York Press, 2001.

Keywords: day laborers, Japan, working class, social conditions

This book concentrates on the theme of Japan's day laborers, the urban labor markets where the men gather to find work, and the cheap lodging districts where many of them live. These day laborers tend to live outside the two dominant institutions of contemporary Japanese society: the nuclear family and the company. The author, by focusing mainly on the day-laboring districts of Yokohama and five other cities, discovers a large group of individuals that has opted out of their traditional, communal way of life. As a result, issues such as their lifestyle, the exclusion from mainstream society, the absence of family life, and a career that can easily lead to homelessness and an early death on the street are analyzed.

210. Giordano, Lorraine. *Beyond Taylorism: Computerization and the New Industrial Relations*. New York: St. Martin's Press, 1992.

Keywords: automation, QWL, labor process

This book explores the specific ways automation and Quality of Work Life (QWL) programs affect the labor process through a detailed case study of a U.S. defense plant. The author argues that computerization and QWL strategies represent two of the most powerful current industrial attempts to reorganize production methods. QWL programs and automation are examined in this sociological analysis as significant forms of both organization and control of the labor process.

The features that distinguish computer automation from its predecessors are outlined, and the effects of micro-computer based automation on employment and employee skills are also analyzed. Moreover, the relationship between computerization and the decision-making process of an industrial organization is considered.

The book is divided into two main sections: "Automation and the Organization of the Labor Process" and "The New Industrial Relations and QWL." See part 1, chapters 3 through 8 for a description and analysis comparing workers' experiences with conventional and computerized equipment. Part 2 of the text examines organizational changes underway that are designed to increase flexibility in the production process and gain workers' cooperation in that process.

211. Glendon, A. Ian, and Eugene F. McKenna. *Human Safety and Risk Management*. London: Chapman and Hall, 1995.

Keywords: mental health, psychology, stress, stress management, coping, shift work, burnout

This book provides a comprehensive framework for "some of the major psychological issues which may be subsumed under a human resource management (HRM) heading—one which is oriented toward risk management (RM)." In this work, the authors attempt to stretch psychology from a basis of existing empirical and theoretical knowledge into new areas—mental health and accidents, for example, issues that "can be validly and usefully informed by input from applied psychological knowledge." The authors also seek to analyze the changing nature of approaches to managing risk as it applies to individuals and groups in the workplace.

See especially part 3 of the book on "The Work Environment." Within this section, chapter 7 explores issues of risk management and human health on the group level. Chapter 8 "Stress, Stress Management, and Psychological Health" is the strongest chapter in terms of preventive work strategies and healthy work models. A wide range of topics are covered including: job stressors (such as working conditions, shiftwork, job overload, underload, burnout and unemployment); personality and health issues, stress and lifestyle, coping strategies (individual and organizational), health promotion programs, social support, and human resource management approaches to stress management. Also see chapter 10 "Managing Human Risks." This chapter explores a systems approach to work health and safety culture, providing an extensive and practical safety audit methodology and other techniques for risk assessment. Chapter 11, the final chapter, sets out "a prescriptive program of action based on current knowledge" with implications for the area of healthy work.

212. Godnig, Edward C., and John S. Hacunda. *Computers and Visual Stress: How to Enhance Visual Comfort while Using Computers*. Charlestown, RI: Seacoast Information Services, 1990.

Keywords: computers, health, stress, eye strain, ergonomics, work, job design, video display terminal, health risks

The purpose of this brief volume, written by an optometrist specializing in behavioral optometry, is to explore visual stress—an increasingly prevalent health concern resulting from the computer age. Chapter 1 introduces the range of eye problems associated with computer use and outlines the direct and indirect signs and symptoms of video display terminal (VDT)-induced visual stress. Chapter 2 presents background information on the functioning of both visual and computer systems. Chapter 3 describes the visual stress problems in terms of symptoms and causative factors, and chapter 4 gives suggestions on creating an ideal workstation environment. Chapter 5 provides information on an optometric approach toward reducing visual stress. The chapter covers the following subjects: key visual skills needed for VDT viewing; requirements of a proper eye examination for computer workers; visual training procedures that are useful for conditioning the eyes for the demands of VDT use; and stretching exercises for general relaxation. Chapter 6 summarizes the book and suggests possible long term solutions to the VDT visual stress problem. The authors make the important point that the emergence of the post-industrial information-based society has greatly increased the demand on the eyes for close-up work. Data entry clerks, computer programmers, airline reservation agents, telephone operators, word processors, and many other workers are obliged to focus on computer terminals at very close range, we are reminded. However, "we must remember that our eyes are adapted for distant viewing. . . . The change in emphasis on our visual system from distance viewing to close-up viewing has occurred in less than 50 years. Our visual system is unable to handle this increased use of near vision naturally. Instead we must actively adapt by modifying our work environment and work behavior."

The authors take a holistic approach toward improving vision, encompassing areas as diverse as visual training procedures, diet, work organization, and education. Vision is viewed as a complex process that includes learning, and that can be altered and improved by following the proper regimen.

213. Goetsch, David L. *Occupational Safety and Health in the Age of High Technology for Technologists, Engineers and Managers*. 2nd ed. Englewood Cliffs, NJ: Prentice Hall, 1996.

Keywords: industrial hygiene, industrial safety

This comprehensive text covers all of the fundamental health and safety topics, with a particular emphasis on health and hazard issues in the context of modern (high technology) workplace environments. It is intended primarily for use in universities, colleges and corporate training settings, by educators in such disciplines as industrial technology, manufacturing technology, industrial engineering, occupational safety and management.

See especially chapter 1 for a historical overview of the Health and Safety Movement, chapter 2 on "Accidents and Their Effect on Industry," and chapter 6 "Roles of Health and Safety Personnel."

Also see chapter 7 for a discussion of "Stress and Safety" (topics here include sources of workplace stress, human reactions to stress, shift work and stress, techniques for reducing workplace stress, etc.). Chapter 22 deals with "Promoting Safety" and chapter 23 with "Health and Safety Training." Chapter 25 examines health issues, computers and automation. Chapter 26 focuses on ethics and safety. Chapter 31 "TQM and Safety Management" includes a discussion of the relationship between TQM and safety. Each chapter is followed by a thematic summary, review questions and a listing of key terms and concepts.

214. Goldberger, Leo, and Shlomo Breznitz, eds. *Handbook of Stress: Theoretical and Clinical Aspects*. 2nd ed. New York: Free Press, 1993.

Keywords: stress, workload, burnout, coping

This is a sourcebook on a variety of subjects regarding stress such as the history of the stress concept, decision making under stress, effects of stress on neurochemistry, stress and the immune system, measurement of stress and coping, psychiatric and somatic conditions, extreme stressors, treatments, and supports. There also exists a section on common stressors that contains three chapters of relevance to healthy work. Chapter 19 on occupational stress outlines the history of the field, types of occupational stress, effects of occupational stress, moderator variables and theories. Chapter 20 reviews the empirical evidence regarding two of the factors that affect the health of workers: psychological workload and the social environment at work. The long-term and short-term effects of high workload are examined. Evidence for and against the demand-control model is presented. The section on the effects of the social environment on health discusses direct effects on mental and physical health and the buffering effect of social support. Burnout is the subject of chapter 21, which explains its costs, measurement, causes and coping strategies.

215. Golden, Lonnie, and Deborah M. Figart, eds. *Working Time: International Trends, Theory and Policy Perspectives*. Advances in Social Economics. New York: Routledge, 2000.

Keywords: hours of labor, labor supply, working time and public policy, innovations in working time

The trend toward longer or more differential hours, underemployment, overwork, and the "time squeeze" among many workers in post-industrial countries is the main theme explored by all of the authors. Within work there are relevant matters, such as: duration (observed either daily, weekly or annually, by family or individual); distribution (the extent to which workers are getting the amount of work they desire) among workers by gender, race, or job type; the degree of flexibility and control workers may possess regarding its duration, timing and pace; and the implications of worker well-being, productivity, or equity. This work reveals that the level, distribution, and alterations in individuals' hours of work reflect their responses to trends in wages, inequality, consumerism, or balance of power. Working time is becoming ever more determined within the web of evolving culture and social relations as well as traditionally conceived market, technological, and macroeconomic forces, and institutions such as collective bargaining and government policy. Trends in working time are also presented, and alternative theoretical and historical perspectives are provided to restructure work, either to allow a better balance between work and nonwork life or to promote employment opportunities.

216. Golembiewski, Robert T., Robert A. Boudreau, Robert F. Munzenrider, and Huaping Luo. *Global Burnout: A Worldwide Pandemic Explored by the Phase Model*. Greenwich, CT: JAI Press, 1996.

Keywords: stress, burnout, organizational behavior, industrial relations

This comprehensive text, written from an organizational behavior and industrial relations perspective, details the results from strain-related research conducted in over thirty countries. The research deals with stress as well as burnout in various global work settings.

Despite a rather technical and statistically-oriented theoretical approach, the book provides a wealth of information on the estimated incidences of burnout and its persistence, and the costs for both individuals and organizations. Social and health consequences are also highlighted. The methodological foundation of the research is referred to as the "phase model" of burnout, an index comprised of an extensive inventory of items designed to tap into the phenomenon of burnout, including measures of depersonalization, emotional exhaustion, personal dissatisfaction, etc.

Preventive approaches to the problem of burnout are not addressed specifically, but a brief section on the issues of "ameliorating burnout" is enlightening (see chapter 7 "Open Issues in Approaching Burnout"), particularly because it reveals the almost total lack of research literature dealing with the question of "solutions." See especially chapter 4 "Human Costs of Burnout: Health-Related Indicators around the World."

The substantive conclusion of this work is very clear and emphatically presented. All research in the field suggests that an increasing number of people worldwide are experiencing advanced burnout and that the condition has a strong tendency to persist over extended periods of time.

217. Goodman, Paul S. and Associates, eds. *Designing Effective Work Groups*. Jossey-Bass Social and Behavioral Sciences Series, Jossey-Bass Management Series. San Francisco: Jossey-Bass Publishers, 1986.

Keywords: work design, work groups, quality circles, sociotechnical systems

This collection of writings offers theoretical perspectives on the design of effective work groups. "New models are presented on leadership in groups, technology and group performance, intergroup relations, and so on." As a study of groups in organizations, the book has direct relevance for the development of quality circles, labor-management participation teams, and autonomous work groups.

Chapter 2 explores group decision making and group effectiveness in the context of self-regulating groups such as quality circles and sociotechnical work systems. See also chapter 4 "Impact of Task and Technology on Group Performance." Limitations of current usages of task and technology are identified, and then a new interdisciplinary perspective is provided. Of special interest for the promotion of healthy work concepts is chapter 11 "Studying Groups at Work: Ten Critical Needs for Theory and Practice."

218. Göranzon, Bo, and Ingela Josefson, eds. *Knowledge, Skill and Artificial Intelligence*. Springer Series on Foundations and Applications of Artificial Intelligence. London: Springer-Verlag, 1988.

Keywords: artificial intelligence, skill, tacit knowledge, knowledge embedded in experience, anthropocentric

This volume is the outcome of a conference (held in London in March 1987) sponsored by the Swedish Center for Working Life on the topic "Knowledge, Skill, and New Technology." The book examines "the long term effects of new technology on the way people acquire their skills in working life." The issue of skill formation and the question of how skills can be developed and maintained are central to the text. The concept of tacit knowledge is also explored. These issues are illustrated by "case studies concerning professional groups with experience of advanced computer technology." Consideration is given to programs for education and training in society and in working life.

Section 2 of the text deals with "Tacit Knowledge and Apprenticeship," by looking at case studies on nursing, weather forecasting and automated factory production. Chapter 6, on "Tacit Knowledge, Working Life, and Scientific Method," examines the role of tacit knowledge in the workplace and its implications for understanding the place of expert systems in working life. Chapter 7 considers the conditions necessary for the transfer of skills, and chapter 8 focuses on the education and training of workers in the context of creative participation. A human-centered approach is also emphasized. See especially chapter 12 by Mike Cooley on "Creativity, Skill, and Human-Centered Systems." Cooley analyzes advanced computer systems as part of a historical continuum and considers the implications of humans being rendered more and more passive as machines become more active. Chapter 13 explores the "Limits of Automation in Administration" and chapter 16 looks at "Expert Systems, the Division of Labor, and Division of Knowledge."

219. Goumain, Pierre, ed. *High-Technology Workplaces: Integrating Technology, Management and Design for Productive Work.* New York: Van Nostrand, 1989.

Keywords: technology, work design, management, productivity

This book examines the design and management problems of high-technology workplaces in an integrated way. The editor of the volume notes that "work processes and the social environment of organizations are being redefined . . . as a result of the introduction of new information technologies." Because the impacts of information technology have many systematic implications, some of which have implications for the physical work environment, "this book favors a holistic approach that looks at the technological, social, and environmental aspects together."

The editors argue that in order to foster productive work environments in high-tech workplaces "it is critical to maintain a fit between changing information and telecommunication technologies, changing work processes, changing organizations and people, and changing physical environments."

Part 1 of the text explores major societal trends and developments in the information-based society; knowledge-based industries; and new patterns of manufacturing. Part 2 considers the planning aspects of developments for high technology. The contributors focus on high-quality work environments and settings as essential for high-quality knowledge workers. Part 3 examines the managing and designing projects for high-technology workplaces. Technological means, organizational requirements, and the role of management are given close attention. Part 4 provides specific examples of design strategies in practice.

220. Graham, Laurie. *On the Line at Subaru-Isuzu: The Japanese Model and the American Worker*. Ithaca, NY: ILR Press, 1995.

Keywords: case study, lean production

The debate about the Japanese model of management rages on: is the cooperation between management and workers genuine or coerced? However, what concerns Graham is the American experience with the Japanese model. How do

American workers view the Japanese model? This ethnography of American non-union workers at the Subaru-Isuzu Automotive (SIA) plant near Lafayette, Indiana, seeks to understand the experience of Americans within the Japanese lean production model. Graham worked on the line at SIA for six months and covertly compiled observations and experiences. She comments on the seven dimensions of organizational control exercised there: (1) worker selection, (2) orientation and training, (3) the team concept, (4) the philosophy of *kaizen*, (5) the culture of cooperation through egalitarian symbols, (6) the computerized assembly line, and (7) just-in-time production. In addition, Graham chronicles the gradual decrease in worker morale in this informative case study.

221. Grandjean, Etienne. *Ergonomics in Computerized Offices*. London: Taylor and Francis, 1987.

Keywords: video display terminal, ergonomics, human factors

This volume, written by a leading European ergonomics specialist, offers a comprehensive analysis of the computerized office environment from the perspective of human factors engineering. The author explains how the proper introduction and use of automated equipment can prevent problems for workers, creating a work situation that is more comfortable, more productively efficient, and less stressful. Information provided in the book is intended to help ergonomists and engineers design workplaces that conform to human needs and human capabilities. Basic design and planning principles are introduced against a detailed background of relevant human physiology and psychology.

The text would also make a good introduction to the subject for students of industrial engineering and design, computing and occupational psychology.

The following chapter titles indicate the scope of the work: (1) "The Present Metamorphosis of Offices"; (2) "VDT Jobs Seen through Ergonomic-Tinted Spectacles"; (3) "Physical Characteristics of VDTs"; (4) "Vision"; (5) "Ergonomic Principles of Lighting in Offices"; (6) "Visual Strain and Photometric Characteristics of VDTs"; (7) "Ergonomic Design of VDT Workstations"; (8) "Noise"; (9) "Radiation, Electrostatic Fields, and Alleged Health Hazards"; (10) "Occupational Stress, Work Satisfaction, and Job Design"; and (11) "Recommendations for VDT Workstations."

222. Green, Eileen, Jenny Owen, and Den Pain, eds. *Gendered by Design? Information Technology and Office Systems*. London: Taylor and Francis, 1993.

Keywords: information technology, gender relations, sociology, anthropocentric

This book brings together two areas of research and debate: "First, sociological analyses of gender relations in the workplace, most specifically in relation to information technology (IT); and second, the body of interdisciplinary research into the design of computer systems."

The papers in this collection establish "new links between empirical and theoretical work in computer science and social science," with an emphasis on the impact of gender relations upon computer systems design processes.

The first section of the book offers a review of existing interdisciplinary approaches to office systems design in relation to IT. Focus is on human-centered systems design, problems and opportunities, etc. Section 2 highlights some of the major theoretical issues that underlie discussions of gender and computer systems. Section 3 provides a contemporary view of IT in the office context (i.e., changing trends and working patterns with respect to gendered assumptions). Section 4 examines new initiatives in Europe and Scandinavia, particularly with regard to human-centered design strategies, and guidelines for a gender perspective of IT.

This volume offers a unique gender-perspective on computer-based information technologies. It is well-researched and offers many useful insights on the application of human-centered computer design.

223. Greenbaum, Joan, and Marten Kyng, eds. *Design at Work: Cooperative Design of Computer Systems*. Hillsdale, NJ: Lawrence Erlbaum Associates, 1991.

Keywords: system design, computers, sociology, anthropology, psychology, linguistics, human factors

This book presents a unique approach to the subject of computer system design. The papers included in the collection "bring together a wealth of practical system development experience with a depth of background in pertinent fields such as sociology, anthropology, linguistics, and psychology." The contributors "force computer scientists to recognize the embeddedness of social interactions in their work . . . and to re-examine the conceptual framework and assumptions of their everyday activities."

Although the book deals primarily with computer system development, it also calls attention to "relationships of language to action, and concern for participation and cooperation in design." It is a striking example of "reflection in action."

This book offers a fine balancing of theoretical analysis with practical applications in the field of computer design. See especially chapter 2 "From Human Factors to Human Actors: The Role of Psychology and Human-Computer Interaction Studies in System Design" by Liam Bannon. Also see chapter 6 "Workplace Cultures: Looking at Artifacts, Symbols, and Practices" by Keld Bødker.

224. Greenberg, Edward S. *Workplace Democracy: The Political Effects of Participation*. Ithaca, NY: Cornell University Press, 1986.

Keywords: democracy, case study, socialism, alienation

The author uses the American Pacific Northwest plywood industry to collect empirical data on the relationship between workplace democracy initiatives and political movements. More specifically, he seeks to determine whether workplace democratization leads to democratization of social, economic, and political life. What is the connection to socialism? The author argues that the appeal of workplace democracy, especially of worker self-management, to socialists is due to three intellectual/political traditions: (1) the literature regarding alienation, (2) the encouragement of participatory democracy, and (3) the interest in radical but popular democratic strategies for overthrowing capitalism. These three traditions are outlined in the introductory chapter and serve as the basis of the empirical study and analyses that this book constitutes.

225. Greenlund, Kurt J., Kiang Liu, Sarah Knox et al. "Psychosocial Work Characteristics and Cardiovascular Disease Risk Factors in Young Adults: The CARDIA Study." *Social Science and Medicine* 41, no. 5 (1995): 717-23.

Keywords: stress, disease

This large research study, with a sample population of black and white male and female workers "examines the associations of high job demands, low decision latitude, and job strain with cardiovascular disease (CVD) risk factors." The researchers use advanced statistical analysis methods to analyze the associations of these job-related characteristics with blood pressure, total serum cholesterol, alcohol use and cigarette consumption.

The study itself (known as CARDIA) was undertaken to determine the validity of strong claims made in recent years to the effect that psychological stress at work is related to the development of cardiovascular disease, independently of the other known risk factors (the two characteristics of work thought to most affect health outcomes in general being excessive job demands and a lack of control over one's job). Results of this particular study are somewhat surprising. According to the job strain model, "job demands should be positively associated with CVD risk factors, while an inverse relation is expected between job decision latitude and CVD risk factor levels."

In fact, contrary to the job strain model, low job strain and higher decision latitude were associated with greater alcohol use among white women workers. Confounding variables intervening in this particular result may have been due to women entering traditionally male dominated management and white collar occupations where they experience stressors such as sexual discrimination or harassment.

The authors of the study also point out that their participants were a relatively young group with limited exposure to the work environment "and thus may not yet have succumbed to the effects of work life on either their health or their lifestyle."

226. Grenier, Guillermo J. *Inhuman Relations: Quality Circles and Anti-Unionism in American Industry*. Labor and Social Change. Philadelphia: Temple University Press, 1988.

Keywords: unions, quality circles, QWL, industrial relations, participation, case study

This book is about "how the new humanized management 'manages' power and how workers yield to it, not from lack of courage but from lack of choice." The author argues that the so-called new managerial humanism often disguises employee manipulation and control, and sometimes even union-busting.

The book presents an exploratory case study of the teamwork concept as applied by the Johnson & Johnson Corporation, in one of its non-unionized American industrial plants. The author examines "the control and manipulation of workers by company managers and consultants" during a period in which the team concept was proposed as an employee organization alternative to unionization. The focus is on the methods used by management to regulate information, interaction and attitudes of workers in its attempt to introduce mechanisms of control via a reorganized work structure. The book does not cover, to any significant degree, many of the generally positive ideas coming from management concerning the new humanism in management. Although the author acknowledges the contribution of union quality of work literature to an increased understanding of work participation, his firsthand experience cautions him against "accepting new human relations schemes at face value."

227. Grint, Keith, and Rosalind Gill, eds. *The Gender-Technology Relation: Contemporary Theory and Research*. London: Taylor and Francis, 1995.

Keywords: information technology, gender, computers, sociology, feminism

This volume offers a selection of new articles by sociologists and organization theorists who have made significant contributions to a relatively new field of research—feminist studies of technology. Through a series of case studies, the chapters focus first on the issues raised by different technologies (e.g., computing, domestic and reproductive technologies, education and work) and second on developing a theoretical understanding of the gender-technology relation. Basic questions considered are as follows: "What is the relationship between gender and technology? Are technologies inherently masculine? What sort of assumptions about gender go into their design production and use? Are technologies implicated in women's oppression or could they play a part in women's liberation? Do the rapid changes we are witnessing in medical, industrial and information technologies pose threats to or offer opportunities for women?" The contributors also explore one of the major theoretical debates of the 1990s—the relationship between feminism and social constructivism. In addition, the book discusses eco-feminism, liberal feminism and the more historical perspective that sees technology as masculine culture. See especially "Competition and Collaboration in Male Shaping of Computing: A Study of a Norwegian Hacker Culture" by Tove Håpnes and Knut H. Sørensen. Also see "Negotiating a Software Career: Informal Work Practices and the 'Lads' in a Software Installation" by Margaret Tierney and "On Some Failures of Nerve in Constructivist and Feminist Analyses of Technology" by Keith Grint and Steve Woolgar.

228. Grundy, A. F., and D. Köhler, eds. *Proceedings of the 6th Annual International IFIP Conference on Women, Work and Computerization*. Bonn, Germany: Springer-Verlag, 1997.

Keywords: women, computers, automation, feminism

This comprehensive volume discusses how different areas of society are being transformed by computer technology, with particular emphasis on changes in women's work and life and how these have come about. "Such transformations include the transition from women's traditional work to work based on modern technology; from communicating within personal communities to communicating within virtual communities; from traditional job gendering to new perspectives on 'who does what.'"

The contributors to this collection of essays interpret the word "computerization" broadly to include the organizational and social context in which computer systems are designed and used. Both empirical and theoretical research is presented. The contributions are oriented around the following six topics: "1) Information Society, Multimedia, and Networking (Can women's request for interpersonal networking be realized by new information technology?) 2) Creating Models and Tools (Which paradigms and metaphors have contributed to the construction of computer software and the theory of computer science?) 3) Not Without a Body? Bodily Functions in Cyberspace (Is the body represented in space/virtual reality and to what end?) 4) Labor and Living: Apart or Together? (Do public and private space merge?) 5) Education (What should be the elements of an informatics curriculum that represents informatics as a mode in the web of other disciplines?) 6) History-Herstory (Has feminist criticism changed women's strategies for gaining access to and influencing new technologies?)."

Sample essay titles from the six topic areas include "Sex, Age, and the Desirability of Computers," "The Moral Order of an Information System," "The Physical Body in Cyberspace: At the Edge of Extinction?," "Formation of the Global Office: Women and the Globalization of Information Labor," "Girls and Computer Science: 'It's Not Me. I'm Not Interested in Sitting Behind a Machine

All Day'" and "Gender Segregation in IT Occupations." This is an outstanding collection of research papers and an invaluable tool for further investigation of the subject.

229. Guest, R. H. "Quality of Work Life: Learning from Tarrytown." *Harvard Business Review*, July-August 1979: 76-87.

Keywords: QWL, case study, industrial relations

When business people and researchers talk or write about the beginnings of the human relations era in management today, the name Hawthorne is invariably mentioned. In the future, when they talk about quality of work life, they will refer to Topeka, Kalmar, and Tarrytown. Each plant's experience with a quality of work life effort, essentially a structured program to involve workers in decisions affecting how they work, is unique. Each plant had different problems and different reasons for beginning a quality of work life program. Tarrytown, a GM car assembly plant in New York State, is perhaps the plant with the greatest number of people ever to have undergone such a program and is perhaps one that had the most to gain, for it was in a fairly poor economic state when the program began. This is the story of the developing and ongoing quality of the work life program at Tarrytown, recounted in many cases by the words of the people involved.

230. Guillen, Mauro F. *Models of Management: Work, Authority, and Organization in a Comparative Perspective*. Chicago: University of Chicago Press, 1994.

Keywords: comparative management, United States, Germany, Spain, Great Britain, organizational sociology

By exploring different historical patterns in the adoption of three major models of organizational management—structural analysis, human relations, and scientific management—the author observes how managers have used the models in four countries (the United States, Germany, Spain, and Great Britain) during the twentieth century. The study involves two different types of societies. The first type is liberal-democratic societies consisting of United States and Great Britain and the second type is corporatist societies consisting of Germany and Spain. The study reveals significant differences in the way that ideas, independent of interests and technology, can cause organizational change. Thus, the contrasts between Protestant and Catholic religious backgrounds, as well as between modernist-technocratic and liberal-humanist mentalities, emerge as key factors in determining managerial practice and ideology. Also explored are larger issues such as the impact of the state and the professions on managerial behavior, the role that managers play in modern societies, and the interaction of government, labor, and managerial elites.

231. Gustavsen, Björn, Bernd Hofmaier, Marianne Ekman Philips, and Anders Wikman. *Concept-Driven Development and the Organization of the Process of Change: An Evaluation of the Swedish Working Life Fund*. Dialogues on Work and Innovation. Amsterdam: John Benjamins Publishing Company, 1996.

Keywords: case study, QWL, organizational change

The authors summarize their work as follows: "The Swedish Working Life Fund—a temporary organization functioning from 1990 to 1995—distributed 10 billion Swedish crowns for workplace development and initiated 25,000 projects. More than half of the total labor market was affected. This evaluation study, that is built on case studies as well as a survey of a representative sample of the project population, describes the emergent characteristics of organization development in Swedish enterprises and services. In order to locate the efforts of the fund within an explanatory context, the study draws on the idea of concept-driven change, of participation in development processes, of development coalitions, of infrastructure for change, and of a society that is supportive of change."

232. Gustavsen, Björn, and Gerry Hunnius. *New Patterns of Work Reform: The Case of Norway*. Oslo: Universitetsforlaget, 1981.

Keywords: democracy, labor relations, sociotechnical systems, participation, case study

This book examines working life reform programs and the industrial democracy movement in Norway. The authors provide a detailed account of new forms of work organization, emphasizing their political background and actual impact on working life and health and safety. The reforms discussed are of relevance for all countries with aspirations for meaningful workplace change. The focus throughout the text is on practical strategies for improving the quality of working life.

Chapter 1 offers an overview of labor relations in Norway. Chapter 2 explores industrial democracy programs (topics here include the reorganization of work, the sociotechnical perspective, participatory strategies, and case study material). See chapter 3 for a discussion of work reform and productivity, worker involvement, conflict resolution and the role of research. See chapter 6 for a good critique of the "conventional approach to safety and health in work." Chapter 7 provides an analysis of the "merger between work assignment and participatory democracy." Topics discussed include "freedom, competence, and worker control" and "job characteristics, work environment, and safety."

233. Haak, Agnes T. *Dutch Sociotechnical Design in Practice: An Empirical Study of the Concept of the Whole Task Group*. Assen, The Netherlands: Van Gorcum, 1994.

Keywords: sociotechnical systems, case study

The diffusion of sociotechnical systems design from the Tavistock Institute in London to other places resulted in different versions of sociotechnical work design. The Dutch design has unique objectives and methods and is described in chapter 2. The linking of practice and theory is the main concern of the author and is addressed in chapter 3, focusing on areas of improvement in the sociotechnical approach. The remainder of the work consists of a detailed case study of a Philips semiconductor plant that underwent the sociotechnical redesign process. The whole task groups on the shop-floor are the focus of the study. The similarities and differences between the actual whole task groups and the theoretical characteristics are noted. From this, the relative importance of different group characteristics is determined. Problems with the management of whole task groups are also considered. The book goes on to describe a new measuring instrument that translates the ten design principles for whole task groups into measurable characteristics.

234. Hackman, J. Richard, et al., eds. *Psychology and Work: Productivity, Change and Employment.* Washington, DC: American Psychological Association, 1986.

Keywords: psychology, productivity, organizational behavior

The contributors to this volume explore core issues in psychology and work and develop "a sophisticated perspective on issues that range from the individual in systems, to innovation and change, to new approaches to management and career patterns, through employment and its effect on family systems." The editors begin the text by noting that the problems associated with productivity, economic competition, unemployment, and the adoption of new computer-based information technologies "will require very different approaches and solutions to which psychology has major expertise to contribute. . . . National discussions and policy processes that do not include psychology's systematic approach deprive our society of a critically valuable source of talent, represented by the implications of psychology's knowledge base." Considerable attention is given to the implications of psychology's insights for the organization of productivity and work systems.

See especially "Work as a Human Context" by Rudolph Moos. The author examines "the relationship between a traditional emphasis on human relations that leads to concerns with organizational development and quality of life. The synthesis becomes an emphasis on the reciprocal interaction between the impact of work and employment and the impact of the social context of work as illustrated and examined throughout a series of settings." In "Technological Change and the Structure of Work," Louis G. Tornatzky presents the implications of new computer-assisted technology and notes the resulting implied revolution for organizing systems of work and management. "The processes of change and integration of these new technologies has major implications for preparing the work force and for training at individual, group, and management levels." See also "Career Issues through the Life Span" and "Work, Family, and the Child."

235. Hakken, David. *Computing Myths, Class Realities: An Ethnography of Technology and Working People in Sheffield, England.* Boulder, CO: Westview Press, 1993.

Keywords: computers, technology, case study, manufacturing, deskilling, skill

This volume is about the extensive change—on the job, where people live, in social relationships—taking place in contemporary societies. "The book examines whether this social change is caused by the introduction of computer-based new technology or 'computerization.' To answer this question, computerization is examined culturally, through the holistic approach of anthropology." The conclusions presented in the book were reached through extensive ethnographic fieldwork carried out in an industrial area in the north of England experiencing extensive computerization.

The major theoretical issues addressed by the study are as follows: "Can the bulk of the social change *associated with* computing be said to have been *caused by* computer technology, developing as a largely independent force having an internally generated direction? Conversely, should the changes be viewed as more fundamentally determined by other, nontechnological, social forces?"

The authors detail the forms of computerization taking place in Sheffield and how the physical act of production (in terms of food, clothing, energy, etc.) has changed with the introduction of computers. They also explore the specific impact of computing on both service workers and employees in the manufacturing sector (especially with regard to skilling/deskilling).

In addition, the book focuses on "the ways that direct human action, as opposed to structures (such as the national state and media) shapes computerization and social reproduction—especially the actions of working-class people."

See especially chapter 4 "Computerization of Work," chapter 7 "Theorizing Computerization," chapter 12 "Computing and Gender," and chapter 13 "Class, Culture, Computing, and Politics."

236. Halpern, Norman. "Sociotechnical Systems Design: The Shell Sarnia Experiment." 31-75 in *Quality of Working Life: Contemporary Cases*, edited by J. B. Cunningham and T. H. White. Ottawa: Labour Canada, 1984.

Keywords: sociotechnical systems, case study

This is a case study of the development of the Shell Canada chemical plant in Sarnia. The project illustrates a sociotechnical systems design. Management and labor work in collaboration on the design of all the jobs at the plant as well as the design of the organization itself. The chapter reports how this led to higher productivity as well as a much happier workforce.

237. Ham, James M. "Work and Health." Speech delivered to Workers' Compensation Board, St. John's, Newfoundland, 1990.

Keywords: health, stress, disease

In this important speech delivered to Workers' Compensation Board members, James Ham clearly and convincingly urges his audience to broaden their perspective. To a group who is normally only concerned with industrial hygiene and workplace hazards, he suggests that dysfunction and disablement due to the psychosocial conditions of work be included in their consideration of "industrial disease." These psychosocial effects should be included under the definition of ill-health "arising out of and in the course of employment."

The first part of the lecture explores the determinants of health using a socio-epidemiological perspective. The entire "social and physical context of work, family, leisure, and society" must be taken into account. Ham refers to the World Health Organization's definition of health and he adopts this for use in this speech; it is urged that this definition be used at all times by Workers' Compensation Boards. Next, Ham calls upon evidence linking life expectancy, mortality and rates of coronary heart disease to types of jobs, social classes and psychosocial conditions of work such as autonomy, decision latitude, social support and psychological demand.

Ham goes on to probe the existing challenges to changing Workers' Compensation's attitudes. One obstacle is the clinically individualistic approach currently in use and not in agreement with the social epidemiological perspective. He calls attention to the need for more context-based research. This revolutionary attitude toward work will, he claims, not only improve worker health, but also social health and productivity, and will result in a more just society.

238. Hammarstrom, Olle, and Russel D. Lansbury. "The Art of Building a Car: The Swedish Experience Reexamined." *New Technology, Work and Employment* 6, no. 2 (1991): 85-90.

Keywords: manufacturing, automotive industry, comparative

The Swedish automobile industry has recently encountered significant difficulties. This article reviews a major study of the relationships between production, technology, and work organization in Volvo and Saab. It compares the Swedish approach to automobile production with those of the American and Japanese companies and speculates on whether the Swedish industry will survive in the coming decade.

239. Hammer, M. "Reengineering Work: Don't Automate, Obliterate." *Harvard Business Review*, July-August 1990: 104-12.

Keywords: computers, work design, case study

Hammer argues that American companies have not realized the real powers of computers because they still adhere to old notions of work and work organizations. The introduction of new information technologies requires that the old rules pertaining to job design be discarded and new ones engineered to make work and technology more compatible. The article includes brief case studies of Ford Motor Company and MBC.

240. Hamper, Ben. *Rivethead: Tales From the Assembly Line*. New York: Time Warner Company, 1991.

Keywords: blue-collar workers, United States, biography, automobile industry workers, General Motors Corporation, employees

As a former assembly-line worker, the author brings insight into the world of blue-collar work in the automobile industry. His life experiences are chronicled, from his drinking and drug-taking, to pulling double shifts, to General Motors' idea of quality control, just to name a few. This book deals with how workers cope within a world of crashing noise, suffocating boredom, and other tragic realities of assembly-line work.

241. Handy, Charles. *The Future of Work: A Guide to a Changing Society*. Oxford: Basil Blackwell, 1984.

Keywords: trade unions

This is a rather personal view of the changing world of work that grew out of the author's discussions with managers, union leaders, politicians and voluntary workers. It is not intended as a comprehensive review of the futurist literature, nor as a scholarly work for professional scientists—though much of its content is certainly relevant to specialists in the sociology of work. Rather, "it is an attempt to stimulate the thoughtful person at home or in the office."

The basic argument in the book "starts from the assumption that what we are experiencing is more than a cyclical adjustment—we are seeing the gradual tapering off of the employment society, a society in which jobs are the measure and means of most things." Given this disintegration of the traditional concept of employment and everything it entails, the author undertakes to question "the assumptions with which we have lived so comfortably for over three hundred years."

Topics explored are as follows: changing patterns of employment as related to new technology, structural options for new concepts in employment (shorter work week, work sharing, etc.), marginal work and the "underground" economy, education and the reorganization of work, individual and societal choices for new work lifestyles, etc. See especially chapter 4 "Reorganizing Work," chapter 5 "The New Agenda," and chapter 7 "Choices (for the future)."

242. Handy, Charles. *Beyond Certainty: The Changing Worlds of Organizations*. London: Hutchison, 1995.

Keywords: organizational change

This collection of loosely-structured essays reflects a rather broad range of interests on the part of the author. He discusses economic trends in market economies, work culture, organizational change in large organizations, the role of management, and general social trends and their impact on individuals. Chapter 2 examines the restructuring of corporate organizations and emerging employment patterns. Chapter 3, entitled "Balancing Corporate Power: a New Federalist Paper," considers the foundation of integrated organizations, global networks and leaner work structures. The author sees the concept of federalism as an appropriate one "since it offers a well-recognized way to deal with paradoxes of power and control: the need to make things big by keeping them small; to encourage autonomy but within bounds, etc." In Chapter 4, the author asks the question "What Is a Company For?" Issues of social responsibility, environmental stewardship and community involvement are discussed. Chapter 5 explores the subject of lifetime employment, offering a number of reasons for its being a disadvantageous proposition, both for employers and employees. Chapter 6 considers the post-employment period of life, retirement. The responsibilities of employment organizations in this regard are examined. Other topics discussed in this book are as follows: the place of integrity and ethics in organizations; the Japanese work ethic; "flat" organizations; flexible work schedules; and global market competition.

243. Handy, Charles. "Trust and the Virtual Organization." *Harvard Business Review*, May-June 1995.

Keywords: computers, virtual organizations

This article suggests that it may be easy to be seduced by the technological possibilities of the virtual organization, but "the managerial and personal implications may cause us to rethink what we mean by an organization." At its simplest level, the author notes, "the managerial dilemma comes down to the question, How do you manage people whom you do not see? The simple answer is, by trusting them, but the apparent simplicity disguises a turnaround in organizational thinking." The rules of trust are both obvious and well established, according to the author, but they do not sit easily with a managerial tradition that believes efficiency and control are closely linked and that you can't have one without a lot of the other. "Organizationally, we have to wonder whether a company is, in the future, going to be anything more than the box of contracts that some companies now seem to be." Handy asks whether a box of contracts is a sustainable basis for getting the work done in our society, or "is it not, in fact, a recipe for disintegration? For society as a whole, the challenge will be to make sure that virtuality brings benefits to all and not just to a favored few. Organizations and, in particular, business organizations, are the linchpins of society. That gives them responsibilities beyond themselves, responsibilities that virtuality throws into high relief." Much of this article discusses the particular implications for management of placeless organizations that exist as activities but not as buildings, of e-mail communication, of videoconferencing and of personal places that are not attached to a place. The personal consequences of not having a room of one's own, or at least a desk of one's own, are assessed in light of research that cites the importance of a sense of place, face-to-face contact, and even office politics and gossip.

See especially "The Managerial Dilemmas." In this section, the author notes that "for trust to work (in virtual work environments) large organizations need fairly constant, smaller groups." Also see the "Seven Cardinal Principles of Trust" that are outlined as well. Paradoxically, the author reports, "the more virtual the organization, the more its people need to meet in person."

244. Harpaz, Itzhak, and Raphael Snir. "Workaholism: Its Definition and Nature." *Human Relations* 56, no. 3 (March 2003): 291-319.

Keywords: working hours, demographics, employee attitude, correlation analysis, organizational behavior

The term "workaholism" is widely used, but there is little consensus about its meaning, beyond that of its core element: a substantial investment in work. Following Snir and Zohar, workaholism was first defined in the present study as the individual's steady and considerable allocation of time to work-related activities and thoughts, which does not derive from external necessities. Subsequently, it was measured as time invested in work, while controlling the financial needs for this investment. The relation between workaholism and possible attitudinal, demographic, and situational variables was examined through two representative samples of the Israeli labor force. The following predictor variables were significantly related to workaholism: work centrality; economic orientation; occupation types; employment sector; and gender. For those variables, gender was found to be the strongest predictor—that is, men, in comparison with women, have a higher likelihood of being workaholics. Moreover, married women worked fewer hours per week than unmarried women, while married men worked more hours per week than unmarried men.

245. Hartman, Heidi, ed. *Computer Chips and Paper Clips: Technology and Women's Employment.* Vol. 2, *Case Studies and Policy Perspectives*. Washington, DC: National Academy Press, 1987.

Keywords: computers, automation, women, policy, case study

This is an examination of the changes that have taken place in the participation of women in the labor market, with particular emphasis given to the role of new office technologies. Part 1 of the book provides an overview of these changes and offers policy prescriptions regarding research and development, improved training and education in computer use, enforcement of equal opportunity laws, etc. Part 2 consists of four case studies describing the impact of information technology in the insurance industry, among bookkeepers, among secretaries, and in computer-related occupations. Part 3 offers a historical perspective of "Technology and Trends in Women's Employment," with a focus on the restructuring of work (temporary, part-time, and at-home employment) and the impact of computerization in the workplace. Part 4 provides an analysis of "Policy Perspectives" and technological change. Attention is given to new office and business technologies, the role of governments and trade unions, and quality of employment issues.

246. Hartman, Heidi, Robert E. Kraut, and Louise A. Tilly, eds. *Computer Chips and Paper Clips: Technology and Women's Employment.* Vol. 1. Washington: National Academy Press, 1986.

Keywords: computers, automation, women, policy

This volume identifies and analyzes the effects of technological change on both the quantity and quality of women's paid employment. It focuses particularly on innovations in computerized information processing and telecommunications and their applications in offices in the past, present, and likely future. The interest of the Panel on Technology and Women's Employment is in determining whether women may be differently affected by these technological innovations relative to men, and, if so, how; to what extent women of different ages, educational backgrounds, and race and ethnic groups may be affected differently, and what factors may be shaping these effects. The authors focus on new technologies in clerical occupations such as secretaries, typists, file clerks, interviewers, telephone operators, dispatchers, mail carriers, insurance adjusters, bank tellers, etc.

This volume seeks to identify the positive and negative aspects of technological change in the office setting and considers how employers' decisions to adopt and implement computer technologies and workers' participation in these processes can affect outcomes. The book also recommends private and public policies that can alleviate negative effects, promote improvements in women's employment opportunities, and produce a more human work environment for all. Chapter 1 discusses the measurement and characteristics of technological change and explores in a schematic way the economic and social context of technological change and the employment effects that can result. Chapter 2 looks at selected examples of technological change in communications and information processing and considers especially its effects on women's employment levels, absolutely and relative to men, and on the content and quality of work. Chapter 3 analyzes the content and quality of work. Chapter 3 analyzes the current and future effects of technological change on the levels of employment and the structure of occupations and considers changes in both the supply and demand of workers. Chapter 4 analyzes the current and likely future effects of technological change on employment quality and examines how job content changes in terms of autonomy, responsibility and knowledge. Chapter 5 offers recommendations to facilitate the mutual adaptation of technology and employment.

247. Harvey, Carol D. H., ed. *Walking a Tightrope: Meeting the Challenges of Work and Family*. Hampshire, UK: Ashgate Publishing, 2000.

Keywords: work and family, family policy, unemployment and family, gender and work

It is becoming more and more common for family members, especially women, to walk a tightrope between the demands of work and family. The chapters of this book demonstrate how modern families both respond to workplace changes as well as provide cultural continuity. The chapters examine this dual role of family in countries such as Finland, Sweden, Denmark, Belgium, Spain, South Africa, Taiwan, China, and Canada. Examples of issues investigated include the following: the changing nature of gender relationships amongst Finnish fathers of young children; Sweden's unemployment and family life including household division of labor and well-being; the differences in work and family ethos between Denmark, Belgium, and Spain; white South African men in dual-earning households; the family status of Taiwanese and Chinese women and how their job influences their role in the family; and the effect of workplace location on how Canadian families use time in balancing their employment and household work. These examples illustrate both the power of the culture to perpetuate patriarchy as well as the influence of market forces, particularly labor force participation of women.

248. Haslegrave, Christine M., John R. Wilson, and E. Nigel Corlett, eds. *International Occupational Ergonomics Symposium*. Zadar, Croatia: Taylor and Francis, 1989.

Keywords: work design, ergonomics, stress, health, participation, preventive

Specialists in ergonomics and work design from twelve countries contribute to this collection of thirty-three papers that make a significant contribution to healthy work concepts. Even though the primary focus of the overall work is on the practical implementation of work design initiatives, including job redesign, the wider contextual issues of work environment, work load, stress at work, and overall organizational design are also discussed.

An overview article on ergonomics practice in industry is generally accessible and the case studies are illustrative of some of the do's and don'ts of successful design. A subsequent article critically assessing current methodologies for workplace analysis and evaluation is somewhat more technical and requires a grounding in ergonomic theory to be fully grasped. However, many other articles make a salutary contribution to the literature on healthy work: "An Integrated Approach to the Design of Work" examines strategies whereby various contextual features may be incorporated into design. A summary of work and health issues is provided in "Factors Affecting Health in the Workplace." "Job Evaluation Procedures to Identify Ergonomic Stress," "Stress and Health in Self-Paced Repetitive Work," "Participative Work Design: A Systematic Approach" and "New Technology and the Quality of Work" are other articles with a preventive orientation.

249. Hassard, John, and Ruth Holliday, eds. *Organization-Representation: Work and Organization in Popular Culture*. London: Sage Publications, 1998.

Keywords: working life in the popular media, organization, social relationships

The complex social relationship between organization and its representation are unraveled, offering new insights into the interaction between popular images and the power relations governing society, working life, and culture. Insights are offered into the relations between culture, power, and work. More importantly, it goes beyond such purely ontological questions, thus demonstrating a critical analysis of the relationship between popular culture and the nature of organizational life. It thereby enhances the reader's understanding of both.

250. Hathway, Gloria J., Nick H. Proctor, James P. Hughes, and Michael L. Fischman, eds. *Proctor and Hughes' Chemical Hazards of the Workplace*. 3rd ed. New York: Van Nostrand Reinhold, 1991.

Keywords: occupational health and safety

This standard reference book on hazardous workplace chemicals contains entries on 542 chemicals in alphabetical order. Each entry lists the chemical formula, synonyms, threshold limit value (TLV), physical form, uses, route of exposure, and toxicology. The toxicology information given includes signs and symptoms of overexposure, carcinogenicity, mutagenicity and fetotoxicity. As much as possible, dose-response relationships are shared with the reader. Clinical effects, hints for emergency clinical evaluation, recommendations for occupational safety and health standards, exposure prevention and treatment are also discussed. When information regarding human health effects is lacking, results of animals tests are presented.

Aside from this reference section, the book also contains four chapters that pertain to occupational health practice. Chapter 1 deals with how exposure limits are set. How to handle medical situations in the workplace is the topic of chapter 2. When to suspect occupational disease, how to present complaints, and some physical clues to occupational poisoning are deliberated. Chapter 3 is devoted to the diagnosis of occupational disease. Chapter 4 "Industrial Hygiene Aspects of Occupational Chemical Exposure" concludes this section.

The appendices provide coverage of the following three topics: National Institute of Occupational Safety and Health (NIOSH) recommendations for occupational safety standards, neurotoxic chemical agents, and basic concepts of risk assessment.

251. Hattery, Angela. *Women, Work, and Family: Balancing and Weaving*. Understanding Families, edited by N. Bert and David M. Klein Adams. Thousand Oaks, CA: Sage Publications, 2001.

Keywords: working mothers, women's labor force, history

Women, Work, and Family examines the juggling act performed by working mothers who balance their obligations to both work and family. The author describes women's conflicts of interest as well as the decision-making process through which they accomplish this balancing. By interviewing thirty married women, all with children under the age of two, the author uncovers a remarkable range of ways in which these women weave together the complex strands of their lives. The data is examined from a number of theoretical standpoints, including structural theory, motherhood theory, and feminist theory; however, the key variable that runs through all the data is economic need, which has an obvious effect on work patterns.

252. Haworth, John T. *Work, Leisure and Well-Being*. London: Routledge, 1997.

Keywords: mental health, unemployment, leisure, sociology

Many different psychological and sociological theories on the relationship between work and leisure have been formulated. This book reviews the various models proposed to date and continues the scholarly debate. The author is also interested in how well-being is determined by various aspects of work and leisure. After providing an overview in the introductory chapter, chapter 2 argues that social institutions can both support and restrict independence and well-being. The experience of the unemployed is the subject of the third chapter. The next two chapters deal with principal environmental influences on mental health. The importance of enjoyment to well-being is examined in chapter 6, which cites various studies, including some that suggest that the majority of enjoyable experiences come from work rather than leisure. The implications of the "practice theory" on work and the quality of life are the subject of chapter 7. The remainder of the book consists of five guest chapters by leading scholars who analyze the characteristics, costs and rewards of "serious leisure," the importance of leisure for health, leisure and work for young people, retirement and future trends and scenarios.

253. Heap, Nick, Ray Thomas, Geoff Einon, Robin Mason, and Hughie Mackay, eds. *Information Technology and Society: A Reader*. London: Sage Publications, 1995.

Keywords: information technology, forecasting, labor process

This volume (suitable for use as a textbook) examines many of the social, political, and technological impacts of information technology. "It explores both the social and technological issues associated with IT developments, and asks, How are these developments controlled? By whom? Are they inevitable? Are IT innovations driven by technology or by social factors? Who has access to the technology? Who benefits?"

The collection is divided into five subject areas. In part 1 "Differing Perspectives," the authors adopt a critical attitude to developments in IT. They discuss the "social influences that determine both the design and implementation of IT innovations" and examine the ways in which this social shaping of technology occurs.

Part 2 "IT in the Workplace" presents "contemporary ideas in industrial sociology which have developed from studies of the uses of IT in manufacturing." These ideas challenge the Marxist and Taylorist theses of the nature of the labor process that see the role of automation as being to increase control over labor and, through deskilling, to reduce labor costs. Here a broader and more pragmatic approach is taken to explanations of the role and effect of IT at work.

The readings in part 3 "IT and Learning" address the question of why IT is used in education and training. Themes discussed in this section include the following: resource-based learning; collaboration and interactivity; the effectiveness of IT; access for the disabled and remote learners; and humanistic vs. mechanistic learning approaches.

Part 4 "IT and the Home" introduces a range of issues and debates about IT in the home that have been developed in cultural and media studies. Two of the readings focus on specific technologies: the home computer and the telephone.

The final part "IT Futures" offers a disparate collection of essays that touch on a number of issues relating to future developments of IT. Teleworking and virtual reality are two of the topics discussed.

254. Heller, Frank. "Sociotechnology and the Environment." *Human Relations* 50, no. 5 (May 1997).

Keywords: sociotechnical systems, environment, pollution

This paper makes a theoretical case for the extension of the sociotechnical model as a heuristic device to include those aspects of the environment that are directly or indirectly affected by technology. The author refers to this as the sociotechnical model. It is noted that "the founders of the sociotechnical model perceived its relevance at the macro level of the community, at the meso level of whole organizations, as well as at the micro level of the primary work systems, but it is at the primary work system that most applications have been carried out." Nevertheless, "an efficient micro level sociotechnical solution may still cause the technology to have a harmful impact on the environment." The author suggests that the development of a systemic heuristic device (called the socio-ecotechnical model) allows for both intra- and extraorganizational factors to be jointly assessed and optimized. The paper develops the argument in five stages, starting with a brief historic review of the sociotechnical concept. The first stage also shows that an extension of sociotechnology was given serious consideration by the founders of the model. Second, "the extension of the model derives from two of the roots that characterized the original concept, namely contingency rather than generalistic theory and decentralized democratic decision making rather than the division of labor and hierarchy." Third, it is argued that "as a consequence of the dominant emphasis of the traditional model on the micro level of organizational design, its relevance for modern open system organization theory is diminishing. Fourth, by underemploying or omitting meso and macro level applications, the sociotechnical model has not engaged itself with debates initiated by economists although they can be shown to be relevant."

In the final stage of the argument, two examples of possible applications are given, one concerning the intracompany and external measures to reduce pollution, the other relating to a research project on raising energy consciousness in secondary schools.

255. Heller, Frank, Eugen Pusic, George Strauss, and Bernhard Wilpert. *Organizational Participation: Myth and Reality*. New York: Oxford University Press, 1998.

Keywords: organizational behavior, organizational sociology, industrial relations

The authors examine the changing forms of—and changing debates around—organizational participation. They review an extensive literature of experiments and practical experiences through a critical evaluation of the available data to reach several conclusions about the importance and utility of organizational participation for organizations in the present and in the future.

256. Heller, Frank A. "The Technological Imperative and the Quality of Employment." *New Technology, Work and Employment* 2, no. 1 (1987): 19-26.

Keywords: sociotechnical systems, work design

This article challenges the widespread concept of a technological imperative that is alleged to lead to greater economic efficiency. The sociotechnical model, supported by evidence from past research and recent cases, undermines the validity of the imperative and presents an alternative based on choices.

257. Herbst, P. G. *Sociotechnical Design: Strategies in Multidisciplinary Research*. London: Tavistock Publications, 1974.

Keywords: sociotechnical systems, democracy, organizational design, organizational change, sociology

This classic volume represents one of the most outstanding contributions to the field of sociotechnical design. Written by a long-time associate of the Tavistock Institute of Human Relations, the author conveys a thorough understanding of sociotechnical research and a closely-related program of study known as the Industrial Democracy Project.

The introduction to the book provides a succinct history of research in sociotechnical design that is invaluable for those wishing to appreciate the evolutionary advances in the field, as they are related to technological innovation and change in the workplace.

The author notes that an early discovery made by the sociotechnical model was that "the technological system determines the characteristics of the social system (through the allocation of work roles and the technologically given dependence relations between tasks). Performance is a function of the joint operation of the social and technical systems." The author continues by pointing out that a fundamental principle began to emerge from early studies—a principle that remains critical to all contemporary strategies and progress related to the design of healthy work environments—"if the technological system is optimized at the expense of the social system, the results achieved will be sub-optimal." From this basic truth came the realization that a truly effective and humane work organization would necessitate "the joint optimization of the technical and the social systems."

The author also discusses the implications of the sociotechnical approach for other disciplinary areas such as architectural planning and town planning, etc.

Much of the material in this text illustrates the many ways in which "industrial organizations . . . induce or require changes in the environment of which they form a part," changes that, if not accompanied by adequate knowledge of societal consequences, may well produce "a weakening of the social structure on which industrial development depends."

A profound understanding of "the social ecology of industry" is clearly evident throughout the book. As noted by the author, "changes introduced within any one organizational sector or a lack of adjustive change can have an almost immediate influence, directly or indirectly, on other sections of the ecology."

See also chapter 2 "Approaches to Sociotechnical Design" and chapter 3, which offers an excellent case study illustrating the application of sociotechnical principles to ship organization.

258. Herington, Thomas N., and Linda H. Morse, eds. *Occupational Injuries: Evaluation, Management, and Prevention*. St. Louis: Mosby-Year Book, 1995.

Keywords: occupational health and safety

This is a comprehensive but conventional approach to work-related injuries and illnesses. It is a practical, clinically-oriented guide for treating workplace injuries. The preface notes that what the front-line caregivers need to know is how to perform a thoughtful examination, which variables to consider, how to treat the injury, when to refer the patient to another health care worker and how to consider the context of the patient's workplace.

Four sections comprise this book. The introductory section provides an overview treatment of the following topics: epidemiology of work injury, worker's compensation, occupational health clinics, administrative aspects, information management (computers), legal issues and ethical issues. Section 2 "Occupational Injuries" contains chapters on specific injuries and disorders of the hand, wrist, elbow, shoulder, neck, low back, knee, foot, ankle, brain, eye, skin, chest and abdominal area. Section 3 "Special Issues" addresses patient management, pain management, psychiatric issues (stress, somatization, violence, suicide) and disorders related to the building, temperature, vibration, radiation and other aspects of the work environment. Finally, Section 4 explores methods for prevention and control of injuries. But the approach presented here is not truly preventive—it simply stresses the importance of personal protective equipment, ergonomics and rehabilitation.

259. Herzberg, Frederick. "The Wise Old Turk." *Harvard Business Review*, September-October 1974: 70-80.

Keywords: QWL, work design, participation, knowledge embedded in experience, job enrichment

Whenever a manager recognizes the need for a job enrichment or motivation in his own organization, he is immediately faced with a problem unrelated to implementing the program in his company. He has to decide which of the many available approaches to enrichment he should adopt; the differences between them are not always clear. In this article an expert in the field of motivation discusses four different approaches to job enrichment, outlines their major features and purposes, and then puts them into perspective regarding organizational development in general. He concludes that orthodox job enrichment, that is based on the notion that individual growth is the key to organizational health, is the approach that most often results in happier employees and higher productivity. He also suggests that one of the primary causes of current worker dissatisfaction is that, in the name of efficiency, most jobs have been robbed of meaning. The author feels that some of the old richness could be restored to jobs if managers would check with the "wise old Turks" in their companies to find out what that richness encompassed.

260. Herzberg, Frederick. *The Managerial Choice: To Be Efficient and to Be Human*. 2nd ed. Salt Lake City: Olympus Publishing Company, 1982.

Keywords: case study, job enrichment

The book discusses the various approaches to work improvement along with their unique advantages and disadvantages. Its strength lies in its practical application of theories on the relationship between workers and their work environment, with special emphasis given to the role of management. See especially chapter 3 of the text. It provides a comprehensive treatment of job enrichment programs and their place in the humanization of work. The author calls for a reversal of traditional industrial engineering practice (that tends to result in high worker direction and poor motivation) by suggesting that we "enrich jobs rather than denude them."

Research topics examined include the following: alienated workers and company costs; coping with job boredom; orthodox job enrichment; ingredients of a good job; sociotechnical systems; participative management; industrial democracy; employee motivation; steps to job enrichment with case study results of various programs; motivating job enrichment efforts; and barriers to job enrichment programs. There is considerable case study material provided here, with details on the results of individual programs. Although somewhat dated, the empirical findings are still of use in developing healthy work strategies.

261. Herzenberg, Stephen A., John A. Alic, and Howard Wial. *New Rules for a New Economy: Employment and Opportunity in Postindustrial America*. Ithaca, NY: Cornell University Press, 1998.

Keywords: employment forecasting, labor market, service industries workers, supply and demand, forecasting, manufacturing industries, employees

During the 1980s there was a widely shared assumption that good jobs, at least for those without higher levels of education, were to be found only in auto plants and steel mills. Many people were not even willing to consider seriously whether the service sector could even generate good jobs and improve the living standards for the majority of Americans. Nowadays, more people tend to give the services that employ the vast majority of American workers more serious consideration as they are viewed with a sense of possibility and promise as well as continuing trepidation. This book aims to encourage that sense of possibility and promise by seeking to understand the dynamics of today's service industries and jobs and use that understanding to map out a set of public policies that will benefit workers as well as businesses and consumers.

262. Heymann, Jody. *The Widening Gap: Why America's Working Families Are in Jeopardy and What Can Be Done about It*. New York: Basic Books, 2000.

Keywords: work and family, impacts on children, economic inequalities, gender inequalities

In today's workforce employees have learned to keep quiet about their family needs. It is more accepted to leave the office early for a meeting or a medical appointment than it is to tend to a family matter. In many cases, this problem is compounded by outdated working conditions and inadequate social support. Many parents lack paid leave, and those who receive no paid sick or vacation leave often have to let their sick children stay at home alone or send them to school sick. Children's education also suffers as a result of a lack of parental involvement. Often parents do not have time to help children with homework or to attend parent-teacher interviews. These problems are even more evident in poor families where children with special needs do not receive the required community based services and where public policy has failed to address the issues in this area. Low income families suffer more than others because income limitations further restrict the options available to their children. In many cases the only option is for grandparents to help in the care of the children. There has been a failure to adapt workplaces and social institutions to the needs of working families, and this has led to an ever increasing degree of inequality in the United States.

263. Himmelweit, Susan, ed. *Inside the Household: From Labor to Care*. Capital and Class Series. New York: St. Martin's Press, 2000.

Keywords: family, family services, households, economic aspects, home economics, intergenerational relations, feminist theory

Social scientists are beginning to analyze and talk about the household as a key economic and social institution. As households change, the expectations of what men and women do within the households change, and as a result gender employment expectations change, all of which have profound effects on the structure of modern economies. The first article sets up the rest by introducing the question of the family wage, which entails the issue about the household and its division of labor. The next article attempts to fit the analysis of domestic labor into existing Marxist categories designed for the analysis of paid commodity-producing labor. The article recognizes that the centrality of childcare, both as the main contribution that domestic labor makes to the continuation of capitalism and as the main barrier to women's participation in paid work. The following article examines the result of a study done in England on how domestic tasks were allocated in households where the man was unemployed and the women were employed. The fourth article was written in response to the previous one, where again high male unemployment was combined with a significant growth in female part-time employment. However, by looking at a wider range of households and using a broader survey, this article was able to account for and study a wider variety of people. The following three articles provide critiques of the original domestic labor debate and examine areas they see as important absences in the other writings. The two concluding chapters raise a different issue altogether: how women's experiences, attitudes and behaviors differ and the effects these differences have.

264. Hinshaw, John, and Paul Le Blanc, eds. *United States Labor in the Twentieth Century: Studies in Working-Class Struggles and Insurgency*. Revolutionary Studies. Amherst, NY: Humanity Books, 2000.

Keywords: working class, United States, history, twentieth century, labor movement, industrial relations, industrial mobilization

The history of workers is an important but poorly understood aspect of American life. This book offers an overview of the hidden history of American workers by examining questions that deal with ethnic, racial, and gender diversity, the history of labor radicalism, the effects of affluence and consumerism on workers, and where workers are headed in today's economy. The authors argue that the weaknesses of the current labor movement will not result in the end of class conflict but the development by workers of new strategies to deal with the changing work environment.

265. Hirschhorn, Larry. *Beyond Mechanization: Work and Technology in a Postindustrial Age*. Cambridge, MA: MIT Press, 1984.

Keywords: computers, work design, division of labor

The image of the computer as the ideal machine is refuted in this classic book about the transformation from the mechanized to the cybernetic manufacturing system. In order to understand the new technology and its potentials and limits, Hirschhorn examines three areas: (1) the technical foundation of mechanical machines, (2) the differences and tensions between cybernetic machine systems and older job design and management strategies, and (3) experiments with workplace designs that are suited to cybernetic systems. From the examination, he concludes that there are critical discontinuities in machine design, the relationship between workers and machines, and the relationship between people at work. Each section thus focuses on one of these three discontinuities to describe the history and a potential system of technology and work.

266. Hirschhorn, Larry. *The Workplace Within: Psychodynamics of Organizational Life*. MIT Press Series on Organization Studies. Cambridge, MA: MIT Press, 1988.

Keywords: machinery, work design, psychology, sociology

Hirschhorn (a seminal figure in behavioral science and industrial sociology management research) presents a "comprehensive psychodynamic" approach to work life with direct, profound implications for the development of preventive strategies and healthier workplaces. The author explores the "normal psychological injuries of work," the organizational intricacies of bureaucratic/corporate culture, programs for effective management training, the effects of the postindustrial milieu on work and the psychosocial effects of modern technology on workers.

Chapter 1 reveals how "organizations create 'normal' psychological injuries as people face the anxiety of taking their work roles." Chapter 2 examines "the links connecting anxiety, organizational boundaries, and feelings of aggression." Chapter 3 considers "the details of these connections by assessing how people take and violate roles."

These three introductory chapters provide a foundation for the author's psychodynamic conception of work. After that he moves away from a focus on individual psychology to an examination of group behavior in various organizational settings. The relationships between workers and between workers and managers are then considered with emphasis given to various strategies employed and whether they promote or reduce workers' anxieties.

Much of the remainder of the book makes use of case studies to further assess the "management" of workplace anxieties and the social defense mechanisms used to cope with stressors.

In the final section of the book Hirschhorn links his psychodynamic approach to broad social/cultural trends. He argues that "people may find it difficult to value the work they do and understand its purpose if the society as a whole has no coherent sense of what it values." He further argues that if companies "do not train workers to manage new sociotechnical systems . . . the new technologies and the more integrated sociotechnical domain will create more anxiety."

267. Hirschhorn, L., and T. Gilmore. "The New Boundaries of the 'Boundaryless' Organization." *Harvard Business Review*, May-June 1992: 104-15.

Keywords: organizational design, work design, knowledge embedded in experience, management

In an economy founded on innovation and change, one of the premier challenges of management is to design more flexible organizations. One method of meeting this challenge has been the concept of the "boundaryless" corporation, where traditional boundaries are removed and new boundaries emerge that are psychological (and hence invisible) in nature. How can these new boundaries be used productively? Many ways are discussed and implicit notions of mental-maps and knowledge embedded in experience (KEE) emerge.

268. Hlatky, A., Lai Choi Lam et al. "Job Strain and the Prevalance and Outcome of Coronary Artery Disease." *Circulation* 92, no. 3 (1 August 1995).

Keywords: stress, disease

In responding to the hypothesis that high job demands and low job decision latitude can lead to coronary disease, the researchers in this study aim "to test whether job strain is correlated with the pressure of coronary disease at angiography or with long-term outcome in patients with angiographic coronary disease."

In the study, "employed patients under the age of 65 years undergoing diagnostic coronary angiography completed a self-administered questionnaire about their job duties and work environment. Job strain was measured by the method of Karasek. Statistical analyses were performed using logistical regression."

The authors conclude, "This study provides no support for the hypothesis that job strain, as measured by the method of Karasek, leads either to the development of coronary atherosclerosis or to the precipitation of coronary events in individuals with angiographically documented coronary artery disease."

The authors indicate that further research is required in order to determine whether other measures of stress (especially in the workplace) can better predict the development of cardiac disease.

269. Hochner, Arthur, Cherlyn S. Granrose, Judith Goode, Elaine Simon, and Eileen Appelbaum. *Job-Saving Strategies: Worker Buyouts and QWL*. Philadelphia: W. E. Upjohn Institute for Employment Research, 1988.

Keywords: QWL, participation

The closing of A&P supermarkets in Philadelphia created the perfect opportunity to compare worker buyouts and quality of work life (QWL) programs. Some stores reopened as Super Fresh stores with QWL while other stores were bought out by workers and renamed O&O. Using interviews with employees and employers, the authors address questions regarding the effectiveness of worker buyouts and how they compare to other job saving methods. Do they lead to meaningful power distributions, increased worker control and more effective organizations? The authors summarize the structure of the book as follows:

"First, here in chapter 1, we place worker buyouts in the context of employee ownership and worker participation, theoretically, historically, and practically. In Chapter 2, we present a theoretical framework of the organizational processes involved in employee-owned firms and the expected outcomes for organizations and individual workers. The framework will attempt to explain in theory how worker buyouts function and how they affect the organizations' operations and the individuals in them. Chapter 3 presents the research design and methods of data collection used, namely semistructured interviews and systematic questionnaire surveys. In chapter 4, the formal structures of the O&O and Super Fresh stores are described. Chapter 5 reports data primarily from interviews concerning the personal experiences of the workers and the informal social structures of the stores. Chapters 6 and 7 present quantitative tests of hypotheses derived from theoretical framework. Worker-level perceptions, attitudes, and economic outcomes are included in chapter 6. Store-level functioning and outcomes are examined in chapter 7. The final chapter, 8, draws conclusions and translates them into policy-relevant recommendations for future research and practice."

270. Hochschild, Arlie Russell. *The Time Bind: When Work Becomes Home and Home Becomes Work.* New York: Henry Holt and Company, 1997.

Keywords: dual-career families, work and family, sex role, working mothers

In this book the author interviewed everyone at a Fortune 500 company, from top executives to factory hands. It was discovered that none of the working parents were taking the company up on chances for flextime, paternity leave, or other "family-friendly policies." Instead, parents were fleeing homes that had been invaded by the pressures from work, while the workplace seemed transformed into a quasi-surrogate home. The author portrays spouses as efficiency experts, children as emotional bill collectors, and parents who mentor mainly their workmates. This book reveals that our current way of life isn't working in an age where time is becoming increasingly scarce.

271. Hodson, Randy. *Dignity at Work.* New York: Cambridge University Press, 2001.

Keywords: work and dignity

The ability to establish a sense of self-worth and self-respect and to enjoy the respect of others is necessary for a fully realized life. Work plays a large part in this, yet the workplace often poses challenging obstacles because of mismanagement or managerial abuse. It is equally important for organizations to insure the dignity of employees as they attempt to make effective use of their human capital. In this book, the author applies ethnographic and statistical approaches to this topic, and thus obtains a clear idea of the causes, consequences, and patterns of workers' efforts to maintain dignity. He also uses his findings and analysis to reevaluate contemporary workplace theories, including those based on the traditions of Weber, Marx, Foucault, Durkheim, and feminist theories of the workplace.

272. Hoerr, John, and Michael A. Pollock. "Management Discovers the Human Side of Automation." *Business Week*, 29 September 1986: 70-5.

Keywords: sociotechnical systems, work design, technology, productivity, teams

The reorganization of work for the well-being of employees results in productivity gains for the company. This is the discovery reported upon in this article. After noticing that large investments in technology did not seem to be paying off, some American corporations began shifting their focus away from purely technical solutions. Companies such as Shenandoah Life Insurance Co. have begun to integrate workers and technology in sociotechnical systems. The authors predict that this trend will revolutionize workplaces. They also conclude that these changes are not occurring quickly enough. New attitudes toward labor-management relations are reviewed as well. They criticize the old practice of scientific management and describe the new approach that involves teamwork, the recombination of the brain and the hand, flatter organizations, profit-sharing and worker responsibility. The history of sociotechnical systems is traced from the Tavistock Institute in the 1940s to Volvo plants in Sweden in the 1970s. Team work and semi-autonomous work groups receive considerable attention.

273. Hoffman, Lois W., and Lise M. Youngblade. *Mothers at Work: Effects on Children's Well-Being*. Cambridge: Cambridge University Press, 1999.

Keywords: working mothers, husband-wife relationships, maternal employment, father's role

The effects of the mother's employment on family life and children's well-being is the main topic examined in this book. It begins with a review of previous research on this topic and then reports the results of a study designed to answer the key questions that had emerged. The focus of the study is based on 369 families with an elementary school child, living in an industrialized city in the Midwest. The one or two parent families cover all bases in terms of race and economic circumstances. The analysis reveals how the mother's employment status affects the father's role, the mother's sense of well-being, and child-rearing patterns and how these, in turn, affect the child.

274. Hood, Jane C. *Men, Work, and Family*. Newbury Park: Sage Publications, 1993.

Keywords: gender relations, women, men, family, fathers

With the growing number of career women, traditional gender roles are being transformed. Whereas women were once primarily nurturers, they are now often juggling work and family responsibilities; and where men were once primarily providers, they are now accepting more responsibilities in the home. This book examines the diversity and complexity of men's work and the roles they are holding within family life. Part 1 "Fathering and Providing" explores stereotypes of family men in general, the work demands and family roles of Japanese fathers, and the work and family patterns of elderly Mexican American men. In the second part of the book, there are six studies on role allocation and role change with a look into the priority of work versus family orientations of contemporary adolescent boys and girls; the resistance to change from college men toward family and work in the 1980s; differences in household labor time for White, Black, and Hispanic men; the reluctant compliance within work-family roles allocations in dual-earner Chicano families; the balancing of work and single fatherhood; and the meanings of housework for single fathers and mothers. Part 3 of this book is particularly relevant to healthy work as it examines links among policy, workplace organization, and family roles. It begins with a chapter that asks the question: "Are 'family-supported' employer policies relevant to men?" In this chapter, the author believes that there is a rise in work/family stress and more time spent by men on family work than is thought to be true. The next chapter examines the changing gender roles in Sweden resulting in nurturing fathers and working mothers; although it further discusses the reasons behind the reluctance by working family men to make use of the paid parental leave benefits. In the last chapter, two models of linking work and family are presented. It was found that at first women had a harder time juggling work and family, but that later it was the men that had more difficulty.

275. Horner, David, and Peter Day. "Labor and the Information Society: Trades Union Policies for Teleworking." *Journal of Information Science* 21, no. 5 (1995): 333-41.

Keywords: teleworking, telecommuting, technology, unions

This paper examines the implications of teleworking for trades unions and offers a historical perspective by comparing current developments in teleworking with the "micro-electronics revolution" debate of the late 1970s and early 1980s. The author suggests that the interest today in teleworking is seen as "the focal point of a wider debate relating to the diffusion of flexible work patterns facilitated by the networking of information communication technology and the development of the Information Society." The evolution of telework as a means of organizing work is mapped out and the trade union response outlined. Arguments pertaining to new technology are assessed as well. The paper concludes "by promoting a legislative framework to ensure best employment practices, and by urging trades unions to develop policies that meet both the challenges and opportunities of the Information Society." The authors note that for trades unions, the widespread diffusion of teleworking has implications both for the employment status of their members and for the very nature of trades union organization itself. "The flexibility for workers offered by telework may be a Trojan horse for further casualization of work and the undermining of the power of trades unions. Flexibility for the employer and flexibility for the teleworker may have quite different meanings." For example, the authors quote several reports that focus on the use of teleworking schemes as integral parts of managerial strategies aimed at cost reduction and the maintenance of competitive advantage. However, according to one trade union spokesperson, "computer home-work . . . particularly for unskilled female labor, represents a retrogression to the conditions of a nineteenth-century cottage industry, undermining pay levels, job security, quality of work, child care services, and occupational health and safety standards."

276. House, James S. *Occupational Stress and the Mental and Physical Health of Factory Workers*. Ann Arbor: Institute for Social Research, University of Michigan, 1980.

Keywords: stress, factory work, mental health

This comprehensive work focuses on the psychosocial effects of job stress (both objective and perceived characteristics) among factory workers in a large American industrial plant. Most of the data is collected from an extensive self-administered questionnaire that taps into a variety of stress-related measures including job satisfaction, occupational self-esteem, social support mechanisms, physical and emotional health indicators, etc. Both qualitative and quantitative methods are used to assess research results.

Research findings suggest a broad range of perceived occupational stressors ("e.g., excessive workload, role conflict, responsibility, lack of intrinsic rewards") associated with "reported symptoms and medical signs of ill health."

Social support was found to be a significant mediating factor: "Among workers with high levels of support, stress had little impact" on health outcomes, while "among those with low support, stress had substantial adverse effects on health."

Part 3 of the text "The Impact of Job Stress on Mental and Physical Health" is especially useful in terms of highlighting the particular job characteristics that correlate with significant levels of stress-related dysfunction—socially, psychologically, and physically. The implication in this study for workplace redesign and stress-prevention are alluded to but not dealt with explicitly.

277. Howard, Ann, ed. *The Changing Nature of Work.* San Francisco: Jossey-Bass Publishers, 1995.

Keywords: industrial relations, forecasting, psychology, sociology

Both work and workers are undergoing a fundamental change, raising the question of whether these two sets of changes will result in a major mismatch. The book is written mainly from an industrial/organizational psychology perspective. It anticipates change as well as analyzes how workers must change to meet future challenges.

Part 1 is concerned with the connections between the workplace and its social-political-economic milieu. Part 2 explores the factors driving change, with a particular focus on the factors related to manufacturing and office work. Chapter 3 consists of two relevant articles. The first is Jan Van der Spiegel's history of the microelectronics revolution. He foresees more humane computing in the future. In the second article, Don Davis observes that human capacities are being stretches as the boundaries around work are now less defined. Just-in-time (JIT) inventory control, total quality management (TQM) and advanced manufacturing technology are the three technology-related initiatives studied by Toby Wall and Paul Jackson in chapter 4. They stress that psychological factors need to be considered when implementing these strategies. Chapter 5, another useful chapter, examines what is known about technology's impact on office work, the possible impacts of new computer-supported cooperative work systems and augmented realities and implications for human resources management. In part 3, the focus is on workers, particularly American workers. How do they measure up against what is needed in the future? The process of work is scrutinized in part 4. Of particular interest is Sue Mohrman and Susan Cohen's chapter 10. They reflect upon how people will relate to and depend on each other in lateral organizations of the future. The fifth and final section summarizes the conclusions and themes regarding working in a post-industrial society.

278. Howard, Robert. *Brave New Workplace.* New York: Viking Books, 1985.

Keywords: QWL, technology, organizational change, corporate culture

This book critically examines the wholesale transformation of working life that is occurring in the advanced industrial societies. The author questions the utopian claims made by harbingers of "the brave new workplace"—those who envision the emerging (corporate) work environment as one that promises a "caring community," a " realm of self-fulfillment and meaningful work," and "social renewal with economic prosperity."

"Part one examines the managerial assumptions and values motivating the use of new computer technology . . . the contradictions for both workers and the corporation itself when managers try to put those assumptions into practice; and the psychological costs of those contradictions for the workers who experience them." (See especially chapter 2, "Contradictions of Control"; and chapter 3, "Personal Costs.")

In part 2, the author "shows how recent attempts by the corporation to 'humanize' technology and work are fundamentally flawed and how the ideas behind the new management styles . . . far from encouraging self-development, can engender a new kind of dependence on corporate power." (See especially chapter 4, "The Human Connection" and the case study material on Silicon Valley regarding implications for occupational health.)

Part 3 of the volume considers "the deterioration of other institutions, that, historically, have mitigated the worst effects of the corporate control of work." Recent changes in the trade union movement are explored here.

Throughout the text, the author reveals a concern for developing new strategies and institutions dedicated to the social control of technology and work.

279. Hughes, Gordon, and Ross Fergusson, eds. *Ordering Lives: Family, Work and Welfare*. An Introduction to the Social Sciences: Understanding Social Change. New York: Routledge, 2000.

Keywords: family, tradition to diversity, certainty to flexibility, welfare, security to responsibility

Family, work, and welfare are three familiar and influential social institutions, and this text looks at their role in maintaining social order and promoting social change in the United Kingdom from the 1950s to the beginning of the twenty-first century. It shows how everyday life within these social institutions is constantly affected by processes of power and resistance and charts the ways in which wider social changes have influenced these processes.

280. Hughes, John, Dave Randall, and Dan Shapiro. "CSCW: Discipline or Paradigm? A Sociological Perspective." 309-23 in *Second European Conference on Computer-Supported Cooperative Work*, edited by L. Bannon, M. Robinson, and K. Schmidt. Amsterdam: Kluwer Academic Publishers, 1991.

Keywords: work design, computers

The authors argue that there is still much confusion about what is meant by cooperative work, and therefore what is meant by CSCW (Computer-Supported Cooperative Work). It does not arise simply where more than one person is involved, and other attempts to delimit the field do not succeed. Since all work is socially organized, it would seem that all work potentially falls within the CSCW domain. If so, then (1) it would not be confined to a particular class of system ("groupware"), (2) it would not be a small specialism but would extend virtually throughout system design, and (3) its interdisciplinary character would affect large areas of its contributing disciplines. The authors defend these consequences, and argue that CSCW is therefore more akin to a paradigm shift for its contributing disciplines than a particular subdiscipline in itself. They also consider not what CSCW is but how it has arisen in terms of a political economy—the interests of researchers, funding institutions and clients—and a set of ideologies. This sets out a position for contributing disciplines but leaves open the detailed content of interdisciplinary relations.

281. Hughes, Marija Matich. *Computer Health Hazards*. Vol. 2. Washington, DC: Hughes Press, 1993.

Keywords: computers, health, video display terminal, radiation, repetitive strain injury, monitoring

This volume is a comprehensive study on computer health hazards, mostly in the form of annotated bibliographic entries classified by subject and identified by author, title, publisher, and date and place of publication. The publication is intended for lawyers, physicians, librarians, health researchers, employers, legislators, labor unions, and other concerned citizens. It is designed to assemble the current knowledge about computers as they affect health. This includes: "making the general public aware of the existing scientific literature on the problem, making that literature easily accessible to facilitate legal research and to be useful to attorneys and legislators involved in legislation and litigation on computer hazards. It also informs physicians who are dealing with little understood illnesses resulting from exposure to electromagnetic radiation, and people who are documenting their worker's compensation claims and product liability cases." Entries are divided into eight chapters alphabetically; all of the information on computer issues is in books, articles, pamphlets and government documents from the United States, Canada, Great Britain, Sweden, Japan, Italy and five other European countries. The first chapter deals with radiation, as well as with computer radiation emissions. The second chapter deals with electromagnetic radiation (EMR) effects on health. (This section covers male breast cancer, cancer in police officers, brain cancer in computer operators, cardiovascular problems, and pregnant women using VDTs.) Chapter 3 deals with EMR litigation concerns, and chapter 4 discusses legislative and regulatory issues. Electronic monitoring of employees is considered in chapter 5, and noise concerns are raised in chapter 6. Chapter 7 discusses prevention, and chapter 8 looks at general safety concerns relating to VDTs.

282. Hunnicutt, Benjamin. *Work Without End: Abandoning Shorter Hours for the Right to Work.* Philadelphia: Temple University Press, 1988.

Keywords: economics, work, leisure

From the early to middle decades of the nineteenth century to the Great Depression, the American work week became shorter and shorter. This struggle for shorter hours was a major movement involving labor unions, governments, and philosophers. However, since the conclusion of the Depression, the work week has remained stable at approximately forty hours and the shorter work week is no longer a political or labor issue. Very little research has been done regarding why such a broad-scale and enduring trend suddenly stopped. Hunnicutt seeks to remedy this situation by providing a first attempt at answering this question. He uses historical narrative to describe and analyze the factors that accounted for the success of the shorter-hour movement and those forces that extinguished it. Hunnicutt considers both the historical and economic "answers" to the question. Important in the discussion, of course, is the issue of the tradeoff between leisure and work and how people decide between them. Other factors that led to the abandonment of the trend are identified as a reduction in fatiguing work, the availability of consumer credit, easier work, employment stability, the rising price of recreation, and advertising and better marketing.

283. Huws, Ursula. *The New Homework: New Technology and the Changing Location of White-Collar Work.* London: Low Pay Unit—Public #28, 1984.

Keywords: teleworking, computers, skill

This brief volume looks at the experience of teleworking in four countries and offers the results of a survey on homework. The technological developments that have made the phenomenon possible are reviewed (i.e., innovations in computer and telecommunications equipment), and the factors that have limited its spread are considered as well. In the sample population surveyed here, "average pay levels were found to be significantly lower than going rates for similar work on-site, and some homeworkers also lacked a number of benefits available to comparable on-site workers. . . . A majority of the homeworkers felt that they had no promotion prospects." The author also reports that "isolation was found to be a major problem in most cases, in many being cited as the main reason for preferring on-site work should circumstances permit it." Despite the problems associated with teleworking, it was felt by many of the sample to have considerable advantages, particularly flexibility and the opportunity it provided to combine work with childcare. For employers, the main advantages of using home-based workers were increased productivity, lower overheads, and flexibility. Disadvantages included problems of remote management and monitoring—although developments in the technology were rapidly eliminating the latter difficulty for many types of work. The report concludes with a list of points for further consideration, including a code of good practice for the employment of homeworkers. In sum, the findings presented here suggest that despite high qualifications and skills, most new technology homeworkers are isolated and undervalued, earning substantially less than the going rates in their industry.

284. Hyman, R., and W. Streeck, eds. *New Technology and Industrial Relations.* New York: Basil Blackwell, 1988.

Keywords: work design, Fordism, neo-Fordism, deskilling, technology, general

This comprehensive anthology includes material on flexible specialization, Fordism, neo-Fordism, the deskilling debate, new technology and trade unions, information technology, industrial relations, and other related topics. See chapter 2 for an analysis of Piore and Sabel's "flexible specialization" thesis as advanced in *The Second Industrial Divide* (1984): While Fordism calls for the separation of conception from execution and rigidly defined job categories and skills, "flexible specialization" requires flexibility within the workforce and collaboration between designers and skilled producers to make a variety of goods with general purpose machines. Employees must possess the readiness and ability to perform a variety of functions and to acquire new skills as techniques and products evolve.

285. Illich, Ivan, ed. *Shadow Work.* Boston: Marion Boyars, 1981.

Keywords: sociology, anthropology, subsistence economy

This collection of essays by the noted philosopher and historian deals with the rise of what the author refers to as the "shadow economy." As he states in the introduction, "I have coined this term to speak about transactions that are not in the monetized sector and yet do not exist in pre-industrial society. With the rise of the shadow economy I observe the appearance of a kind of toil which is not rewarded by wages and yet contributes nothing to the household's independence from the market . . . (it is) a necessary condition for the family wage earner to exist."

The book constitutes a major historical and sociological analysis of modern humanity's economic existence. Illich traces and analyzes options that surpass the conventional political "right-left" alternatives and presents the concept of the "vernacular" domain—a domain that includes the shaping of language, the preparation of food, childbirth and recreation, etc. In this volume, Illich presents a provocative assessment of the "controlling uses of language and science and the valuation of women and work." Once again, he excels at seeing through the social ordering that affects industrial culture.

286. International Labor Office, ed. *Automation, Work Organization and Occupational Stress*. Geneva: International Labor Office, 1984.

Keywords: automation, machinery, stress, skill, policy

Although we have learned a great deal in the years following this work's publication, it nevertheless addresses many serious and broad questions. Recognizing that automation was rapidly changing work and working conditions, this Meeting of Experts on Automation, Work Organization, Work Intensity and Occupational Stress sought to determine the impact on skills, worker responsibilities, careers, and occupational stress as well as the implications for work organization and job design. The conclusions regarding these matters are conveniently summarized. The book also contains informative working papers divided into the following four categories: (1) legislation and collective agreements in industrialized countries; (2) policies and practices in market economy countries; (3) policies and practices in centrally planned economies; and (4) work organization and occupational stress.

287. Irving, R. H., C. A. Higgins, and F. R. Safayeni. "Computerized Performance Monitoring Systems: Use and Abuse." *Communications of the ACM* 29, no. 8 (August 1986): 794-800.

Keywords: monitoring, stress, management

The purpose of this article is "to provide empirical evidence on the perceived effects of computerized monitoring and control systems." To accomplish this, individuals in organizations with computerized monitoring systems were compared to individuals in similar jobs but without computerized monitoring.

The authors introduce their article by noting that "the increasing computerization of office functions provides management with new opportunities to monitor, assess, and control employee productivity. By designing software packages that automatically record counts of production, error rates, and time taken to process items, organizations are now obtaining accurate, quantitative data on worker performance." The study reported on here reveals both positive and negative effects. "Results indicate that computerized monitoring is associated with perceived increases in office productivity, more accurate and complete assessment of workers' performance, and higher levels of organizational control. Respondents indicate that managers overemphasize the importance of quality in evaluating employee performance. Workers perceive increased stress, lower levels of satisfaction, and a decrease in the quality of their relationship with peers and management as a consequence of computerized monitoring. The relevance of existing models of performance monitoring is examined in light of these findings."

See especially section 2 "Literature Review" and section 5 "Summary and Conclusions."

288. Iwata, Noboru, and Kazuo Suzuki. "Role Stress—Mental Health Relations in Japanese Bank Workers: A Moderating Effect of Social Support." *Applied Psychology: An International Review* 46, no. 2 (1997): 207-18.

Keywords: stress, mental health, support

The authors summarize their article as follows: "The relationship between role stress at work and mental health status, and the moderating effect of social support, were examined in a sample of Japanese bank workers. Hierarchical moderated multiple regression analyses revealed that role overload had the largest association with mental health status and its interaction with co-worker support was also significantly associated with mental health status. Visual inspection indicated that this interaction should be regarded as a convergent relationship; i.e. high co-worker support would be effective to keep mental health status at low to medium levels of role overload, but become less effective at a higher level of role overload. This relationship was replicated for male clerks, but varied for female clerks, and was not significant for male chief clerks or higher. This might suggest that contradictions in the moderating effects of social support reported in earlier literature from Western countries could, at least in part, be explained by differences in the types of stress, strain, and social support, as well as the situational context of the samples."

289. Jackson, Paul R., Sean Mullarkey, Sharon K. Parker, and Toby D. Wall. "Advanced Manufacturing Systems and the Changing Nature of Work." 590-3 in *Advances in Agile Manufacturing*, edited by P. T. Kidd and W. Karwowski. Amsterdam: IOS Press, 1994.

Keywords: work design, work performance, worker control

Here, the important variable of worker control is related to the uncertainty of manufacturing systems. The first longitudinal study compares two groups of operators whose jobs were redesigned (from specialist control to operator control) to enhance their control over AMT systems. The group that worked on low uncertainty systems experienced little change. However, the high uncertainty group experienced a sharp reduction in overall downtime and the incidence of downtime. The second longitudinal study took place on a very uncertain robotics line. Operator control was increased by allowing them to perform maintenance and fault-finding instead of calling in an engineer in the case of a problem. Increasing problem-solving demand and task control reduced downtime as predicted by Karasek and Theorell's model.

The authors conclude, "Where there is high technological or environmental uncertainty, specialist control of AMT systems harms performance, while devolving control to shopfloor workers themselves allows them to manage uncertainty effectively and leads to substantial performance benefits. Operator control of high-uncertainty systems benefits performance because active system management by operators allows them to generate new knowledge that they are sanctioned to use in their status as local experts." The development of multi-skilled operators, defining new interdisciplinary work roles, reduction of functional specialization and more decentralized organizational structures are recommended.

290. Jackson, Paul R., Toby D. Wall, Robin Martin, and Keith Davids. "New Measures of Job Control, Competitive Demand, and Production Responsibility." *Journal of Applied Psychology* 78, no. 5 (1993): 753-62.

Keywords: employee satisfaction, stress, mental health

The authors expand the traditional Job Characteristics Model that was used in the 1970s and 1980s to measure employee satisfaction and well-being. The old model that described jobs in terms of five core dimensions—skill variety, task identity, task significance, autonomy and feedback—from the job itself is seen to be problematic in the 1990s. The authors contend that "recent research on employee job design for advanced manufacturing technology (AMT) clearly illustrates the limitations of the job characteristics approach."

The research findings reported in this article suggest that new technologies such as numerically controlled machine tools and flexible manufacturing systems require the addition of new job dimensions or constructs in order to fully assess employee well-being and performance. These five new constructs include: timing control—"the individual's opportunity to determine the scheduling of his or her work behavior," method control—"individual choice in how to carry out given tasks," monitoring demand—"the extent of passive monitoring required," problem-solving demand—"the active cognitive processing required to prevent errors," and production responsibility—"the cost of errors in terms of both lost output and damage to expensive equipment."

In conclusion, the researchers maintain that there are solid empirical grounds for establishing new indicators of employee well-being and performance, although further research is required to clarify and broaden these measures. Despite the technical, statistical methodology involved in the study, the implications for further study of worker psychological health are significant.

291. Jacobsen, Joyce P. *The Economics of Gender*. 2nd ed. Malden, MA: Blackwell Publishers, 1998.

Keywords: women, economic conditions, social conditions, sex roles in the work environment, sex discrimination

The second edition of this work gives an introduction to the differences between women's and men's economic opportunities, activities, and rewards. The primary focus is on contemporary U.S. patterns. The author devotes four chapters to cross-societal comparisons and also takes a close look at the evolution of contemporary patterns over time and the impact on them in terms of race, ethnicity, and class. Also, throughout the book the pros and cons of various policies, including "comparable worth" and welfare programs are discussed.

292. Jacoby, Daniel. *Laboring for Freedom: A New Look at the History of Labor in America*. Armonk, NY: M. E. Sharpe, 1998.

Keywords: labor, history, labor movement, labor policy, labor laws and legislation

The book's central theme is an interpretation of the quest for freedom by the average worker in the context of the history of the labor movement in the United States. It describes the conditions in which workers lived and worked, and shows that labor protests against these conditions were based on the American tradition of the primacy of alienable rights. It examines how protests that stemmed from this tradition clashed with the equally American tradition asserting a nearly absolute liberty of individual contract.

293. Jansen, Arild. "Editor's Introduction: Technology and Working Life." *Futures*, December 1991: 1011-8.

Keywords: organizational design, CIM, policy, technology

This is a review article introducing a special issue of *Futures* on technology and working life. It summarizes the papers contained in the journal, grouped into subject areas such as the question of whether we are entering the information age, technology policies, the workerless factory, organizational change and human capital, and economic development. The articles have been abstracted and entered separately into this annotated bibliography.

294. Jarl, Ann-Cathrin. *Women and Economic Justice: Ethics in Feminist Liberation Theology and Feminist Economics*. Uppsala Studies in Social Ethics 25. Uppsala, Sweden: Uppsala University Library, 2000.

Keywords: market economics, feminist economics, feminist ethics

The focus of this work is on women, justice, and economics, analyzed with regard to economic justice. The present situation for poor women is that they have access to very few possibilities in providing for their own basic needs through wage labor, access to and control of arable land, or opportunities to obtain an education. Essentially they are denied equal rights. The book argues that the right to life is a universally recognized right supported by international law, feminist ethics and feminist economics, and everyone who is willing and able should have the option to provide for their basic needs of clean water, food, housing, elementary education, elementary health care and sanitation in a sustainable manner.

295. Johansen, Shawn. *Family Men: Middle-Class Fatherhood in Early Industrializing America*. New York: Routledge, 2001.

Keywords: fatherhood, history, nineteenth century, fathers and husbands, fathers and children's transition to adulthood

By examining the letters and diaries of a number of fathers, the author abandons the simplistic yet often commonplace notion that men in the first half of the nineteenth century had little interaction with their children. The "separate spheres" are demonstrated not to be so separate after all. In fact, there are many cases of fathers anxiously awaiting the birth of their children, raising their sons and daughters, and worrying about their families. This book helps to break down many of our contemporary myths and stereotypes about the role of fathers in the nineteenth century.

296. Johnson, Jeffrey V. "Empowerment in Future Worklife." *Scandinavian Journal of Work, Health and Environment* 23, supplement 4 (1997): S23-S7.

Keywords: power, health, management

The author uses epidemiological evidence to examine the relationship between power and health. It is noted that "a large number of studies have demonstrated that health may indeed be strongly related to power differentials—those in the upper class have the best health profile, while those in the working class and those who are marginally employed have the worst health." The paper further points out that "the differences in health status across social class groups may be explained with reference to the relative inequality in access to social resources, such as power and control over critical aspects of daily life. It is in this context that understanding the role of the workplace becomes essential. Epidemiological and psychobiological research on the work environment has shown that low levels of empowerment in daily worklife, measured in relation to few possibilities to control work content and process, is strongly related to neurohormonal arousal, drug and alcohol use, mental distress, excess chronic disease, and even risk of early death." On the other hand, "efforts to increase levels of power and control at the rank-and-file level of modern industrial organizations have resulted in improved health behavior, greater activation, participation in occupational health and safety activities, and reduced levels of self-reported stress." It is argued that the concept of control—both individual and collective control—is essential in order to understand the structural and historical determinants of empowerment at the workplace. Johnson also turns his attention to a more critical assessment of the term "empowerment" by addressing the question: "Empowerment for whom?" Several recent definitions of empowerment are offered from a public health perspective, and the community health empowerment perspective is summarized as well (see page 24).

Finally, the author takes issue with some of the new ways in which the term empowerment is now being used. "One perspective that is popular in some managerial circles owes much to Japanese production methods and it is becoming associated with the term 'lean production.' This approach to empowerment focuses on increasing the degree of participation on the part of the rank and file in task level decision making, supervision, and job changes; yet it is often accompanied by downsizing and results in work intensification within the surviving work force. This type of empowerment has been criticized by some in the labor movement as a form of 'management by stress.'"

Johnson concludes that "occupational and environmental health scientists, in their professional activities, need to ask themselves continually the questions Who do my actions serve? Empowerment for whom? What is our role as professionals in the empowerment process? First, and most importantly, we must do no harm."

297. Johnson, Jeffrey V., Walter Stewart, Ellen M. Hall, Peeter Fredlund, and Tores Theorell. "Long-Term Psychosocial Work Environment and Cardiovascular Mortality among Swedish Men." *American Journal of Public Health* 86, no. 3 (1996): 324-31.

Keywords: stress, disease

Here is the authors' abstract of the article: "*Objectives*. This study examined the effect of cumulative exposure to work organization—psychological demands, work control, and social support—on prospectively measured cardiovascular disease mortality risk.

"*Methods*. The source population was a national sample of 12517 subjects selected from the Swedish male population by Statistics Sweden in annual surveys between 1977 and 1981. Over a 14-year follow-up period, 521 deaths from cardiovascular disease were identified. A nested case-control design was used. Work environment exposure scores were assigned to cases and controls by linking lifetime job histories with a job exposure matrix.

"*Results*. Conditional logistic regression analysis was used in examining cardiovascular mortality risk in relation to work exposure after adjustment for age, year last employed, smoking, exercise, education, social class, nationality, and physical job demands. In the final multi-variable analysis, workers with low work control had a relative risk of 1.83 (95% confidence interval [CI] = 1.19, 2.82) for cardiovascular mortality. Workers with combined exposure to low control and low support had a relative risk of 2.62 (95% CI = 1.22, 5.61).

"*Conclusions*. These results indicate that long-term exposure to low work control is a risk factor for cardiovascular disease mortality."

298. Jones Jr., Harold B. "The Protestant Ethic: Weber's Model and the Empirical Literature." *Human Relations* 50, no. 7 (1997).

Keywords: capitalism, Protestant ethic

In this article, "empirical research concerning the Protestant ethic is reviewed in relation to Max Weber's model of the part a specifically religious ethos played in the rise of capitalism." For Weber, the author reminds us, Western legal and commercial changes were not in themselves an adequate explanation. "Essential also was the set of values emphasized by ascetic Protestantism: self-discipline, hard work, the careful use of time, the reinvestment of one's gains, personal honesty, creative innovation, and faith in the rewards of a just God. Empirical research has found positive correlations between Protestant ethic values and internal locus of control (self-discipline), hard work, honesty, and belief in a just world. Findings with regard to the use of time and money are inconclusive. The relationship with creative innovation has not been examined. There is a need for empirical study of the relationship between the Protestant ethic and personal religious orientation."

The author suggests that there is one sentence that is probably the best possible one in summarizing the Weber thesis: "Economic individualism had its roots in religious individualism." Jones asks: "Is this sentence descriptive only of something that happened centuries ago, or does it point to a basic fact of human psychology? Spiritual concerns may not in our time weigh as heavily on the mind of the believer as they did when Calvin thundered from his pulpit. . . . There may nevertheless be a strong relationship between certain types of religious conviction and the values of the Protestant ethic. Considering the emerging interest in the relationship between spirituality and work values . . . this may be suggested as an area that deserves serious empirical research."

299. Jones, Jacqueline. *A Social History of the Laboring Classes: From Colonial Times to the Present*. Problems in American History. Malden, MA: Blackwell Publishers, 1999.

Keywords: working class, United States, history, social conditions, labor classes

Work, being one of the most important aspects of every American's life, is studied from colonial times to the present. Beginning with the seventeenth century, the experiences of different groups of American workers—urban and rural, waged and unwaged—within the context of the economic transformations that have occurred at regular intervals throughout American history, are examined. Also, the denigration of women's housework, technological advances, the transition of slavery to free labor, and the rise of the global assembly line are major themes used to demonstrate how, in response to these changes, workers have reconditioned themselves according to their ethnicity, gender, race, and task. The majority of the book concentrates on the history of the American labor movement, based initially in antebellum trade shops, then in sprawling industrial complexes, and lastly in workplaces similar to those of Las Vegas hotels and casinos.

300. Jones, Susan. *The Human Factor: Maximizing Team Efficiency through Collaborative Leadership*. London: Kogan Press, 1992.

Keywords: participation, teams

This book on organizational theory and practice emphasizes the central role of the "human factor" in achieving effectiveness and efficiency in working and learning environments. The superiority of the participatory approach as opposed to the traditional authoritarian model is demonstrated in both educational and workplace settings. The author argues that despite the growing "human resource/participation" rhetoric—the true value of the "human factor" is still often ignored in practice.

Part 1 of the text focuses on "Collaborative Leadership and Organizational Success." Topics discussed include the following: human relations and quality of performance; collaborative leadership, participation motivation; ethics and success, etc.

Part 2 explores "The Core Collaborative Skills and Business, Educational, and National Cultures." Topics discussed include the following: skills and team roles; the role of management; organizational culture; employee involvement and caring for the employee; and the role of education and training.

Part 3 examines "Developing the Core Collaborative Skills of Leadership and Teamwork." Topics include the following: learning by collaborative doing; a core collaborative skills checklist; and basic team format.

301. Joseph, Antoine. *Skilled Workers' Solidarity: The American Experience in Comparative Perspective*. States and Societies. New York: Garland Publishing, 2000.

Keywords: labor movement, history, skilled labor, solidarity, comparative industrial relations

It is argued in this work that national labor movements are shaped by the interaction of specific structural factors during the industrializing era. The first couple of chapters provide a theoretical and comparative framework, developing a causal explanation of labor solidarism based on specific variables. The key idea of these beginning chapters is to show that specific historical structural variables are responsible for molding social, political, and economic environments in ways that directly affect the development of labor movements within capitalist democracies. The following three chapters assess the empirical evidence for the development of class factions, as well as elaborate the political, social and economic environment that led to the emergence of a strongly particularistic labor movement. This is concluded by the final two chapters that apply the model and analysis to certain formative features governing the emergence of the American welfare state, as well as providing a summary and a conclusion.

302. Kahn, Robert L. *Work and Health*. Wiley Series on Organizational Assessment and Change. New York: John Wiley and Sons, 1981.

Keywords: health, stress, coping

This volume offers an intensive treatment of employee health in organizations. While all aspects of health are considered, primary attention is given to mental health and to the role of work and work environments in fostering increased well-being on the part of employees. The author examines the meaning of work to people in various life circumstances, summarizes what is known about the characteristics of jobs that can affect health, and describes the sources and effects of occupational stress and strain. The final chapters review alternative strategies for promoting healthful employment in ways compatible with organizational effectiveness.

Chapter 1 offers an overview of "Work in Industrial Societies" and chapter 2 discusses "Occupational Differences in the Meaning of Work." Chapter 3 considers "The Context of Jobs" and chapter 4 looks at "Stress and Strain: The Evidence." Chapters 5 and 6 explore the effects of job loss on physical and mental health. See also chapters 8 and 9 for "Strategies of Coping and Adaptation."

303. Kanigel, Robert. "Taylor-Made." *The Sciences*, 1997: 18-23.

Keywords: Taylorism, comparative

Even after Taylor's death and the denouncement of his beliefs by most people, the influence his ideas exert is enormous. He transformed, of course, factory work as described in detail by Kanigel. But Taylor's ideas were applied to other fields including offices and hospitals. The article goes on to chronicle the spread of Taylorism to other countries, especially Japan, where it had a big impact. Even today, Kanigel points out, evidence of Taylorization is present everywhere, most notably in the almost sacred principle that efficiency is desirable and waste is shameful. Also, the separation of mind and body in work and the notion that humans and machines should work together efficiently are widespread. The article is basically a summary of Taylor's life, work and ubiquitous influence.

304. Kaplan, Marty, and Tom Rankin. *Quantitative Measures from Organizations Undergoing Major Change in the Way Work is Performed: A Survey of Eighteen Canadian Workplaces*. Prepared for the meeting of the Premier's Council on Economic Renewal. Ontario: Task Force on the Organization of Work, 1993.

Keywords: quality, productivity, human resources, industrial relations

New forms of work organization such as self-managing teams and employee participation will make a major contribution to the economic renewal of Ontario. This is the conclusion reached by the Task Force on the Organization of Work that studied fourteen Canadian workplaces before and after the introduction of such strategies. Four other companies were studied that had a new form of work organization from the start. These companies were compared with similar companies with a traditional organizational structure. Five aspects, namely quality, productivity, costs, human resources and labor management relations, were measured and analyzed. For the most part, organizations reported gains for all five indicators. This report for the Premier's Council on Economic Renewal therefore provides some evidence, albeit from a very small sample, that workplace democratization benefits both employees and the corporation.

305. Karasek, Robert. "Labor Participation and Work Quality Policy: Requirements for an Alternative Economic Future." *Scandinavian Journal of Work, Environment and Health* 23, supplement 4 (1997): S55-S65.

Keywords: health, participation, work design, skill, policy

In this outstanding paper, the author endeavors to outline the prerequisites for a new social policy approach known as the "work quality approach." This new approach is first differentiated from the others "and then relinked to them via bridges constructed in the extension of this paper." After outlining the fundamental principles of traditional market-oriented policy and welfare state policy and noting the increasing prevalence of a prevention focus in social policy making, Karasek introduces his version of a work quality basis for social policy. "The work quality perspective also claims that the market model covers too narrow a range of social behavior to describe the whole of current social reality. Instead, it claims that many of the costs and benefits of work activity are also transferred through non-market, social relation processes which link work experience to life inside and outside the job—which can be called work quality effects." The author maintains that "work quality issues now have major effects on (i) the innovation capability of companies and workers, (ii) community and family stability, (iii) health and mental well-being, and (iv) the strength of democratic institutions. These effects are both desirable and undesirable, and they have reached a size of dramatic—not peripheral—importance." Karasek further points out that "a social policy, based on work quality need not limit itself to overlooked 'costs,' but can focus on generating overlooked 'benefits' of the production system as well, thereby addressing productivity issues: organization of innovative production and creation and distribution of output to support social stability." The author also argues that "the full potential of a work quality organization perspective cannot be understood until it is viewed comprehensively as the basis for a new model of economic activity." See especially the four requirements for a new model of economic activity that could resolve some current dilemmas—listed at the end of the paper on pages 64-65.

306. Karasek, Robert, and Töres Theorell. *Healthy Work: Stress, Productivity and the Reconstruction of Working Life*. New York: Basic Books, 1990.

Keywords: stress, demand-control model, social support, illness

This is a classic book that first brought attention to the now famous "demand-control" model of analyzing work situations and their outcome on the health of the employees. The work is based on a ten year study of nearly 5,000 workers and clearly demonstrates a relationship between work related illness (especially cardiovascular and problems with blood pressure) and workers' lack of participation in the design and outcome of their labors. This book is an invaluable resource for anyone who is interested in improving the organization of work to make it healthier.

307. Kaufman, Bruce E., and Morris M. Kleiner, eds. *Employee Representation: Alternatives and Future Directions*. Madison, WI: Industrial Relations Research Association, 1993.

Keywords: industrial relations, participation, unions, work councils

This is an excellent collection of essays in the (sub)field of industrial relations known as employee representation. The introduction to the book points out that the concept first arose in the 1920s and quickly evolved into a scientific exercise intended to resolve many of the common problems in the workplace created by inequity, authoritarianism, and inefficiency. The authors contend that all "progressives" in the field today recognize that the creation of a win-win situation for employers and employees (one that results in higher productivity and profits as well as more harmonious relationships between employers and employees) requires "some form of employee representation, or 'industrial democracy.'"

After defining the characteristics of industrial democracy, a brief review of historical trends in the American industrial relations system is provided. This is followed by a systematic analysis of "various discussions of employee representation written by leading experts in the field." Topics discussed in the eleven chapters include the following: "A review of empirical studies on the economic impact of employee representation" that concludes that this impact is often positive; "Factors behind the decline in union density in the United States economy"; "Alternative forms of employee representation" (beyond the traditional practice of collective bargaining); "Evolving models of work force governance"; "Employee representation through the political process"; "Case studies on 'Work Councils'—The German Experience"; and "Co-management Strategies: The Saturn Partnership" (in the auto industry). These chapters represent an outstanding and diverse collection of research articles. The case study material is particularly useful in the context of preventive work models.

308. Kelly, John E., and Chris W. Clegg, eds. *Autonomy and Control at the Workplace: Contexts for Job Redesign*. London: Croom Helm, 1982.

Keywords: work design

The aim of the authors represented in this book is to understand the meaning and impact of job redesign at the organizational level. The twin concepts of autonomy and control provide the theoretical foundation for a range of analyses that examine "the organizational process surrounding the development, implementation, and subsequent evaluation of job redesign." A variety of social science perspectives are included, all sharing a particularistic/empirical orientation. Case study material is also extensively used throughout the text. The need for collaboration between managers, trade unionists, psychologists, sociologists and economists is stressed, although much of the material presented remains on a micro level, which does little to build bridges across discipline boundaries. Although somewhat dated, this volume makes a definite contribution to the literature in the field. However, there is a shortage of content that deals explicitly with preventive action, the notable exception being chapter 5 "The Process of Change: Practical Paradigms for Redesigning Jobs."

309. Kemp, Donna R. *Mental Health in the Workplace: An Employer's and Manager's Guide*. Westport, CT: Quorum Books, 1994.

Keywords: mental health, industrial relations

Although many of the topics covered in this book are not of direct relevance to healthy work (general discussions on mental health problems, employee selection and mental health issues, employment law, placement and supervision of workers with mental health problems, psychological testing, drug screening, genetic testing, managing the substance abusing employee, personality, grievances and termination, violence, relocation, layoffs, retirement, the impaired manager and financing mental health care), other sections are useful.

Chapter 6 "Creating a Mentally Healthy Work Environment" concludes that workplaces can be made more healthy by changing the corporate culture. More specifically, employers should empower workers, make the workplace friendlier, and lead, not manage. The chapter begins with an overview of the movement toward a better quality of worklife. End-of-pipe solutions and issues such as organizational policies regarding family leave, childcare, elder care, flexible work schedule, substance abuse, smoking, discrimination and surveillance, their importance and recent improvements are discussed. The next section provides information on how to design a healthy working environment. The physical environment, management development and organizational development are the areas that are explored. Workplace stress is the next subject of study. The causes of stress, individual differences in dealing with stress and how employers can decrease stress in the workplace are investigated. As well, emotional health programs and wellness programs to prevent and to deal with mental and physical problems are considered, with plenty of examples from American companies. The importance of mediation techniques during conflict resolution and reduction is stressed. This chapter is basically an easy to read collection that summarizes the research into the above mentioned topics.

310. Kenney, M., and R. Florida. "Beyond Mass Production: Production and the Labor Process in Japan." *Politics & Society* 16, no. 1 (1988): 121-58.

Keywords: flexible specialization, labor process, Fordism, knowledge embedded in experience, knowledge separated from experience

A political economy approach is used to examine the production and labor process in Japan. Traditional labor process theories are applied and rejected. The authors examine Toyotism, Fujitsuism, and flexible specialization as well as various forms of corporate organization.

311. Kenney, M., and R. Florida. "Japan's Role in a Post-Fordist Age." *Futures*, April 1989: 136-51.

Keywords: work design, labor process, forecasting

What will supersede the Fordist model of industrial organization as industry shifts from mass-production technology to new information technologies? Possible alternative models are presented. Of the several models that have been suggested, the authors state that the only viable model is the one that can be learned from Japanese industrial organization. This post-Fordist model "replaces the specialization and deskilling of the Fordist model with a new industrial organization based upon integrative and flexible work organization, shopfloor learning, and net-worked production complexes." This model is referred to as Fujitsuist, after Fujitsu Ltd. Fujitsuim as a new mechanism for sustained economic growth is described and analyzed. This is done after the four alternative models ("neo-Fordism," "global Fordism," "post-Fordism" and "flexible specialization") are outlined and their weaknesses noted.

312. Kenney, M., and R. Florida. "How Japanese Industry Is Rebuilding the Rust Belt." *Technology Review*, February-March 1991: 25-33.

Keywords: manufacturing, knowledge embedded in experience, policy

The revitalization of the American Rust Belt by the Japanese spurred this inquiry into Japanese production organization methods. The article lays out why their methods work for them. Unlike their American counterparts, the Japanese invest heavily in their own plants in order to maintain state-of-the-art manufacturing systems, and they set them up for close linkages between manufacturing, management, R&D and suppliers. Together with this there is less of a separation between "hand and brain" by comparison with U.S. industry. The article analyzes the auto industry, focusing on the track records of United States-Japanese collaborations. The just-in-time approach, the steel industry, tires and rubber, and the drawbacks of Japanese-owned factories are examined in the remainder of the article.

313. Kingsolver, Ann E., ed. *More Than Class: Studying Power in United States Workplaces*. SUNY Series in the Anthropology of Work. Albany: State University of New York Press, 1998.

Keywords: industrial sociology, United States, business anthropology, minorities, employment, case study, social classes, power (social sciences)

By focusing on work sites ranging from security booths to bedrooms to mining shafts, instead of the traditional shop floor, this book examines the changing texture of power relations in American workplaces. Class analysis is seen as a powerful tool for thinking about addressing inequalities at the very center of American social and economic organization. The use of new approaches are also examined—for example, the analysis of the intersections of identity and empowerment or disempowerment through constructions of gender, ethnicity, and race—so that the subtle and not so subtle power relations in workplaces can be studied.

314. Kirby, J. Philip. "A Sociotechnical Approach to Reducing Manufacturing Cycle-Time: A Case Study." Technical paper MM85-721. Society of Manufacturing Engineers, 1985.

Keywords: manufacturing, sociotechnical systems, case study

"'Just-in-time' manufacturing strategies that aim at reducing excess materials, time and space to expose quality problems will not fulfill their total promise as a response to off-shore competition, without implementing complementary organization redesign efforts as well. Quality improvement requires that we adopt a new participatory industrial management model in manufacturing; that is, a model that gives authority, skills and information to the employees to respond to quality problems that surface, when they occur, at the time they occur. A sociotechnical systems model, provides a diagnosis and implementation process that pushes the decision-making and problem-solving capability to the shop floor where quality problems will be increasingly evident as we 'lower the waterline' by implementing reduction inventory programs." This thesis is tested in a case study of the Electronics, Control and Distribution Products Division of Westinghouse Canada Inc.'s Airdrie, Alberta, plant.

315. Kirp, D. L., and Douglas S. Rice. "Fast Forward: Styles of California Management." *Harvard Business Review*, January-February 1988: 74-83.

Keywords: organizational behavior, comparative

The innovative and distinctive Californian style of doing business is explored. Pool side meetings, gourmet cafeterias, and the blurring of the line between work life and private life make Californian organizations unique. Their encouragement of innovation to the extreme makes the companies extremely successful. Because of their differing styles, mergers between Californian companies and traditional American companies often pose problems. Recently, however, Californian-Japanese joint ventures such as NUMMI (New United Motor Manufacturing, Inc.) seem to have been able to combine the best of both worlds. This Toyota-GM joint venture has increased productivity and reduced absenteeism. The article, while not preventively oriented, provides a glimpse of successful Californian organizational styles.

316. Klein, J. A. "The Human Costs of Manufacturing Reform." *Harvard Business Review*, March-April 1989: 60-6.

Keywords: participation, just-in-time, case study, statistical process control

The manufacturing reforms referred to here are just-in-time (JIT) approaches and statistical process control (SPC). The article revolves around a case study of an engine plant that shows that these reforms do not necessarily empower or provide autonomy to employees. JIT and SPC often claim to empower the workforce by demanding that workers schedule their own work, determine how to carry it out, and manage their own daily activities. However, in the case of this engine plant that already valued worker participation, autonomy and morale, the implementation of JIT and SPC brought along with it employee complaints.

They felt a loss of team autonomy because under JIT, team activities had to be coordinated with the activities of other teams. Loss of individual autonomy was also experienced as slack time was lost, more pressure was felt, and time for team meetings and self-management was reduced. SPC, with its strict procedures, limited workers' creativity when solving problems or making decisions.

The article continues by asking, What can be done about this? The author recommends rethinking zero inventory, emphasizing flow (not pace), focusing on task design (not execution), giving workers the right to move, and allowing for workplace management of quality and resources. The article concludes with the statement that managers should not promise workers autonomy if they actually want cooperation, revealing that the orientation is not preventive.

317. Kling, Rob, ed. *Computerization and Controversy: Value Conflicts and Social Choices*. 2nd ed. San Diego: Academic Press, 1996.

Keywords: computers, general

This excellent critical anthology (an update of the 1991 edition; see Dunlop, Charles, and Rob Kling, eds.) examines many of the key value conflicts and social choices surrounding the issue of computerization. A lead article for each part of the book provides an integrated overview and places each article in context within the various debates. This edition includes a large number of articles that focus on current issues and contexts as they appear in the mid-1990s.

Controversies and questions explored in this collection include the following: "How appropriate are technologically utopian and anti-utopian scenarios for understanding the future? Does computerization demonstrably improve the productivity of organizations? Should computer systems be designed to empower workers? How do computer systems designers often ignore the complexity of women's work? How can computerized system designs incorporate social principles? Does electronic mail facilitate the formation of new communities, or does it undermine intimate interaction? Is computerization likely to reduce privacy and personal freedom? What risks arise from computerized systems in health care?"

The contributors to this comprehensive volume are scholars in computer science, information systems, sociology, psychology, law, management, and journalism. Excellent articles by Langdon Winner, Rob Kling, Sven Birkerts, Andrew Clement, Judith Perrolle, and Peter Neumann are contained.

318. Knights, David, Hugh Willmott, and David Collinson, eds. *Job Redesign: Critical Perspectives on the Labor Process*. Aldershot, UK: Gower, 1985.

Keywords: work design, labor process

This collection of essays (mostly by specialists in industrial relations and management science) adopts a critical perspective on job redesign, questioning "the view that the redesign of jobs in practice as primarily motivated by a humanistic ideology of improving job satisfaction and the quality of working life."

Considered an important text in the sociology of work and occupations, this work can be seen in the context of Marxist-inspired theories of work organization. Writing out of the tradition of labor process theory, many of the contributors to this volume are skeptical of "widespread claims that job redesign can provide a true reconciliation of the 'needs' of individuals (employees) and the 'needs' of organizations (employers)."

Consequently, the primary interest in developing prescriptions for humanizing reforms, through strategies such as job rotation, job enlargement, job enrichment, quality circles and autonomous work groups, etc. is replaced here by "an interest . . . in developing *radical* critiques of the theories and practices associated with job redesign."

In short this work is non-prescriptive and non-psychological in its approach, focusing instead on the historical, political, economic and sociological contexts of job redesign. This book offers a healthy corrective to some of the conventional approaches in this area that often have a naive faith in the humanistic and productive virtues of job redesign. Nonetheless, the lack of attention given to possible solutions or at least some positive reference to the growing literature on healthy workplace design would seem to be a drawback to this collection.

319. Kobayashi, Audrey, ed. *Women, Work, and Place*. Montreal and Kingston: McGill-Queen's University Press, 1994.

Keywords: women

Just as the title suggests, the book explores the complex relations between women, work, and place. It is the result of a symposium of the same title that provided scholars of different disciplines a forum for exchanging ideas. The differing experiences of working women are tied together by the theme of place. Women from the fields of geography, history and sociology each contribute a chapter focusing on topics such as the transformation of the workforce in nineteenth-century Montreal, the feminization of skill in the British garment industry, the work-family relationship for Japanese immigrant women in Canada, a labor dispute situation in Ontario, the restructuring of the United States labor force, restructuring in an urban context, gentrification and women's work roles, inequality at work and theoretical issues regarding women in the city.

320. Kobayashi, Fumio. "Japanese Perspective of Future Worklife." *Scandinavian Journal of Work, Environment and Health* 23, supplement 4 (1997): S66-S72.

Keywords: health, lifetime employment

The author reports the results of a study on the influence of the traditional lifetime employment system in Japan on the health of workers, on perspectives of the future worklife of Japanese workers, and on possible measures for promoting the health of workers. It is reported that Japanese workers enjoy an extremely high standard of health relative to all other workers internationally due to such factors as a well-balanced diet, the Japanese educational and employment system, and even the distribution of wealth. However, while it is pointed out that the traditional Japanese employment system has brought a very satisfactory health condition to Japanese workers on the one hand, it has caused several health problems related to long work hours on the other. The author offers statistical data relating to the phenomenon of *karoshi*, or death from overwork, and provides information on the psychosocial/physiological effects of long work hours. The paper also discusses how the Japanese work environment will unavoidably be changed in the future, by such factors as the rapid growth of the aged population, the increasing participation of women in the labor force, changes in the style of work due to the introduction of high technology (such as computers) into the workplace, and the restructuring of organizations. Finally, the author examines health promotion strategies in the workplace, including those conducted by companies themselves and others sponsored by the government's health and labor ministries. It is concluded that "in the future, integrated health promotion programs in the workplace will need to be conducted both individually and comprehensively, and the activities should be expanded to even smaller scale enterprises."

321. Kochan, Thomas A., Harry C. Katz, and Robert B. McKersie. *The Transformation of American Industrial Relations*. New York: Basic Books, 1986.

Keywords: industrial relations, QWL, case study, history

As the title suggests, this volume is a historical overview of the American system of industrial relations and collective bargaining. The authors address the question of whether changes triggered by the deep recession of the early 1980s are fundamental ones reflecting "deep-seated environmental pressures" and evolving organizational strategies or whether they are merely temporary adjustments. Industrial relations are examined in unionized and non-unionized settings, along with changes in the process of labor negotiations. Quality of working life (QWL) approaches are assessed, as are changing worker expectations and values. In addition, the evolving market and technological conditions are considered, especially in relation to the serious problems posed by economic restructuring and technological adaptation for workers. Limited case study material is also included, but there is little emphasis on health-related concerns and preventive strategies for change in the workplace.

322. Kochan, Thomas A., and Michael Useem, eds. *Transforming Organizations*. Oxford: Oxford University Press, 1992.

Keywords: organizational change, comparative, skill, management

This collection of essays written from the perspective of organizational and management theory endeavors "to develop creative and useful models of organizational change" by challenging managers to "rethink their assumptions about their roles, their organizations, and the values, motivations and talents of their employees." Once again, the bottom line for the authors, in terms of the necessity for such changes, rests on "contemporary concerns over the ability of firms to adapt to and compete effectively in today's global economy." The contributors to this volume are all involved in "a debate over the organizational practices that can best serve advanced industrialized economies and societies in the future." Toward this end the book explores a number of fundamental questions, through the use of extensive empirical research, cross-cultural comparisons, and a number of different theoretical models. The basic questions probed in this work are: "What is the new model of organizations that underlies the changes being advocated? Do these changes fit together in a coherent internally-consistent fashion? What evidence is there to suggest this new model or these new practices are superior to the traditional approach? Finally, how are systemic changes . . . in organizational practices to be achieved?" See especially chapter 9 "Using Human Resources in Skill Formation: The Role of Training" and chapter 12 "Changing the Conditions of Work: Responding to Increasing Work Force Diversity and New Family Patterns."

323. Kohler, C., and K. Schmieri. "Computer-Integrated Manufacturing (CIM): Technological and Organizational Change in the West German Capital Goods Industry." *Journal of Manufacturing Systems* 10, no. 1 (1991): 21-31.

Keywords: CIM, manufacturing, computers, automation

This article investigates the actual diffusion of CIM technologies and related developments in the organization of production and work. The results of a survey in West Germany (before reunification in 1990) show that the utilization of CIM components and their integration is limited, yet promises dynamic growth and extensive dissemination in the near future. As far as organizational change is concerned, different paths of development are observed. The majority of companies pursue traditional Taylorist strategies of functional and task specialization. A strong minority experiments with alternatives in limited areas, and a small minority integrates functions and tasks throughout production. A large number of contextual factors influence these developments. The chosen strategy for implementing CIM components and systems plays an important role in determining the direction of technological and organizational change in companies.

324. Kohn, James P. *The Ergonomic Casebook: Real World Solutions*. Boca Raton: Lewis Publishers, 1997.

Keywords: workplace design, case study

This book takes on the challenge of applying occupational health and safety theory to actual workplace practice. The author is particularly concerned with overcoming the difficulties associated with "the difference between how the workplace should be ideally designed and the limitations that occur in pre-existing facilities." Applications of the book, as well as implications for preventive work strategies and healthy work concepts, are plentiful. The book uses a case study approach to illustrate sound ergonomic practices in heavy industry, the service industry, agriculture and the office work environment. In these case studies, methods are described for identifying ergonomic problems. Specific causes—referred to as ergonomic stressors—are then reported, and recommended strategies for the elimination of identified stressors are indicated. Strategy effectiveness and evaluation of results are discussed as well. See especially section 2.7 "Office Environments Case Studies" and section 2.9 "Utility Industry Case Studies."

325. Koike, Kazuo. "Human Resource Development and Labor-Management Relations." 289-330 in *The Political Economy of Japan*, edited by Kozo Yamamura. Palo Alto, CA: Stanford University Press, 1987.

Keywords: skill, knowledge embedded in experience, labor-management relations, Japan

This chapter examines human resource development and labor-management relations in Japan in detail. In particular, it evaluates the higher productivity of Japanese labor and the cooperation of labor unions. The author suggests that Japanese shop-floor workers have intellectual skills similar to white-collar workers—though perhaps developed differently—and that these skills are frequently used by them to solve unusual problems.

326. Koslowsky, Meni. *Modeling the Stress-Strain Relationship in Work Settings*. New York: Routledge, 1998.

Keywords: job stress, psychology

Stress is a means by which events, internal and external to the individual, produce an effect that is psychologically, and often physically, debilitating. Case-controlled, retrospective data to help understand the variables and associations between elements of stress has yet to be made abundantly available. In response to this dearth of information concerning stress, this book seeks to identify specific examples of the stress-strain process and offers multivariate techniques such as multiple regression analysis and structural equation modeling to help interpret data.

The book addresses common stress related problems such as cardiovascular disease, hypertension, back problems, depression, anxiety, absenteeism, and others, and covers theories of organizational stress, stressors themselves, extra-organizational stressors such as cultural values, environment and home/familial stressors, as well as stress assessment instruments, psychological and physiological reactions to strain, behavioral consequences of stress, mediators and moderators, modeling the stress-strain process, and general methodological issues.

327. Kozik, T. J., and D. G. Jansson, eds. *The Worker in Transition: Technological Change*. New York: American Society of Mechanical Engineers, 1989.

Keywords: technology, automation, computers, health, mental health, alienation

This is one of the best sourcebooks on the impact of automation on workers; almost no workplace that has computers or automated processes is left unanalyzed. The studies range from the work of control room operators in large scale plants to computerized administrative work. Machine paced work and its consequences are examined in detail as are the new demands placed on skills, concentration, quantitative and qualitative output, and physical resources. In terms of healthy work, the article by R. B. Pipe, "Work, Madness, and Powerlessness: The Mental Health of Workers in the Technological Workplace," is particularly insightful in terms of the alienating effects of automation. Policy implications, the need for radical work redesign, and a change in corporate culture are consistently spelled out for every work situation. Considerable use of case study material enhance the value of this book.

328. Kraemer, Kenneth L., and James N. Danziger. "The Impacts of Computer Technology on the Worklife of Information Workers." *Social Science Computer Review* 8, no. 1 (Spring 1990): 592-613.

Keywords: information workers, job enrichment, support, computers

Given the fact that there has been more than a decade of empirical study on the social impacts of computer technology that has produced a significant body of research, the authors suggest that "it is feasible to attempt serious efforts to synthesize the research findings in order to advance toward grounded theory on various issues addressing social impacts of computing." In that context, "this article assesses recent research that examines the impacts of computing on the worklife of information workers. It uses a broad analytic framework to organize discussion of research since 1985, to assess the consistency and coherence of the research, and to suggest where systematic comparative analysis is needed in the future. Research findings are summarized with regard to the impacts of computing on decision-making, control, productivity, social interaction, work environment, and job enhancement."

The authors note that four essential concepts from organizational theory guide the selection of key variables for empirical research on the impacts of computer technology on information workers. See figure 1, which presents a framework for a general theory of the effects of computing on work. Variables used include people (information workers), tasks (information processing), technology (computers) and impacts (control, social interaction, job enhancement, etc.). Also see the subsection entitled "Toward More Comparative Analyses of Computing Impacts" that highlights seven general, metatheoretical observations that emerge from the authors' assessment of empirical studies.

329. Krahn, Harvey J., and Graham S. Lowe. *Work, Industry, and Canadian Society*. 2nd ed. Scarborough: Nelson Canada, 1993.

Keywords: general, sociology

This comprehensive and well-researched volume is written by two leading Canadian specialists in the sociology of work and occupations. It would make an excellent textbook, given the fact that it is both highly readable and covers a vast range of subject matter with precision and clarity.

The authors "synthesize key theoretical debates in the sociology of work and industry and, at the same time, document emerging labor market, technological, industrial, and workplace trends." The major theme linking the diverse subjects addressed in the book is that "a clear understanding of the factors affecting work and of the alternatives to existing workplace arrangements are essential preconditions for diverting changes that could benefit Canadian workers." Major topics examined in the text include the following: the rise of flexible employment; changing skill requirements in both the goods-producing and service sectors; automation and its implications for workers; the transformation of work in relation to the global economy; the post-industrial society debate; and classic material on alienation and the labor process and technology and job satisfaction. See especially chapter 2 "Industrial Capitalism, Post-Industrial Society, and Social Theory" and chapter 10 "Job Satisfaction and the Quality of Work." This final chapter provides a good overview of the literature on job satisfaction and dissatisfaction with respect to gender, age, race, and education. Moreover, the impact of automation and microelectronic technology on workers is discussed, along with a review of work-stress research and new strategies for personal growth of workers.

330. Kraut, Robert, Susan Dumais, and Susan Koch. "Computerization, Productivity, and Quality of Work-Life." *Communications of the ACM* 32, no. 2 (1989): 220-37.

Keywords: QWL, deskilling, computers, automation

This article offers a detailed examination of what happened to productivity and quality of working life when a large company introduced a computerized record system. The overarching goal of the authors is to illustrate via this case study the methodological and conceptual complexities involved in assessing technological effects.

Before describing the research setting, discussing issues of methodology, and presenting the results, the authors provide a good summary of research findings on the effects of computers and telecommunications technologies on work productivity and quality of work-life.

A number of measures in the study show that "service representatives' jobs became less satisfying, less interesting, and generally of poorer quality following the introduction of the computerized record system . . . [employees] reported that both the overall interest level and enjoyment of the job had deteriorated after the computerized record system was installed." Moreover, "examining the components of job quality in more detail shows that service representatives' work had less variety, was less challenging, and [they] were less able to see the results of their work. . . . [In addition], contact with work colleagues became a less frequent and less satisfying component of service reps' work life."

Other results from the study suggest that the technology effects of the computer system were not unidirectional: for some employees "the technology reduced their job pressure and, surprisingly, increased their happiness and mental health." In other words, some data supports arguments that office automation technology, primarily used to increase productivity, can at the same time upgrade jobs.

331. Kraut, Robert E., ed. *Technology and the Transformation of White-Collar Work*. Hillsdale, NJ: Lawrence Erlbaum Associates, 1987.

Keywords: white-collar work, computers, technology, case study

Computer technology is rapidly and drastically changing white-collar work in the United States. The nature of the changes range from increased work exploitation and routinization of work to increased productivity and higher quality of working life. The contributors seek to understand how the new technologies can be used to achieve the latter and not the former types of changes. Part 1 "Social Impact of White Collar Technology" analyzes the effect of new technology on employees. The concerns of organized labor and the importance of consulting employees in the early stages of change are addressed in chapter 2. The rationalization and feminization of labor at Aetna Life Insurance Company from 1910 to 1930 and the transformation of clerical jobs in the last 100 years are the subjects of chapters 3 and 4. An historical and feminist perspective of the impact of technology on the organization of work is provided in chapter 5. Discussions of software programmers and telework conclude the section. The second part, entitled "Implementing Technology in the Office," stresses that understanding the nature of office work and the process by which technology is adopted is essential for implementing healthy workplace designs. Studies of PC use in offices, the role technology plays in social interaction at the office, sociotechnical design tools, case studies and "Choices En Route to the Office of Tomorrow" are examined.

332. Kugelmass, Joel. *Telecommuting: A Manager's Guide to Flexible Work Arrangements*. New York: Lexington Books, 1995.

Keywords: telework, telecommuting, management

This volume examines, from a managerial perspective, the role of telecommuting and flextime in modern work organizations. The author, conscious of the apprehensions with which many managers and supervisors view flexible work, offers evidence of the ways in which "flexibility actually increases control through managing by objective. . . . It encourages organizations to see how they can use flexible work arrangements to improve productivity and to reduce costs of space and skyrocketing absenteeism with only modest expenditures." The author also shows "how management interested in a more effective and reliable work force can motivate flexibility programs." The book "demonstrates how telecommuting leverages existing technology and personnel investments," while also suggesting how the risks and drawbacks of flexible work can be "managed and minimized." Some of the potential problems discussed in this context include the following: telecommuter isolation, organizational loyalty, workaholism, promotional barriers to telecommuters, union objections, and inequity in allocating flex-work.

While the author of this work views flexible work as primarily a management strategy for all kinds of organizations (regardless of type of product, level of technology, or type of work force), he also offers considerable insight on how, from a social/psychological perspective, telecommuting transforms modern work relations and the meaning of work itself. See especially chapter 1 "Working in a Changing World," chapter 2 "What Is Flexible Work," chapter 5 "Challenges to Flexible Work," chapter 7 "The Technologies of Flexible Work," and selective chapters in part 2 of the book on "Implementing Flexible Work." The books also includes some case study material and suggestions for problem resolution.

333. Kusterer, Ken C. *Know-How on the Job: The Important Working Knowledge of "Unskilled" Workers*. Boulder, CO: Westview Press, 1978.

Keywords: alienation, knowledge embedded in experience, unskilled labor, Taylorism

Although this volume was written more than twenty years ago, its central insights remain of great relevance to healthy work research and the study of human-centered workplace design. The author notes that despite automation, bureaucratization, the ever narrower division of labor, and the influence of Taylorist industrial engineering, "today's 'unskilled' workers must acquire a substantial body of knowledge to survive and succeed on their jobs." Although this working knowledge is "indispensable to the production process . . . it is informally learned and generally unrecognized by anyone outside the workplace."

The author argues that "the unacknowledged existence of these valuable skills . . . helps to explain why the experience of alienation is a more complex and contradictory phenomenon than theorists have expected." The author concludes from his research that "alienated from management and its cost-minimizing, profit-maximizing goals, yet committed somehow to the workplace community and its goals of use-value production, the consciousness of these workers encompasses contradictory elements, causing a fundamental ambivalence toward their work situation and their own work activity."

These conclusions are derived from in-depth case studies conducted in a bank and a paper products factory and from interviews with a variety of workers, mostly women, in other blue- and white-collar work environments.

See especially chapter 1 "Introduction to the Research," chapter 2 "A Case Study of the Core Department of the Great Eastern Container Corporation," chapter 6 "Workers' Knowledge and Workers' Alienation," chapter 8 "Working Knowledge and Work Control," chapter 7 "Working Knowledge: A Summary Statement," and chapter 9 "Some Implications."

334. Lafferty, William M., and Eliezer Rosenstein, eds. *The Challenge of New Technology and Macro-Political Change*. International Handbook of Participation in Organizations for the Study of Organizational Democracy, Co-operation, and Self-Management 3. Oxford: Oxford University Press, 1993.

Keywords: participation, democracy, organizational change

This volume focuses on the issues of technology and worker participation "and the far-reaching macro-political influences on organizations in the 1980s and 90s. Several articles reflect the clear ideological shift where the values of workplace democracy and participation have been strongly challenged by demands for greater productivity, competition, and effectiveness. New perspectives and research findings are offered in relation to issues such as employment equity, stock ownership schemes, information technology, etc."

Contributions cover a broad spectrum of national contexts. Key papers relevant to healthy work have been abstracted in this annotated bibliography. See especially part 6 on "Participation and Technology."

335. Lammers, Cornelius J., and György Széll, eds. *Organizational Democracy: Taking Stock*. International Handbook of Participation in Organizations for the Study of Organizational Democracy, Co-operation, and Self-Management 1. Oxford: Oxford University Press, 1989.

Keywords: participation, history, democracy, comparative

"The overall objective of this series is to provide policymakers, practitioners and academics with works of reference on significant developments in participative practice in organizations. The fields covered include organization and democracy co-operatives, employee share ownership, job involvement, aspects of job design, codetermination, and the participative part of 'quality of work life' schemes."

This particular volume looks at how trends toward participation fared in the harsher conditions of the 1970s and 1980s after the tide of optimism prevailing in the 1950s and 1960s had ebbed. The contributors examine the economic, sociocultural, technological, and political forces at work over these years and analyze the influence they have exerted in this area. The general conclusion is that organizational democracy has not been balked but has in fact adapted its forms and structures alongside changes in society at large.

Part 1 of the text contains an evaluation and review of the field (i.e., participation models, worker co-ops, etc.). Part 2 looks at participative management in the United States; industrial democracy in Norway; and codetermination in Germany. Part 3 examines recent theoretical developments and research findings.

336. Lansbury, Russell, and Duncan Macdonald, eds. *Workplace Industrial Relations: Australian Case Studies*. Australian Studies in Labor Relations. Oxford: Oxford University Press, 1992.

Keywords: industrial relations, case study, unions

This volume presents the results of Australian case studies focusing on industrial relations at the workplace level. Five main issues are explored: "the influence of arbitration systems on workplace industrial relations, the nature of unionism at the plant level, the extent of management control at the workplace, the degree of incorporation of employees by management, and the extent and impact of recent attempts by management to increase efficiency on the shop floor." The case studies deal with a large paint manufacturer, a metal container company, a large residential hotel, an electronics communications company, an automobile assembly plant, and a large food retailing operation. The concluding essay provides an analysis of the existing literature on workplace industrial relations and integrates the findings from the case studies.

The authors note that in their research "the unions were not as influential as might have been expected in such highly unionized workplaces. . . . With some minor exceptions, neither union organizers nor delegates played a dominant role within the workplace." The authors also contend that "a complete exploration of workplace industrial relations requires and analysis of the impact of decisions made by a variety of parties such as corporate management, union leaders, and government officials who are 'beyond the workplace.'"

337. Lawler III, Edward E. *High-Involvement Management.* San Francisco: Jossey-Bass Publishers, 1986.

Keywords: QWL, management, participation

In changing times, people are looking for new ways to manage their workers. The question of whether participative management approaches can increase organizational performance is examined in this book. Part 1 "The Promise of Participative Management" sets out a framework on which other chapters are built by presenting some basic research on organizational effectiveness and potential advantages and disadvantages of participation. Chapter 3 focuses on the meaning of participative management and presents a way of predicting how effective the use of such approaches will likely be. Part 2 concentrates on what works and what doesn't in participative programs and begins in chapter 4 by describing the most popular participative management approach: quality circles. Chapter 5 looks at the use of attitude surveys as a part of such an approach. Job enrichment is the topic for chapter 6, while teams is the subject for chapter 7; both work toward involving people more in their work. In chapter 8 quality-of-work-life approaches to union-management relations are addressed, while chapter 9 examines gainsharing, and chapter 10 focuses on new design plants. In the last part of the book "High Involvement Management: Creating an Effective Approach to Participation," the author explains how high-involvement management works and describes how to manage the change to high-involvement organization. Although all chapters are informative, chapters 4, 6, 8, and 11 are particularly relevant.

338. Lawler, Edward E., Susan Albers Mohrman, and Gerald E. Ledford. *Employee Involvement and Total Quality Management: Practices and Results in Fortune 1000 Companies*. Jossey-Bass Management Series. San Francisco: Jossey-Bass, 1992.

Keywords: total quality management, participation

Proponents of employee involvement (EI) have long argued that it gives a competitive advantage and superior organizational performance to companies that adopt it. The authors of this extensive collection contend that despite the amount of research on the subject, "little systematic information exists on why companies are adopting EI, what types of practices they are adopting as part of their employee involvement programs, and how effective they think EI is." This volume attempts to answer these questions by assessing the results of EI practices in Fortune 1000 corporations.

This study also reports on changes over time in the adoption rate for employee involvement programs among large United States firms, as well as comprehensive data on who uses the programs. In short, the authors state that "the study provides the first systematic data on what is happening with respect to employee involvement trends in the United States." In addition, the relationship between EI programs and related strategies such as total quality management (TQM) is reviewed in detail. One of the benefits of this book, over and above its myriad of research insights, is that it uses a minimum of jargon, and complex statistical analyses are presented with simplicity.

See especially section 1 "Reasons for Studying Involvement Efforts," section 5 "Redistributing Power," section 10 "Success of Reward System Programs," section 12 "Results of Employee Involvement Programs" and section 20 "Plans for Adopting EI Practices." This is an outstanding book and an invaluable resource tool with many applications for the area of healthy work and prevention.

339. Le Blanc, Paul, ed. *The Working-Class Movement in America.* Amherst, NY: Humanity Books, 2000.

Keywords: working class, United States, history, labor movement, labor leaders

The contributors focus their attention on the conditions of the United States working class and the dynamic labor movement of the 1880s. A clear depiction is formed of the United States labor movement and working class at a time when the United States was becoming the world's leading manufacturing nation. Conditions in numerous workplaces and sectors of the labor force are described, all the while studying other important issues such as race, ethnicity, and gender issues, as well as social and economic realities that were destined to block the socialist developments.

340. Lechner, Viola M., and Michael A. Creedon. *Managing Work and Family Life.* Springer Series on Social Work. New York: Springer Publishing Co., 1994.

Keywords: social work, family

This handbook represents a significant contribution to the emerging field of occupational social work. It focuses on the changing needs of families and caregivers who are also faced with demands and responsibilities at work. The book identifies and discusses family-sensitive corporate- and government-sponsored programs and employee benefits, as well as policies directed toward increased employee satisfaction and well-being. The role of flextime, job-sharing and the compressed workweek in improving worker morale and productivity is also emphasized.

Chapter 1 "summarizes the major demographic, social, and economic changes that affect the work and family domains." Chapter 2 describes characteristics of the working caregivers of children, disabled adults, and elderly persons. Issues discussed include work stress, personal stress, work productivity and employer costs of employee caregiver roles. See chapter 4 for "an overview of family-focused benefits and services that have been adopted by corporations, unions, public, and not-for-profit organizations" (e.g., flexible work arrangements, childcare services, financial assistance programs, etc.). Chapter 5 describes the history, structure and function of employee assistance programs (EAPs) and member assistance programs (MAPs). Also see chapter 7 for a discussion of joint corporate and union responses to work and family issues.

341. Leidner, Robin. *Fast Food, Fast Talk: Service Work and the Routinization of Everyday Life*. Berkeley: University of California Press, 1993.

Keywords: routine work, case study

In the tradition of Barbara Garson's *The Electronic Sweatshop*, Robin Leidner presents a detailed field study of routinized work. The focus is on the service industry and on two companies in particular: McDonald's and Combined Insurance. Before providing a detailed analysis of how work is routinized in these two companies, Leidner sets forth the main obstacles to routinizing interactive service work in general and how to overcome them. For example, a variety of strategies are employed to standardize customer actions. As well, service is provided that appears to personalize routines so that resistance to mass-produced service can be overcome. Following the two case studies is a comparison of the two companies and the differing manager-worker-customer relations within them. The ramifications of routinized work on workers is the topic of the next chapter. What are the effects on workers' sense of self and gender identity? The concluding chapter asks what the routinization of service means to society and culture. Leidner argues that cultural norms, behavior and expectations are altered to work against individual identity and social cohesion.

342. Levi, L. *Stress in Industry: Causes, Effects and Prevention*. Geneva: International Labor Office, 1984.

Keywords: stress, prevention

This is a comprehensive analysis of stress induced diseases in various industrial occupations. The later emphasis in this book is on prevention, using an approach that is holistic, ecological, and systematic.

343. Levi, Lennart. "Work, Worker and Wellbeing: An Overview." *Work & Stress* 8, no. 2 (1994): 79-83.

Keywords: stress

The author summarizes the work as follows: "Work related psychosocial stressors originate in social structures and processes, affect humans through psychological (higher nervous) processes and influence health through four types of interrelated mechanisms—cognitive, emotional, behavioral, and physiological. The health outcome is modified by situational (e.g., social support) and individual factors (e.g., personality, coping repertoire). The work environment- stress-health system is dynamic, with many feedback loops. There is little, but increasing, direct evidence of a causal relationship between work-related psychosocial stressors and the incidence of occupational morbidity and mortality. However, a substantial body of indirect evidence strongly suggests that such associations exist and emphasizes the need to understand better their role. Accordingly, research and health action should aim at being systems-oriented, interdisciplinary, intersectoral, health- (and not only disease-) oriented, and participatory.

"In order to identify and monitor problems, and to evaluate presumably therapeutic and/or preventive action, we need well defined concepts within a theoretical model, and reliable and valid methods of measurement for all key components of this system. Our meeting, and the resulting proceedings (WHO 1991), form an attempt to contribute to this development that is furthered by the publication of this special edition of *Work and Stress*."

344. Levine, David I. *Reinventing the Workplace: How Business and Employees Can Both Win*. Washington, DC: Brookings Institution, 1995.

Keywords: work groups, total quality management, participation, work councils, productivity, job satisfaction

This book uses case studies and extensive empirical evidence "to show that greater employee involvement in the workplace can significantly increase both productivity and worker satisfaction." See Chapter 2 for an illustrative case study of worker participation at the NUMMI automobile plant, a joint venture between Toyota and GM (this chapter discusses the organization of "pilot teams," quality circles and new management strategies). Chapter 3 offers a look at employee empowerment through direct participation, work councils, employee motivation, training and employment security. Chapter 4 explores "Managerial, Union, and Business Partner Support." Topics include the following: Just-In-Time Delivery; Total Quality Management; and integrated employee involvement strategies. Chapter 7 discusses "Employee Involvement in Japan." This chapter offers an analysis of Japanese labor relations and external conditions affecting employee involvement. Also see chapter 8, on "Public Policies," for information on improving the efficiency of employee involvement, enhancing skills, worker training, education of workers and managers, and labor legislation.

345. Lewin, David, and Bruce Kaufman, eds. *New Research on Labor Relations and the Performance of University HR/IR Programs*. Advances in Industrial and Labor Relations 10. New York: JAI, 2001.

Keywords: union representation, airline industry, union wage determination, United States auto industry, grievance procedures, HR practices, education

There are five new studies that are presented on key dimensions of union-management relations. The topics that are examined by them include workplace innovation, financial consequences of unionism, wage determination, union representation, and conflict resolution in unionized enterprises in North America. As well, there are four papers that focus on university degree programs in human resource management and industrial relations and the extent to which programs provide students with the skills and competencies currently in demand by employers.

346. Lewis, P., ed. *Health Protection from Chemicals in the Workplace*. Ellis Horwood Series in Industrial Technology. Chichester: Ellis Horwood Limited, 1993.

Keywords: occupational health and safety

The intended audience of this book is managers and workers in the chemical industry and any other workplace where one may encounter potentially harmful chemicals. This book seeks to inform and give practical advice to these people in order to ensure healthier work environments.

The UK and international regulations regarding chemicals in the workplace are summarized in the first two chapters. The role of nongovernmental organizations in the field of occupational health and chemical safety are described in chapter 3. Four categories of NGOs are considered—major international organizations, international industry-supported organizations, national industry organizations, and academic and similar institutions. The focus of chapter 4 is on occupational health services. The objectives, benefits and preventive aspects of these services are presented. Practical information regarding staffing levels, recruitment methods, remuneration of staff and how to be cost-effective is also provided. Occupational health auditing, hazard assessment and assessment of health risks are covered in the three subsequent chapters. Chapters 8 through 14 deal with details of specific "preventive" health issues such as ventilation systems and personal protective equipment, methodological issues such as occupational exposure limits and sampling strategies, and various health effects including acute poisoning, dermatitis and chronic effects.

347. Lincoln, James R. *Culture, Control and Commitment: A Study of Work Organization and Work Attitudes in the United States and Japan*. Cambridge: Cambridge University Press, 1990.

Keywords: organizational behavior, job satisfaction, comparative, case study

This volume presents the findings of "a major survey investigation of the organizational, job and individual-level determinants of work attitudes, values, and behaviors among Japanese and United States manufacturing employees." As a large-scale, multi-level sociological study, it represents one of the largest and most comprehensive comparative research projects to date.

In the introduction, the author indicates that there has been an overwhelming convergence of interest on the part of industrial psychologists, organizational sociologists, labor process theorists and others regarding the importance of loyalty, identification and commitment in the work environment. To quote from the text, "global shifts in the internal structures and employment practices of companies are inducing fundamental changes in the ties that bind employees to the workplace. These shifts in turn are tied to transformations in worldwide economic and industrial organization."

The first chapter in the volume reviews "theories of work organization and the employment relationship and develops the concept of welfare corporatism as a commitment-maximizing organizational form." It also compares the nature of commitment with alternative attitudinal states such as job satisfaction and work alienation. Chapter 2 offers detailed methodology and research design information on the study, and chapter 3 reviews findings on United States-Japan differences in employee work attitudes and behaviors. Chapter 4 "examines the effects of employee position in the organization (authority position . . . quality circle participation, etc.), job rewards (both intrinsic and extrinsic) and task characteristics, etc." Chapter 5 considers the influences of employee work values and background characteristics such as age, gender, marital status, and education. Chapters 6 and 7 shift to the level of the organization and examine differences in production technologies, organizational structures and management styles between Japanese and United States firms. The final two chapters summarize the results of the investigation and construct a "multi-level model" of the commitment process.

For data related to preventive work strategies, see especially chapter 3 "Commitment and Job Satisfaction in the United States and Japan," chapter 4 "Job Attributes and Work Attitudes," chapter 6 "Technology, Society, and Organization," chapter 7 "Organizational Structures in Japan and the United States: A Plant Level Analysis," and chapter 9 "The Future of Welfare Corporatism in Japan and the United States."

348. Lindenfeld, Frank, and Joyce Rothschild-Whitt, eds. *Workplace Democracy and Social Change*. Boston: Porter Sargent Publishers, 1982.

Keywords: participation, job satisfaction

Job satisfaction is essential for our health, self-esteem and general well-being. However, recent studies show that job dissatisfaction is increasing. This book focuses on the lack of worker control throughout the entire labor process and perceives it to be the main source of the problem. Hierarchical control, under which the people who make decisions are different from those who complete the tasks, is very common in today's workplace. A collection of writings from people who have been able to create work organizations of a different form has been assembled in this book. Workplace democracy is examined both in large corporations as well as small worker-collectives. Topics such as worker participation, economic democracy, size of corporations, efficiency of organizations, institutionalization, community trust, auxiliary support, and many others are discussed. Numerous case studies are included as well.

349. Linder, Marc, and Ingrid Nygaard. *Void Where Prohibited: Rest Breaks and the Right to Urinate on Company Time*. Ithaca, NY: Cornell University Press, 1998.

Keywords: rest periods, hours of labor, employee rights, United States

The struggle for and the societal regulation of rest breaks is the main focus in this book. Issues such as why workers need rest periods, the origins of managerial promotion of rest periods for both sexes during World War I, empirical studies of fatigue, the rise and proliferation of various versions of scientific management in the United States and Europe, harmful physical effects of prohibiting employees from voiding when necessary, an overview of the enactment of special rest-periods statutes for women workers at the end of the nineteenth century, analysis from the 1920s to the 1970s over the effect of gender-specific labor-protective laws on equality between sexes, current rest and meal-period laws in the United States, the extent to which workers in the United States actually receive rest periods based on surveys of firms and collective bargaining agreements, and finally the development of a legal theory that supports a right to rest and void at work are all dealt with.

350. Lipnack, Jessica, and Jeffrey Stamps. *Virtual Teams: Reaching across Space, Time, and Organizations with Technology*. New York: John Wiley and Sons, 1997.

Keywords: virtual work teams, information technology, case study

This volume is about a radically new type of small group emerging within organizations via computer networks. The term "virtual teams" refers to these "boundary-spanning (both space and time) centers of people-to-people activity that are the social cells that make up larger network organizations. They are small task-oriented groups. . . . Webs of interactions and relationships bind them together." Essentially, the authors explore how "this most fundamental organization—the team—is transforming" (or "morphing," to use computer lingo), because of new computer capabilities, "into an extraordinary 21st century version." The book focuses on small groups of people working across boundaries supported by the new computer and communications technologies. The authors argue that while "technology extends our capabilities, organizing to do things together is still a human capability." The people side of the organization/technology relationship is the focus of *Virtual Teams*. See chapter 1 for an introduction to virtual teams, a definition, some examples of how companies use them in both low and high tech "versions," and an overview of the principles. Chapters 2 through 7 provide detailed case studies of six companies that utilize virtual teams. The sections at the end of these chapters offer an integrated conceptual framework for understanding and managing this new form of organization. Chapter 8 is a collection of suggestions for starting and maintaining virtual teams, and chapter 9 discusses some of the wider social implications of virtual teams.

351. Littek, Wolfgang, and Tony Charles. *The New Division of Labor: Emerging Forms of Work Organization in International Perspectives*. Berlin: Walter de Gruyter, 1995.

Keywords: division of labor, comparative, general, case study

This is a very comprehensive compilation of articles concerning the debate on the new division of labor, with contributors from many European countries as well as North America and Japan. The main theme of the book is emerging forms of work organization in international perspective. Some of the keywords that identify this new division of labor are: "skill enhancement, multi-skilling, team work, flexibility, flat hierarchies, trust networking, flexible technology, quality, and organizational learning."

The introduction to the book examines the characteristics of the new division of labor, new forms of work organization, and technology in relation to the new division of labor.

The chapters contained in part 1 deal with basic theoretical concepts and questions in the division of labor debate. Topics include the following: trust and its consequences for the coordination of work processes; the emergence of a new sociology of technology; the diffusion of new production concepts and their impact on new forms of work organization; gender and technology; the implications of globalization; and sociological theory and the concept of division of labor.

Part 2 compares various work structures in different countries. Topics discussed include the following: anthropocentric production systems in Europe, service work and the new division of labor, the role of engineers in the division of labor in France and Japan, and the lean production model.

Part 3 "presents case studies of new focus of work organization in different countries and different branches of the economy" in an effort to add to our theoretical and empirical understanding of the subject, from a comparative perspective. Topics covered in these chapters include the following: development of skilled white-collar work in Germany, the "reversal of feminization" of work in Portugal, cooperative work organization in Spain and Northern Italy, the difficulties of cooperation in the inter-firm division of labor, and changes in the labor process in the Finnish shipbuilding industry (a case study approach).

For implications regarding the development of healthy work concepts and preventive strategies see especially chapters 3, 4, 8, 9, 11, 15, and 18.

352. Littler, Craig R., ed. *The Experience of Work.* Aldershot, England: Gower Publishing Company, 1985.

Keywords: work design, case study, Taylorism, Fordism, forecasting, assembly line

The collection of essays put together for an Open University course ponders the human aspects of various work experiences. Section 1 "Work in Non-Industrial Societies" presents ethnographic studies of the Indian caste system and the Trobirand Islanders who garden and grow food for the community. A chapter is concerned with the introduction of time as a currency during industrialization. Chapter 5 informs readers that contrary to common beliefs, productive labor was not confined to the family.

Section 2 "Work in Modern Societies" is subdivided into sections on agricultural work, industrial work, professional work, housework and unemployment. The subsection on industrial work contains a particularly rich collection of essays relevant to healthy work. Life on the assembly line is described and analyzed. A case study of printers and the problems of deskilling and loss of knowledge embedded in experience that is taking place is also included. A chapter entitled "The Design of Jobs" traces the influences of Taylorism, Fordism and job redesign initiatives of the 1970s.

"Work in Non-Capitalist Societies" is the title of the third section and consists of studies of the U.S.S.R. and China.

Finally, "Working outside the Official Economy" is the focus of the last section. For many unemployed people, this is the answer. However, the informal economy cannot possibly employ all of the millions of people looking for work. The final chapter, "The Future of Work," suggests that the "collapse of work" is eminent because organizations are slimming their workforces and automation threatens to replace human workers.

353. Long, Bonita, and Sharon Kahn, eds. *Women, Work and Coping: A Multidisciplinary Approach to Workplace Stress*. Montreal and Kingston: McGill-Queen's University Press, 1993.

Keywords: stress, women, coping

This is one of a relatively small number of studies of workplace stress and coping that focus on women's experience. The editors argue that since "women face quantitatively more and qualitatively different sources of work-related stress than do men . . . research on this topic is essential if we are to understand the effect of employment of women's well-being." The fourteen chapters of the book range widely among issues concerning the individual, the workplace context, theoretical frameworks, policy and interventions, and research methods, as well as views and research that represent different disciplines, and both quantitative and qualitative methodologies. The contributors examine the sources of stress for employed women, the structural and psychosocial moderators of workplace stress, and the appraisals and coping strategies that mediate the stress outcome relationship.

Some of the major work-related stressors discussed in the book include the following: taking care of children and aging parents (for women who work outside the home), sex segregation of work roles, sex discrimination (in terms of salary and promotion), and sexual harassment. The chapters consider perspectives drawn from psychology, sociology, anthropology, and management sciences about women's ways of coping with work stress and the social and cultural context of women's work lives.

Sample chapter titles include the following: "Examining Gender in Organizational Relationships and Technological Change"; "Social Support and Coping of Employed Women"; "Perceived Control and Employed Men and Women"; "Neglected Methodological Issues in Employment Stress"; and "A Theoretical Integration of Women, Work, and Coping."

354. Lowe, Graham S., and Herbert C. Northcott. *Under Pressure: A Study of Job Stress*. Toronto: Garamond Press, 1986.

Keywords: stress, health, case study

The purpose of the book is to demonstrate that specific working conditions result in stress that causes psychological and physical ill health. After an overview of job stress and health concerns in chapter 1, the authors introduce a case study in chapter 2. Letter carriers and mail sorters in an Edmonton post office are investigated. Chapter 3 reports that the two groups of workers experienced very different levels of job stress. Mail sorting seems to be the more stressful job, and is considered the less desirable of the two jobs. Chapter 4 compares mail sorters who sort by hand and those who operate mechanized sorters in order to test the theory that routine, automated work is more stressful. This theory is clearly upheld in the Canada Post study. The findings of chapter 5 suggest that men and women performing the same jobs report almost identical experiences of stress. However, women are more likely to say that their jobs and families conflict and to experience instances of sexual discrimination and sexual harassment. "How Do Post Office Jobs Compare with Other Jobs?" This is the question addressed in chapter 6. The answer is that the Edmonton post office workers experience more stress and a lower quality of working life than the average worker. This leads to the issue of improving the workplace that is dealt with in the concluding chapter. Rather than settle for end-of-pipe solutions that help workers adjust to or deal better with stress, the authors, drawing on their own case study as well as on the existing literature, call for a fundamental reform of the workplace. This restructuring, they affirm, must involve provision of greater decision-making powers to workers as well as a more participatory role in designing less stressful workplaces.

355. Lundstrom, Eric. *The Psychology of the Physical Environment in Offices and Factories*. London: Cambridge University Press, 1986.

Keywords: work environment

The book provides an overview of current knowledge about the psychosocial influences of the physical environment in offices and factories on the basis of empirical research and relevant theory. Lundstrom proposes that people and their physical environments represent interdependent elements of systems and hence exert mutual influence. Of particular importance to the area of healthy work are chapter 4 "Psychological Processes" on stressors and performance and job satisfaction; chapters 5, 6, and 7 on the effects of lighting, temperature, air and noise; chapter 11 "Symbolic Workplace: Self-Identity and Status"; and chapters 12 and 13 on communication, support systems, and privacy and performance.

356. Lupton, T., ed. *Human Factors: Man, Machine and New Technology*. Bedford, UK: IFS Publishers, 1986.

Keywords: human factors, skills, automation, industrial relations, manufacturing

This book is about the interplay of human beings and machines, with particular reference to human factors and advanced manufacturing/information systems. The authors of this collection of essays maintain that "the particular design of machines and layouts is a highly significant influence on the nature of the jobs of those who operate, maintain, program, or monitor the machines." And, the effective operation of advanced technologies obviously involves human beings, thus the need for a comprehensive analysis of the human-machine interface.

Section 1 of the text considers general social and economic issues from a philosophical perspective. Topics covered include the following: problems of automation, technology trends, the future of control, and CAM production techniques and their effect on workers' skills.

Section 2 examines the human-machine interface. Issues discussed include the following: visual display technology, worker disablement and work organization; human factors considerations in facility maintenance; and modeling human motion.

See especially section 3 on job restructuring for material related to flexible manufacturing systems; information technology and productivity; industrial robots; and car assembly at the Volvo Kalman plant.

Section 4 offers research in the area of management relations and human factors, and section 5 looks at the relationship between new technology and employment policy. Section 6 focuses on industrial relations, trade unions and technological change.

357. Lynch, John, Niklas Krause, George A. Kaplan, Jaakko Tuomilehto, and Jukka T. Salonen. "Workplace Conditions, Socioeconomic Status, and the Risk of Mortality and Acute Myocardial Infarction: Kuopio Ischemic Heart Disease Risk Factor Study." *American Journal of Public Health* 87, no. 4 (1997): 617-22.

Keywords: health

The paper is summarized by the authors' abstract as follows: "*Objectives*. This study investigated whether the association between workplace conditions and the risk of all-cause and cardiovascular mortality and acute myocardial infarction differed by socioeconomic status.

"*Methods*. Prospective data were used to examine these associations in 2297 Finnish men, with adjustment for prevalent diseases and biological, behavioral, and psychosocial covariates, and stratified by employment status and workplace social support.

"*Results*. Elevated age-adjusted relative hazards for all-cause mortality were found for men who reported high demands, low resources, and low income; high demands, high resources, and low income; and low demands, high resources, and low income. Similar patterns were found for cardiovascular mortality. In contrast, elevated age-adjusted relative hazards for acute myocardial infarction were observed only in men who reported high demands, low resources, and low income. These results did not differ by level of workplace social support or employment status.

"*Conclusions*. The negative effects of workplace conditions on mortality and of myocardial infarction risk depended on income level and were largely mediated by known risk factors."

358. Machan, Tibor R., ed. *Morality and Work*. Stanford: Hoover Institution Press, 2000.

Keywords: moral and ethical aspects

Tibor Machan and his fellow contributors examine some of the special ethical dimensions of work. They also offer some controversial alternatives to conventional ways of understanding the labor market, by calling for a conceptual and actual merging of labor and management which would end centuries of pseudoconflict and thus any need for a Department of Labor and national right-to-work legislation. They suggest that minimum wage, subsidies, and price support measures violate freedom of choice for all traders in a free society. This work also reveals mandated employee benefits to be unfortunate labor market restrictions that actually harm workers and undermine the morality of the labor market, as well as show how policies set by federal agencies such as the Food and Drug Administration violate basic property or other individual rights and create a "drug lag" between different markets. *Morality and Work* questions why the right to organize and join labor unions should be one of the basic rights of workers, as well as what is the true purpose of government licensing. It is this licensing that allows vested interests to be favored, with some professions gaining, and others failing to gain, "lawfulness." What is held to be morally questionable is the way that employee legislation diminishes the freedom and responsibility of individuals to make decisions regarding their own welfare.

359. Mackay, Allen. *Team Up for Excellence*. Oxford: Oxford University Press, 1993.

Keywords: teams, work groups, comparative, policy

Teamwork can change the way business is done. It can result in increased customer satisfaction, productivity, revenues, decreased costs, empowerment of staff, and make the company a fun place to work. This conclusion was reached by the author after studying customer-responsive teams in New Zealand, USA, Britain, Germany, and Saudi Arabia. He denounces Taylorism and provides a how-to book on building, developing and rewarding teams. The worksheets and exercises make this a practical implementation tool. After discussing mistakes of the past and why teamwork leads to success, the implementation of teamwork is outlined in detail. The necessary steps are: (1) form a management team, (2) compile a list of current measurements (budgets, costs, office size, etc.) to (3) determine what the company was doing, (4) define what functions and tasks need to be done, (5) determine the type and style of environment, (6) determine the need for the Matrix and the form of the Matrix (a tool to organize tasks, functions and skills), (7) determine the need for the Personal Skills Matrix and determine the roles of team leaders, (8) determine the staff numbers and skills required, (9) determine the need for the tasks and, through the staff, determine the resultant JPGs (Job Performance Guide) for all tasks, and (10) determine training that would be ongoing, and determine the types, responsibilities and impacts of training.

360. Magjuka, R. J. "Survey: Self-Managed Teams Achieve Continuous Improvement Best." *National Productivity*, Winter 1991-1992: 51-57.

Keywords: teams

The author introduces the article as follows: "Managers concerned with enhancing productivity and quality in their organizations want to know how to get the most from employee improvement programs (EIPs). But before they can do so, they need to understand EIP design and purpose. This article reports the findings of a national survey of EIP make-up and goals."

361. Majchrzak, Ann. *The Human Side of Factory Automation: Managerial and Human Resource Strategies for Making Automation Succeed.* Jossey-Bass Management Series. San Francisco: Jossey-Bass Publishers, 1988.

Keywords: automation, job satisfaction

This book outlines a range of strategies critical to the successful integration of automated factory systems with their human managers and operators. The author begins by noting the characteristics that distinguish flexible factory automation from conventional equipment and then emphasizes that "these are characteristics that demand people: to aid the integration process, to ensure appropriate equipment reactions to the feedback and to respond immediately to unpredictable events. Thus, the human infrastructure is an essential element of flexible factory automation."

Chapter 2 provides a framework for identifying and selecting "those components of the human infrastructure that need to be analyzed when considering the implementation of automated manufacturing technology (AMT)"—components such as job design, personnel policies, management responsibilities and organizational structure. This chapter also includes a valuable methodology for systematically assessing the effects of the new technology on the workers, managers and the organization. Referred to as the Human Infrastructure Impact Statement (HIIS), this would appear to be an important tool for determining "the extent of change needed in the human infrastructure" and for guiding "the user's choice of AMT equipment." Appendix A has additional information.

Chapter 3 discusses the specific role of operators involved in flexible factory automation and offers a variety of different strategies that are appropriate for coordinating "direct labor." The utility of the scientific management approach for AMT jobs is discredited, and in its place the author proposes more flexible designs such as systematic human-machine systems and work teams.

Other designs reviewed here include job enlargement, job rotation, ergonomics, and the sociotechnical systems approach.

See also part 3 of the text "Second-Order Effects: Organizational Adaptations to Job Changes" for details on new job skills and various selection criteria.

362. Marcson, Simon, ed. *Automation, Alienation, and Anomie.* New York: Harper and Row Publishers, 1970.

Keywords: alienation, general

Various facets of the debate on the consequences of automation and its relation to alienation and anomie are presented in this classic collection. How accurate are the early theoretical expectations that industrialization would lead to alienated industrial workers living in communities undermined by anomie? The papers in part 1 "Technological Change as an Aspect of Social Change" all agree on the significance of the changes but present a variety of views as to what the consequences of the changes are. Part 2 discusses the principles of automation and its significance to the process of industrialization. One of the consequences of automation is organizational change. The change in automobile plants, white-collar workplaces and the corporation are examined in part 3. Not only organizational changes but also changes in industrial relations are inevitable. This is the point argued in part 4, with an emphasis on clerical and other white-collar work. Part 5 looks at types of changes resulting from automation. It considers "The Impact of Automation on Enterprise, Management, and the Occupational Structure." Part 6 begins with Melvin Seeman's article "On the Meaning of Alienation" that provides an analysis of the various definitions and interpretations of the term alienation. These varying meanings are applied to the study of the relationship between the machine, worker and engineer, of industrialization, of the automobile assembly-line worker and of leisure time.

363. Marsella, Anthony J. "Migration, Ethnocultural Diversity and Future Worklife: Challenges and Opportunities." *Scandinavian Journal of Work, Environment and Health* 23, supplement 4 (1997): S28-S46.

Keywords: migration, population, ethnocultural diversity, poverty, security, status, power

As the title suggests, the author discusses "the relationship of migration, poverty, and ethnocultural diversity to future worklife, especially the challenges and opportunities that emerge when people from different racial and cultural groups are required to work competitively in pursuit of wealth, security, status, power, and survival." Marsella maintains that "major global social, political, and economic forces (such as sizeable world population increases, endless south-north and east-west migration, endemic world poverty, inequities in the distribution of wealth and resources, and scores of low-intensity regional wars) must be considered as we pursue our efforts to understand, clarify, and define 'future worklife' because they will ultimately shape and direct it, and overwhelm in importance the local forces at each workplace." The author further states, "To the extent that we choose to recognize and respond to these global forces, we can perhaps participate in choosing our future. To the extent we avoid them, our future may be determined by a limited number of corporate and government people whose visions and concerns are more narrow and self-serving." The paper makes the point that workers from different racial groups and cultural traditions are encountering one another in the contemporary workplace with greater frequency each day as global forces unfold. "And in each microcosmic racial and cultural encounter, there are the macrocosmic issues of power, equality, opportunity, responsibility, justice, and survival. Ultimately, exploring the interface of migration, ethnocultural diversity, poverty, and future worklife raises some of the most vexing and important political, social, economic, and moral questions of our time. . . . There may be immediate answers to the problems of improving employee productivity, morale, and health in a culturally pluralistic workplace, but there are no easy answers to the larger social and moral questions regarding our responsibilities to one another as world citizens."

364. Marsh, Robert M., and Hiroshi Mannari. *Modernization and the Japanese Factory*. Princeton, NJ: Princeton University Press, 1976.

Keywords: sociology, machinery, industrial relations, Japan

This classic study of complex Japanese industrial organizations seeks to explore the validity of the convergence theory of modernization. The authors contend that the theory, as applied to the level of complex organizations, would predict a convergence in the social organization of Japanese and western firms. "On social structural and technological grounds, theory would lead us to expect large, successful Japanese firms to be relatively modernized in their social organization and to be becoming more so." The authors state that "one widely known model of the Japanese firms—the paternalism-lifetime commitment model of the Japanese firms—denies this, and argues instead for an anti-convergence theory." In an effort to test the validity of one theory or the other, the research study examines and relates three sets of variables at the level of the industrial manufacturing firm—technological modernization, the modernization of social organization, and organizational performance.

The authors' position is that "the paternalism-lifetime commitment model exaggerates the uniqueness, uniformity, and traditionalism of the social organization of Japanese firms; that the most successful firms have in fact moved in the direction of more modern organizational structure; and that those firms that have not moved in this direction will exhibit significant organizational strains."

365. Marshall, Edward M. *Transforming the Way We Work: Power of the Collaborative Workplace.* New York: Amacom, 1995.

Keywords: work ethic, collaboration, management

With the ultimate goal of improving the way we work and the conditions and environment within which we work, the author leads us along a path toward understanding the collaborative workplace. The framework required for understanding collaboration is laid out in part 1 in terms of what it is, how it works and what a collaborative workplace looks like. Also addressed are the changes arising from such a different perspective on workplace design and management regarding all aspects of business. Topics covered are culture wars and their competing values; core values of the collaborative work ethic; creating a responsible work environment; core operating agreements; the operating agreements process; collaborative leadership in terms of roles, responsibilities, behavior, and steps to achieving good leadership; the strategic alignment method and implementation; and creating collaborative teams. Part 2 presents a means to create and manage such a workplace in terms of the power embodied in workplace culture, defining and applying the collaborative method, and managing the transition.

366. Marshall, Judi, and Cary L. Cooper, eds. *Coping with Stress at Work.* Aldershot, UK: Gower, 1981.

Keywords: stress, coping

Although this collection of articles was assembled more than twenty years ago, its insights regarding stress management and reduction are still relevant. "Both preventive and remedial possibilities are covered in this volume."

The first part on training (particularly chapter 1 by Melhuish) focuses on the importance of training management to assist the individual at work by equipping him or her with "more skills or physical resilience to stress as prevention."

The second part "Promoting Good Physical and Mental Health" discusses a variety of methods useful in promoting good physical and mental health, such as exercise, relaxation techniques, etc.

The third part of the book emphasizes remedial action to help the individual cope with stress. Occupational health and counseling are dealt with as effective strategies in several work environment contexts.

The final part of the book, "Changing the Environment," is probably the strongest and most useful in terms of advancing long-term structural change and improved quality of working life. This section moves away from individually-oriented action toward environmental/organizational factors of stress. Two case studies on participative job redesign are discussed, along with the role of legislative action in preventing/reducing work-related stress.

367. Marshall, Victor W., Walter R. Heinz, Helga Kruger, and Anil Verma, eds. *Restructuring Work and the Life Course.* Toronto: University of Toronto Press, 2001.

Keywords: sociological aspects, industrial sociology

The structure of people's lives are changed by the work they engage in due to the combining influence of economic, technological, and demographic forces. The defining features of life, including patterns of entry to and exit from work, are shifting, as is the nature of jobs and careers. This collection of essays examines changes in the organization of work and their impact on people at various stages of the life course. The scholars examine the influence of economic, technological, and demographic forces on public, corporate, and union policies concerning the organization of work. The topics covered include education, labor market change, and transitions in the early and middle stages of the working life course, later life transitions in relation to the restructuring of work and retirement, and various aspects of the relationship between individual biography and social structure with close attention given to family and gender issues over the life course.

368. Martin, T., ed. *Proceedings of the IFAC Workshop.* Karlsruhe: Pergamon Press, 1983.

Keywords: work design, automation, CNC, participation

Small and medium sized firms are the focus of this conference's discussion regarding alternative work designs appropriate for automated manufacturing systems. Many of the papers are case studies of experiments in alternative work design. The papers in session 1 are concerned with computer numerical control (CNC) and work design, while session 2 deals with general work design principles. Alternative work organizations such as flexible automation, flexible manufacturing systems, integrated CAD/CAM systems and consideration of social aspects are pondered in session 3. Session 4 contains a paper each on the autonomous production cell and the autonomous production island. Session 5 contemplates the issue of participation in design. It includes a noteworthy paper entitled "Participatory Job Design and Automation: Unanticipated Side Effects" wherein the relationship between increasing automation at work and participation is examined on the basis of two case studies. The last two sessions discuss robots and trends and effects of flexible automation.

369. Martin, T., J. Kivinen, J. E. Rijnsdorp, M. G. Rodd, and W. B. Rouse. "Appropriate Automation: Integrating Technical, Human, Organizational, Economic and Cultural Factors." *Automatica* 27, no. 6 (1991): 901-17.

Keywords: human factors, sociotechnical design, computers

Automation technology, including digital computer and communication techniques, is being applied in an ever increasing range of private and public spheres; and reaching third world cultures not previously exposed to such technology. It is the responsibility of engineers to consider the direct and indirect effects of this technology. To be able to fulfill this responsibility and make proper design decisions, engineers must both understand "appropriateness" within a given boundary and have decision authority, together with other parties participating in the design. Whereas sound methodologies for user-centered design are appearing, anticipating and considering the cultural effects of automation are concerns that go far beyond traditional engineering. Nevertheless, engineers should be more deeply involved in comprehensive technology assessment. Encouraging experiences show how innovative design approaches and consideration of comprehensive sets of requirements can lead to better overall system performance. However, much research on open questions remains to be done.

370. Matteson, Michael T., and John M. Ivancevich. *Controlling Work Stress: Effective Human Resource and Management Strategies*. Jossey-Bass Management Series. San Francisco: Jossey-Bass, 1987.

Keywords: stress, coping, health, mental health

This book begins by underlining the fact that "managers have come to accept the notion that physical and mental health problems can adversely affect productivity," but, at the same time, "managers tend to ignore or reject the proposition that work itself can have an adverse effect on physical and mental health."

Various strategies are offered throughout the text for managing and mitigating occupational stress. Emphasis is given to preventive strategies and methods of effective control.

Chapter 3 examines the sources of work stress (both from within and outside the organization), not to present a systematic list and analysis of stressors but simply to point out their ubiquitous nature. Chapter 4 discusses how stress affects employee health and job performance. Chapter 7 looks at improving individual-organizational relationships. Topics considered include the following: recruitment and selection processes, socialization programs, and career planning and development. Chapter 8 explores the shaping of organizational policies and programs to reduce stress. Topics include the following: stress management programs, organizational-level programs, work scheduling, and survey-feedback systems. Chapter 9 considers techniques for helping individuals control stress more efficiently.

371. Matthews, Gerald, D. Roy Davies, Stephen J. Westerman, and Rob B. Stammers. *Human Performance: Cognition, Stress and Individual Differences*. Philadelphia: Taylor and Francis, 2000.

Keywords: performance psychology, attention and work, human error, stress, arousal and performance, thermal stress and other physical stressors, health, diet, drugs, age, fatigue in relation to work performance

Four sections are used in this book to provide the reader with a comprehensive and accessible review of both performance in the real world and essential cognitive science theory. The first section outlines varying perspectives on performance offered by contemporary cognitive science, including information processing and neuroscience perspectives. The second section studies human error and the following section is linked by reviewing the impact that stress factors such as noise, fatigue, and illness have on work performance. The fourth section assesses individual and group differences in work performance in relation to aging, ability, and personality.

372. McCann, Michael W. *Rights at Work: Pay Equity Reform and the Politics of Legal Mobilization*. Language and Legal Discourse. Chicago: University of Chicago Press, 1994.

Keywords: pay equity, law and legislation, history, social movements, social problems

In his book, Michael McCann explores the political strategies behind more than two dozen pay equity struggles around the nation since the late 1970s, including the conflicts of city employees in San Jose and Los Angeles, as well as of state employees in Washington and Connecticut. By using interviews with over 140 union and feminist activists, it is shown that even when the courts failed to entirely correct wage discrimination, litigation and other forms of legal advocacy provided reformers with the legal discourse (the understanding of legal rights and their constraints) for defining and advancing their cause. This book allows for insight into the relation between law and social change.

373. McKenzie, Jon. *Perform or Else: From Discipline to Performance*. New York: Routledge, 2001.

Keywords: performance, psychological aspects, cultural/ organizational/ technological performance

In studying the relationships between cultural, organizational, and technological performance, an uncanny relationship was observed: all three paradigms can operate together to create powerful and contradictory pressures to perform. The conclusion states that performance will be to the twentieth and twenty-first centuries what discipline was to the eighteenth and nineteenth centuries. This will, as a result, affect future inquiries into globalized power and knowledge.

374. McLoughlin, Ian. "CAD: 'Taylorisation' of Drawing Office Work?" *New Technology, Work and Employment* 4, no. 1 (1989).

Keywords: Taylorism, CAD

Computer Aided Design has been described as a Trojan horse through which drawing office work will be deskilled. This article rebuts the crude Taylorisation thesis that underlies such views and offers an alternative analysis of the effects of CAD.

375. McLoughlin, Ian, and Jon Clark. *Technological Change at Work.* 2nd ed. Buckingham: Open University Press, 1994.

Keywords: human resources, technology

The specific focus of this book is on "technological change in its most pervasive and significant contemporary guise: new computing and information technologies." The central argument starts from the assumption that the process of technological change in organizations involves a number of distinct stages. "At each stage issues arise which involve actors in making choices that are likely to be constrained by a range of 'extreme' factors and also contested and modified over time by other organization members." In other words, say the authors, "technological change involves a process of choice and negotiation."

Chapter 1 explores the significance of computing and information technologies. It also assesses the changes in some of the principle sectors of employment in which this technology is being introduced. Chapter 2 considers four contrasting perspectives that have been applied to the analysis of technological change at work. These are "contingency theory," "labor process" theory, the "flexible specialization" thesis, and the "social action" or "strategic choice" approach. Chapter 3 examines the role of management decision making when new technology is introduced. Chapter 4 looks at the role of trade unions in the innovation process, in particular the extent to which the introduction of computing and information technology has been subject to collective bargaining. Chapter 5 analyzes in detail the influence of new computing and information technologies on the core of work: tasks and skills. Chapter 6 delves into job content and work organization. Chapter 7 explores the manner in which choice and negotiation have shaped forms of control and supervision around computing and information technology.

376. Menzies, Heather. *Whose Brave New World? The Information Highway and the New Economy*. Toronto: Between the Lines, 1996.

Keywords: unemployment, technology, Canada

This is a well-researched Canadian account of technological restructuring and its social and economic effects. After documenting the various implications of advanced computer technology for employment/unemployment patterns, power and control in the workplace, and the individual's experience in society, the author "offers positive suggestions for reviving public debate on the new economy and the information highway, pointing the way to meaningful employment and participation."

Part 1 of the text sets out the main argument—namely "that social spending cuts and deficit reduction are not the key issues of the day . . . restructuring . . . is geared to the interests and needs not of the people, but of corporate economic renewal and global expansion." The introductory chapters describe the disintegration of society being caused by technological restructuring. Topics discussed here include deskilling; the demeaning of work; computers and the centralization of control; and the creation of a global system economy.

Part 2 provides background and critical evidence about "the link between restructuring and a high unemployment rate, jobless economic growth, and a two-tiered labor force with a new near-underclass of people who work only as operatives of computer systems that control and monitor everything they do."

Part 3 of the book offers suggestions for positive future change that will foster human-centered technological systems that are responsive to human social and economic needs.

377. Milkman, Ruth. *Farewell to the Factory: Auto Workers in the Late Twentieth Century*. Berkeley: University of California Press, 1997.

Keywords: automotive industry, lean production

The situation of factory auto workers has improved somewhat over time, although unions are still fighting for better working conditions, better treatment by management, more respect, and a larger decision-making latitude. This book describes the situation of the past and present directly from the experience of the workers themselves. The introduction gives a brief presentation of the ongoing struggle to change the way American plants work their assembly lines, and how those involved have felt and responded along the way. Chapter 2 leads the reader back into the past to get a feel for life as an auto worker in the postwar period under the traditional system at GM-Linden. In chapter 3, the role of the United Auto Workers Union (UAW) in the postwar system is addressed, as well as how this union was affected by the dramatic transformations of the 1980s, many of which were adversarial in nature. Chapter 4 examines cases like those of two GM workers who left the factory itself, at Linden's workforce, and how the new technology and industrial relations introduced in the 1980s are affecting the workers. Additionally, it should be noted that this book contains a criticism of lean production and work.

378. Mishel, Lawrence, Jared Bernstein, and John Schmitt. *The State of Working America 2000-2001*. Ithaca, NY: Cornell University Press, 2001.

Keywords: family income, wages, gender, age, sex, unemployment/ employment, wealth/poverty

There have been three new developments in the realm of working America that have taken place at the turn of the century: the development of rapid wage growth; an acceleration in the growth of labor productivity, meaning the increase of the value of the goods and services that an average worker produces in an hour of work; and lastly the change in the shape of wage inequality. The main task of this book is to document and explain these important new features of the economy.

379. Moch, Michael M., and Jean Bartunek. *Creating Alternative Realities at Work: Quality of Work Life Experiment at Foodcom*. New York: Harper and Row, 1990.

Keywords: QWL, organizational design, quality circles

The book analyzes the failure and success of QWL programs in terms of the differing cognitive structures of the various parties involved, such as unions and management. It suggests that the potential for organizational change is connected to the idea that all of us, including organizations, have cognitive schemata or paradigms that form and guide our behavior.

380. Moody, Kim. *Workers in a Lean World: Unions in the International Economy*. London: Verso Press, 1997.

Keywords: unions, comparative, labor movement

This volume offers a comprehensive study of current labor relations worldwide, in the context of the global power of transnational capital. The author provides "a measured assessment of multinational management's strategies to downsize, introduce flexible production and compel workers to accept less pay for more work." He emphasizes the need, in the face of these changes, for renewal and international coordination among national unions. Examples from North America, Latin America, Europe, and Asia are presented in terms of the extent to which this has been achieved. The author also gives a compelling argument against the conventional wisdom that accepts the irresistible power of globalization. The author maintains that "[t]his book does not offer some simple formula for creating a full-blown international labor movement. Instead it looks at the roots and structures of globalization, their impact on the working classes of different parts of the world, and the most recent working-class responses to the lean regime in the workplace, the global jobs crisis, government-imposed austerity, and the general decline in working-class living standards around the world. The book also looks at the difficult problems associated with the increased differentiation within the working class that results from massive immigration, older racial conflicts cast in new economic molds, the rise of women as a proportion of the workplace, and the changing stratification of the workplace." The position advocated here by the author, known as "social movement unionism," is pitted against the old argument that "a rising tide lifts all ships." Moody maintains that this "has never been convincing to those trapped in steerage. . . . The rising tide must offer the opportunity to reduce and eliminate the old inequalities."

381. Mowshowitz, Abbe. "Social Dimensions of Office Automation." 335-404 in *Advances in Computers*. New York: Academic Press, 1986.

Keywords: computers, automation, health, QWL, industrial policy, organizational design

This is a classic study of office automation from every imaginable aspect—from basic definitions to costs, skills, career paths, health and safety, computer crime, ethics, QWL, policy and others.

382. Mumford, Enid. *Systems Design: Ethical Tools for Ethical Change*. London: Macmillan Press, 1996.

Keywords: QWL, automation, ethics, technology, organizational design ethics, systems, work design, sociotechnical, human-centered

Work systems should be beneficial to humans as well as technically sound, the author states. How to go about creating such ethical work systems is the subject of this publication. It focuses on the ethical choices that system designers must make. The first chapter provides a historical overview of industry, technology and systems design. Next, Mumford examines the role of the moral leader and strategies to assist in the ethical approach by studying how philosophers and biologists view the notion of ethics. Also contained in this chapter are sets of questions for the systems designer to ask when designing high quality work systems. Chapter 3 "Systems Design in an Unstable Environment" deals with poor employer-employee relationships in recent years and how an ethical systems designer can remedy the situation. Mary Parker Follett was a revolutionary business administrator who wrote about employee participation to improve productivity. Her ideas are the subjects of chapter 4. The fifth chapter provides an excellent history and summary of sociotechnical design. Increased freedom for employees can improve the quality of work life, as argued in chapter 6. The concluding chapter integrates the earlier material to provide practical advice on how to design a human-centered system. Appendix A discusses the ETHICS method that "consists of a set of logical, sequential, and analytical steps that are taken when a new computer-based work system is being designed." Appendix B presents a case study of a sociotechnical design approach being applied to the reengineering of a company.

383. Muntaner, Charles, and Patricia J. O'Campo. "A Critical Appraisal of the Demand/Control Model of the Psychosocial Work Environment: Epistemological, Social, Behavioral and Class Considerations." *Social Science and Medicine* 36, no. 11 (1993): 1509-17.

Keywords: stress

"This paper presents a critique of the demand/control model of the psychosocial work environment" that has long been the dominant construct for explaining the relationship between the psychosocial features of work organization (such as low decision-making power and high work demands) and health (most notably cardiovascular disease). The authors acknowledge the importance of the model "because it provides an integrative conceptual framework for the study of occupational stress."

However, they also discuss the limitations of the demand/control model by introducing "the relevance of the historical development of constructs in the field of social psychology," epistemology, behavioral science and sociology. They suggest that the demand/control model could be improved "through use of objective methods of assessing the work environment, incorporating worker input, and avoidance of a strictly disease-specific approach." Finally, it is argued in the paper that the demand/control model "would benefit from an integration with sociology," through the addition of new determinants of individual health such as social class "and its related historical and global changes affecting the labor process (e.g., 'deskilling' of labor)."

384. Murphy, Lawrence R., Joseph J. Hurrell Jr., and Steven L. Sauter, eds. *Job Stress Interventions*. Washington, DC: American Psychological Association, 1995.

Keywords: stress, coping, unemployment, health, policy

This volume investigates stress management training, the promotion of coping strategies among unemployed workers, and help for workers who experience post-traumatic stress disorder as a result of their job. It also presents some promising new developments that enable interventions to be made at the organizational level and thus promote organizational health. Finally, the book examines policy and legislation issues such as workers' compensation claims, the development of occupational stress standards, and occupational welfare in the European Community.

In part 1 "Stress Management Training," see especially chapter 1 "Effects of Instruction on Stress Management Skills and Self-Management Skills among Blue-Collar Employees," chapter 3 "When Relaxation Is Not Enough," and chapter 6 "Worksite Health Promotion." In part 2 "Coping with Job Stress and Unemployment," see chapter 10 "When Couples Cope with Job Loss" and chapter 11 "Coping with Job Loss and Career Stress." Also see the section entitled "The Work Setting." Sample chapter titles include the following: "Diagnosing a Healthy Organization: A Proactive Approach to Stress in the Workplace"; "Redesigning Work Systems to Reduce Stress: A Participatory Action Approach"; "The Prevention of Job Stress by Redesigning Jobs and Implementing Self-Regulating Teams"; and "Interventions for Building Healthy Organizations." Under "Policy and Legislation," see "Appraising Occupational Stress-Related Disorders" and "Developing an Occupational Stress Standard."

385. Mustard, J. Fraser. "The Economy and Social Equity in a Period of Major Technoeconomical Change." *Scandinavian Journal of Work, Environment and Health* 23, supplement 4 (1997): S10-S15.

Keywords: technology, information technology, health, job security

The author attempts "to integrate some of our knowledge about technological change, economic growth, stability of social environments, work, and the health and well-being of populations." It is argued that one of the best markers of a prosperous and civic society is the overall health and well-being of the population. The author further maintains, "We are currently in a period of major technological change in which some believe that the developed countries of the West could disrupt the social balance and stability of their societies and thus produce unstable intolerant undemocratic societies with adverse effects on health and well-being." After outlining some of the major characteristics of the information (or "chips for neurons") revolution that is changing the socioeconomic character of society, Mustard suggests that it is crucial for a society to integrate its economic and social policies and take into account what we now know about the effects of deep and broad technological change on the determinants of health. This is necessary in order to avoid increased income inequality, deteriorated social environments, and unstable, uncivil societies. An extensive list of measures that can be undertaken now to determine how well we are coping with this period of profound technoeconomic change is offered. A few of the more significant of these suggestions include the following: "Design and use a real measure of economic growth. . . . Put in place policies that create incentives to build the new economy. . . . Develop and use measures that combine estimates of economic growth, new ways to use resources, and changes in social environments. . . . Make the state of children the highest socioeconomic priority during this period of change. . . . Take steps to avoid creating an underclass that excludes individuals from being participants in society. . . . Ensure that government programs help sustain cohesive civic communities."

386. Naschold, Frieder et al. *Constructing the New Industrial Society*. Stockholm: Assen Van Gorcum, 1993.

Keywords: work design, democracy, organizational change

In this volume, chapter 4 "The Kaleidoscope of Workplace Reform" is of the greatest relevance for healthy work issues and the application of preventive strategies in the work environment. The author begins by noting that the objectives of the work reform movement ("the development of both the democratization of work and the economic performance of the enterprise") have remained constant for approximately the last forty years. Research carried out during this period, says the author, has established that "participation and productivity are not mutually exclusive phenomena but are positively correlated."

An overview of workplace reform programs is provided, indicating "milestones and other features in the history of the development of new forms of work organization." Major initiatives discussed include the following: "action research" on different management styles conducted by Lewin, Lippitt and White in the late 1930s; the seminal studies carried out by the British Tavistock Institute in the 1940s; the sociotechnical system approach of the 1950s; the participative design model of the mid-1970s; and the Swedish LOM program (1985-1990) on "participation and efficiency."

Also offered is a summary description of the characteristics that differentiate the "Old and New Organizational Paradigms" (see figure 1 on page 174).

Section 2 of the chapter discusses "Today's Challenges: Ambiguities of Participative Democracy" from the perspective of the individual, the organization and society. The question of whether it is possible to "break through the vicious circle of neo-corporatism and bureaucracy" is also considered. Finally, the author examines the "action research" construct in terms of theoretical and methodological issues and problems.

387. Natale, Samuel M., and Brian M. Rothschild, eds. *Values, Work, Education: Meanings of Work*. Amsterdam: Rodopi, 1995.

Keywords: health, psychology, culture, work ethic, case study

This collection of essays provides a rather novel approach to the subject of work and health. The authors attempt to grapple with the various meanings of work by adopting a much broader perspective than is normally the case in this field of study. Topics related to work ethics and morality, values and work, and the role of education in forming attitudes toward work are examined from philosophical, sociological and psychological vantage points.

The introduction to the volume considers the multiple meanings that derive from both the nature of work and the attitudes of workers toward that work. The authors conclude that "no unified definition appears evident."

A brief historical overview of definitions of work is offered, with an emphasis on the Protestant work ethic and the Judaic tradition.

The major reasons for which people work are discussed, as are the ways in which the role of work has changed, especially since the 1960s. The authors suggest that in the last forty years "an extension of freedom from constraints" and "an expansion of rights . . . has led to a decline in educational attainment, labor productivity, and family stability culminating in social disorder."

Also examined is the challenge of restoring a work ethic that includes "the ideals of thrift, industry, diligence and perseverance." See especially chapter 2 "The Role of Affect and the Role of Unconscious Processes in the Prevention of Work Related Psychosomatic Disorders," chapter 9 "Work Rewards: Complementary and Conflicting Distributive Demands," chapter 10 "United States-Japan Comparative Labor Laws: Question of Ethics," chapter 12 "The Cooperative Association and the Community of Work," and chapter 14 "Values at Work: A Case Study in Business."

388. National Academy of Engineering—Commission on Behavioral and Social Sciences and Education, National Research Council. *People and Technology in the Workplace*. Washington, DC: National Academy Press, 1991.

Keywords: technology, computers, case study, organizational change, automation

This volume examines many of the factors that are critical to the successful introduction of computers and other advanced technologies into the workplace. A wide range of essays by professionals in technological innovation, managers and union representatives, as well as engineers and consultants offers practical information for those interested in effectively merging human and technological resources. Reasons for the United States lagging behind many other countries in the introduction of technology are also considered. "Case studies document successful transitions to new systems and procedures in manufacturing, medical technology, and office automation—ranging from the Boeing Company's program to involve employees in decision making and process design, to the introduction of alternative work schedules for Mayo Clinic nurses, to the United States Forest Service's introduction of one of the nation's largest multifunction computer systems. This volume will be a practical resource for managers, researchers, faculty, and students in the fields of industry, engineering design, human resources, labor relations, sociology, and organizational behavior."

See especially "A Case History of Organizational Change: People and New Technology" by James Hettenhaus, "Integrating New Tools into Information Work: Technology Transfer as a Framework for Understanding Success" by T. K. Bikson and J. D. Eveland, and "Introducing a Computer-Based Human Resource System into the United Way" by Robert Krassman.

389. National Research Council of Canada. *The Social Context of Artificial Intelligence: A Guideline and Discussion Paper*. NRCC no. 30187. Ottawa: Associate Committee on Artificial Intelligence, 1989.

Keywords: artificial intelligence, policy, ethics

This government report examines artificial intelligence (AI) from the social point of view. It provides a protocol for assessing AI applications in the areas of robotics, machine translation, natural language processing, expert systems (such as those used in the diagnosis and treatment of disease, industrial plants, telecommunications, etc.), and operations scheduling and process planning. The authors of the report note, "If the applications of AI become as widespread as some advocates believe, or if even only partially so, its influence will be significant on the daily lives of a large number of people. A purpose of this report is to show in what ways this may happen, and to suggest how the benefits may be maximized while minimizing any undesirable effects." The authors further hope that "our understanding of artificial intelligence will be enhanced, and that the selection and design of AI applications will be undertaken with an improved understanding of the social considerations attached to them in addition to those considerations of a business and technical nature."

See especially section 2 "Social Consequences Arising from Artificial Intelligence." Topics discussed include the following: impact of computers on work; privacy concerns; decision making and AI; AI applications and social organization (with case study examples); regulatory bodies; the accreditation of AI products; codes of ethics, etc. Also see section 3 "Social Considerations Arising from Other Information Technologies." Topics considered here include the following: office and factory automation; organizational changes; and macro and societal changes. Section 4 offers "A Protocol for the Examination of Artificial Intelligence Applications from the Social Point of View" and section 5 provides policy recommendations. See appendix 1 for "A Bibliography of Selected References on AI in the Social Context."

390. Neal, Alan C., ed. *Fundamental Social Rights at Work in the European Community*. Brookfield, VT: Ashgate Publishing Company, 1999.

Keywords: social rights at work, European Community, exploitation/ discrimination, security of employment

Defining and developing an effective structure of fundamental social rights for workers in Europe is the main topic of this book. By using specific cases where proposals were being made to incorporate fundamental rights provisions, this volume examines the responses of European labor court judges to the issues raised. In addressing the practical problems of developing enforceable rights, it also offers a judicial contribution to the general fundamental rights debate as well as a discourse on European social policy.

391. Nelson, Margaret K., and Joan Smith. *Working Hard and Making Do: Surviving in Small Town America*. Berkeley: University of California Press, 1999.

Keywords: family, United States, economic aspects, households, rural families, labor supply, sociology, rural, rural development

The recent economic recovery has brought with it a significant degradation in the quality of work. Jobs historically reserved for the service sector are now becoming part of the manufacturing sector as well. Both a growing service sector and a downgrading of manufacturing jobs have created a wholly new phenomenon: a recovery without benefit to a significant number of Americans. By using a random survey as well as in-depth interviews the authors examine what this has meant for working-class families in a specific rural county. The survival strategies of two groups of working class households in Vermont are also explored: the first in which at least one family member has been able to hold onto good work (i.e., a year-round, full-time job that carries benefits) and, secondly, those in which nobody has been able to secure or maintain steady employment. What is found is that households with good jobs are able to effectively use all of their labor power by relying on two workers to engage in on-the-side businesses or bartering with friends and neighbors. Families without at least one good job are considerably less capable of deploying a complex, multifaceted survival strategy. This finding demonstrates that the widely presumed polarization between the formal and the informal economy is more of a myth than a reality; instead, successful household strategies depend on participation in both sectors. This book also provides a gender analysis of the households' internal dynamics during economic restructuring, and their political implications by taking a closer look at how traditional gender roles are perpetuated and subverted within both "good" and "bad" work families.

392. Neumann, Jean E., Richard Holti, and Hilary Standing. *Change Everything at Once! The Tavistock Institute's Guide to Developing Teamwork in Manufacturing*. Oxford: Management Books 2000, 1995.

Keywords: teams, sociotechnical systems, work groups, production cells, case study

This book is a product of the Tavistock Institute's research program and is designed to "provide methods for introducing, developing, and reinforcing teamwork in manufacturing (TIM)." The title of the book refers to the feeling expressed by people inside organizations regarding the tremendous amount of change with which they must cope and adapt to in the present era of restructuring. In an effort to clarify conceptual understanding, the authors suggest that "a teamwork oriented organization uses the principle of autonomy in the context of responsibility, linked to organization-wide influence." This can be applied to individual, group and organization-wide activities. Examples on the individual level include flexibility, job enrichment, etc. At a group level teamwork may take the form of "semi-autonomous work groups," "production cells," etc. Organization-wide aspects include work councils, employee associations, etc.

This volume emphasizes the point that "organizational leaders often do not understand that changes within a particular function—accounting or production planning, for example—have anything to do with teamwork." Consequently, it is argued that a truly effective teamwork organization is created by making "alterations, simultaneously and sequentially, both within individual functions and in ways that cut across the entire organization."

Six core companies participated in the research that is assessed in the text. Specific case study material is also provided. Chapters 2 and 3 describe the history, context and types of teamwork. Chapters 5 through 9 discuss issues in making changes specific to the five particular aspects of organization implicated in creating a teamwork organization: business and organizational strategy; work design and related training developments; quality manufacturing and engineering systems; business planning and accounting systems; and industrial relations and personnel practices. Chapters 4, 10, and 11 provide frameworks, models and methodologies for the development of teams over time with emphasis on "the interconnections and uncertainties inherent in comprehensive change."

393. Newman, Katherine S. *Falling from Grace: Experience of Downward Mobility in the American Middle Class*. New York: Free Press, 1988.

Keywords: social mobility, middle classes, social conditions, economic conditions

It is becoming a common occurrence for downward mobility to take place in today's society. There are hundreds of thousands of middle-class families in which the loss of employment, a drop in income, and economic hardship have become a reality. By using more than 150 in-depth interviews, the author delves into the damaging effects downward mobility has on people and society, such as the suffering of tremendous disappointment becoming debilitating self-blame, which then leads to a host of anxieties about their own competence and security. This in turn weakens family security, thus taking a toll on society.

394. Newman, Katherine S. *No Shame in My Game: The Working Poor in the Inner City*. New York: Alfred A. Knopf and Russell Sage Foundation, 1999.

Keywords: inner city, poverty, underclass, welfare, low wage

In recent studies of low income neighborhoods, emphasis on the jobless has provided only a partial understanding. The working poor, meanwhile, consistently fall well below the poverty line on a yearly basis, yet studies attend mostly to the unemployed. Fueling the argument that the inner city is in its present state because the incentive to get jobs in such neighborhoods is simply absent, this pervading misunderstanding of American poverty provides a seemingly good reason to pass policy agendas of conservative politicians.

While the economy booms, the stock market soars, and unemployment falls below five percent, the explosion of the service economy has widened the gulf between the educated and the uneducated. Hence, regardless of these national improvements, most low income workers, as a result, do not show great future promise.

Why, in a nation that is in such a phase of prosperity unheard of in most other parts of the world, is there such an ever-growing impoverished working class? Racial segregation conflates the problem of a stagnantly poor underclass, as does the continuous contention with decayed housing, poor diet, lack of medical attention, inadequate education, and perpetual job insecurity.

Newman's research is mostly in the form of interviews with inner city children, school teachers, ministers, community figureheads, and working parents. This book presents an anthropological view on a problem often reserved for economists and sociologists.

395. Nichols, Theo. *The Sociology of Industrial Injury*. London: Mansell Publishing, 1997.

Keywords: industrial accidents, sociology

"This book makes an original sociological contribution to industrial injury from the theoretical standpoint of political economy." Extensive empirical research is presented that centers on manufacturing but also extends to construction and coal mining, drawing upon a variety of research methods.

The need for such an investigation is certainly beyond question. "According to World Health Organization (WHO) and International Labor Organization (ILO) estimates, there are about 120 million workplace accidents and about 200,000 deaths a year worldwide." Moreover, the author points out that the estimated economic cost of industrial accidents is staggering. For British employees alone "it is estimated that the cost approaches a thousand million pounds at 1990 prices."

Part 1 of the book addresses "accident theory." Studies of accidents conducted by the Tavistock Institute of Human Relations are assessed and criticized. There is also a critical account of the literature on accidents/injuries from a social science perspective.

Part 2 reviews safety in British manufacturing with special reference to the (1974) Health and Safety at Work Act. The author also situates industrial safety within reigning forms of political economy, indicating for example a relationship between the Thatcher era and a deterioration in industrial health and safety. In addition, workplace industrial relations are examined in order to address the broader determinants of injury. Three institutional features are explored—health and safety arrangements, trade unionism and the size of the employment unit.

396. Nightingale, Donald V. *Workplace Democracy*. Toronto: University of Toronto Press, 1982.

Keywords: participation, democracy, Canada

This book is about employee participation in decision making. At the time it was published, workplace democracy was not commonly found in work organizations in the West. This text, then, represents a relatively early effort to "explore the effects of workplace democracy on the well-being of organization members." It also considers the question of how the economic imperatives of corporations can be reconciled with the psychological and physical health of workers.

A number of different enterprises are examined in terms of their responses "to the challenge of introducing democratic principles into the decision-making processes of the workplace." The author indicates that "data from 1000 respondents in twenty companies have been collected through standardized instruments and through extensive interviews with managers and trade union officials."

The democratic participative strategies adopted by these companies are contrasted with other organizations that have autocratic and hierarchical management styles. The conclusions drawn are of importance to managers, academics, and others who are interested in promoting both productivity and human values in the workplace.

See chapter 1 for a discussion of the major theoretical issues and challenges of workplace democracy. Topics include the "spreading psychology of entitlement," worker.expectations, the erosion of consent, the individual as citizen and employee, the "pluralist perspective" and the "research" (or "human relations") perspective. Also see the research questions listed at the end of this chapter. See chapter 6 for comparative research on "the nature of work in democratic and hierarchical workplaces." Chapter 9 "Workplace Democracy in Perspective" focuses on such topics as an agenda for reform, the evolution of workplace reform, profit sharing and employee ownership, work reform and productivity, implementing workplace democracy, and government initiatives. See especially appendix 1 "Forms of Workplace Democracy in Canada" for detailed case studies. Though somewhat dated, these studies provide excellent firsthand accounts of employee participation programs in a variety of Canadian companies.

397. Noble, David. *Forces of Production: A Social History of Industrial Automation*. New York: Alfred A. Knopf, 1984.

Keywords: technology, automation, computers, history, capitalism

This well-known work in political economy/social history traces the evolution of the design and use of automatically controlled machine tools "from the point of conception in the minds of inventors to the point of production on the shop floor." The author chooses to focus on machine tools because "they are the guts of modern industry, and automation because it is the hallmark of twentieth-century manufacturing technology." Emphasis throughout the book is on the social foundation of this technological development, and thus "upon the ambiguity of the process: possibilities as well as the constraints, the lost opportunities as well as the chosen path." The author avoids the typical and technologically deterministic approach of showing how social potential is shaped by technical constraints. Instead he examines how technical possibilities are delimited by social constraints. "The aim is to point up a realm of freedom within technological development, known as politics. For when technological development is seen as politics, as it should be, then the very notion of progress becomes ambiguous: what kind of progress? progress for whom? progress for what?" Noble clearly believes that an awareness of this ambiguity reduces the powerful hold that technology has exercised on our consciousness, awakens us to the true range of technical possibilities, and leads us to a broader notion of progress and human fulfillment.

Some of the specific topics discussed in the book include Taylorism and scientific management, deskilling and worker alienation, computers in factory process control, computer-assisted manufacturing, Norbert Wiener and cybernetics, programmable machine tool automation, automation and unemployment, unions in the automated factory, automation and management control, scientism in manufacturing and industry, and the degradation of human skills and implicit knowledge. See especially chapter 4 "Toward the Automatic Factory," all of part 2 on "Social Choice in Machine Design," all of part 3 "A New Industrial Revolution: Change Without Change," and the epilogue "Another Look at Progress."

398. Noble, David F. *Progress Without People: New Technology, Unemployment and the Message of Resistance*. Toronto: Between the Lines, 1995.

Keywords: human resources, deskilling, unemployment

This book is a compelling and rather bleak (but realistic) account of the profound social costs of the so-called information revolution. Noble provides a detailed analysis of the "hegemonic ideology of technological progress" with a particular focus on its implications for employment/unemployment.

In the introduction, the author notes that "in the wake of five decades of information revolution, people are now working longer hours, under worsening conditions, with greater anxiety and stress, less skills, less security, less power, less benefits, and less pay. Information technology has clearly been developed and used during these years to deskill, discipline, and displace human labor in a global speed-up of unprecedented proportions."

Noble demonstrates how particular modes of deskilling and marginalizing the workforce are the direct result of state-corporate power structures, "which seek mastery over the global economy and society."

Part 1 of the text is "an attempt to account for the lack of full-scale labor resistance to the corporate technological offensive by means of a historical analysis of our inherited ideology of technological progress." The Luddite movement, both past and present, is outlined here as well. Part 2 looks at the effects of automation in its mechanized and computerized forms, and also focuses on the "religion of technology, tracing the religious roots of our irrational faith in technological salvation."

399. Nohria, Nitin, and James D. Berkeley. "The Virtual Organization: Bureaucracy, Technology and the Implosion of Control." In *The Post-Bureaucratic Organization: New Perspectives on Organizational Change*, edited by Charles Heckscher. Thousand Oaks, CA: Sage Publications, 1994.

Keywords: virtual organizations, organizational change

The book from which this essay is drawn analyzes the change process in modern organizations from bureaucracy to post-bureaucracy. Nohria and Berkeley propose the notion of the virtual organization as an alternative approach to traditional conceptions of bureaucratic organizational structure. The authors of the essays make the case that "with advances in information technology the classical physical requirements for coordinated effort—proximity and documents—are no longer necessary constraints on organizing." In fact, the old assumptions of *location* and *office* are completely undermined. They also argue that technology has created an "implosion of bureaucratic specialization into . . . cross functional, computer-mediated jobs, such that individual members of the organizations may now be considered holographically equivalent to the organization as a whole." It is suggested that "to speak of a work organization as a virtual system serves to call attention to the enabling role of technology (via such things as personal computers, networked databases, and instant forms of telecommunications such as electronic mail) and to the concomitant transformation of certain organizational fundamentals: personal interaction, the division of labor, and so forth. . . . As the wide-scale introduction of sophisticated information technology erodes these features," one can envision "organizations where the traditional means of coordinating people and resources no longer apply—organizations that cease to exist as the rationalized, physical systems Weber had once sought to describe. See the subsection of this essay entitled "Technology and Society: The Virtual in Context" for a detailed description of the characteristics of the virtual organization.

400. Nonaka, I. "The Knowledge-Creating Company." *Harvard Business Review*, November-December 1991: 96-104.

Keywords: work design, knowledge embedded in experience, Taylorism, participation, management

The article explains the Japanese edge over competitors in terms of their rejection of the Tayloristic and Simonian view of the organization. They view the organization as a machine for information processing relying on quantifiable data and codified and unified procedures where new knowledge is similarly measured in hard quantifiable terms such as increased efficiency, lower costs, and improved return on investment. Instead, the leading Japanese companies such as Honda, Canon, NEC, and Matsushita are knowledge producing companies that realize that new knowledge is not simply a matter of "processing" objective information but depends on tapping the tacit and often highly subjective insights, intuitions, and hunches of individual employees and making those insights available for testing and use by the company as a whole.

401. Noon, Randall. *Introduction to Forensic Engineering*. Boca Raton: CRC Press, 1992.

Keywords: forensic engineering

This standard textbook for forensic engineering aims to provide an introduction to the science, methodology, and engineering principles of the field. Information is organized into the following topics: common accidents, incidents and issues; vehicular accidents; vehicle accident reconstruction using basic energy analysis techniques; application of the classical scientific method to accident reconstruction; motorcycle accidents; photographic documentation of accident-damaged vehicles; vehicular and marine lighting; storm lightning damage; vibration and blasting damage; explosions; combustion; determining the point of origin of a fire; arson for profit; electrical shorting; hail damage; drought and its effects; lighting; slip-and-fall accidents; water pipe freeze-ups; principles of machinery guarding; the engineer as expert witness; and reporting the results of investigative engineering. Standard measurements, information to be collected, and descriptive passages make up the chapters. The book can be used as a reference by nontechnical professionals as well as, of course, engineers and technicians new to the field. The book does not have a preventive orientation but reveals how forensic engineers deal with accidents.

402. Noro, Kageyu, and Ogden Bronen Jr. *Human Factors in Organizational Design and Management III*. Kyoto: Elsevier Science Publishers, 1990.

Keywords: QWL, human factors, organizational change

This interdisciplinary book represents a comprehensive selection of papers first presented at an international symposium in Kyoto, Japan. It offers "insights and understanding in the area of human factors in organizational design and management at both micro- and macroergonomic levels." The editors of the volume indicate that the profound political and economic changes occurring throughout the world (especially in the then-Soviet Union, East European nations and several Asian countries) are reflected "in the organization and management considerations addressed by this symposium." The strong cross-cultural theme to the book is seen in the number of countries represented by the contributors.

See section 3.2 on participatory ergonomics for articles such as "A Matrix Approach to Work Design" and "Participatory Ergonomics in Occupational Safety and Health." See especially section 4 of the book that offers an extensive selection of research essays on "Quality of Work Life and Values." This section is organized into four subsections: "Work Design and Analysis," "Safety, Accident Prevention, and Human Protection," "Health and Fatigue," and "Work Space." Also of interest from a healthy work perspective is section 6 on psychological ergonomics and section 8.3f that offers several case studies exploring various workplace design alternatives.

403. NUTEK, Norflex Group (coordinated by the Department for Industrial Policy Analyses at NUTEK). *Flexibility Matters: Flexible Enterprises in the Nordic Countries*. Stockholm: NUTEK, 1999.

Keywords: hours of labor, organizational change, organizational effectiveness

In the Nordic countries of Denmark, Norway, Sweden, and Finland, modern and flexible work organizations have been studied. Thus, the general purpose of this book is to investigate if there is indeed a "Nordic model" for flexibility. By analyzing the first part of the report, it is shown that there is indeed a "Nordic model" for organizational flexibility that has many common features. It is also shown that there is strong evidence of positive effects from using a flexible work organization on productivity, working conditions, and employment growth in Sweden and Finland, and partly in Denmark. This demonstrates an increased awareness in the Nordic countries for the importance of flexible work organizations.

404. Oborne, David J. *Ergonomics at Work: Human Factors in Design and Development*. 3rd ed. Chichester: John Wiley and Sons, 1995.

Keywords: ergonomics, human factors, anthropocentric

This comprehensive textbook examines the symbiotic relationship between the human operator and the work environment. It explains the fundamentals of ergonomics and its role within the context of modern-day work, with particular attention given to the idea of ergonomics as an evolving concept. The author emphasizes that ergonomics is "a way of looking at the world that requires careful thought about the behaviors of all parts of the working system—people and machines—in order that they can exist and work together effectively."

The book also stresses that "we must emphasize the central component within the working system—people. Within the person-centered view, therefore, we recognize that people bring to the system a collection of individual features that can affect the subsequent interaction. Person-centered ergonomics, that this edition discusses, 'weights' the effects of the individual components according to the potential of the person in the system." The author gives significant attention to the psychological aspects of the field of ergonomics in this edition as well.

See especially chapter 1 "Ergonomics: Its Scope and Future," chapters 2 and 3 "The Structure of the Body I and II," chapter 7 "Workspace Design," and chapter 12 "Ergonomics and Safety."

405. O'Driscoll, Michael P., and Cary L. Cooper. "Coping with Work-Related Stress: A Critique of Existing Measures and Proposal for an Alternative Methodology." *Journal of Occupational and Organizational Psychology* 67 (1994): 343-54.

Keywords: stress, coping

This is a rather technical research paper that addresses the issue of how individuals deal with or manage the stress they experience. In particular, it explores effective methods of coping with work-related stress (rather than emphasizing the factors that contribute to stress). In addition, the authors provide an overview of "some of the major methodological difficulties encountered in research on stress coping," noting the limitations of existing procedures, and also proposing "an alternative framework for the assessment of coping with work-related stressors." This alternative model is referred to as "critical incident analysis" or CIA.

Applied to the stress-coping process in work settings, "CIA entails asking individuals to describe stressful transactions in term of three elements: (i) the antecedents or circumstances in which the stress occurred; (ii) their responses in that situation, along with the responses of other people; and (iii) the consequences of both their own and other individuals' behavior." The authors believe that "this approach offers a methodology for linking coping behaviors to sources of stress in work settings, hence providing more comprehensive information about the stress-coping process."

406. Okuda, Kenji. "The Role of Engineers in Japanese Industry and Education: An Industrial Sociologist's View." 83-9 in *Context and Complexity: Cultivating Contextual Understanding*, edited by Magoroh Marayama. New York: Springer-Verlag, 1992.

Keywords: engineering, education, sociology, knowledge embedded in experience, Japan

This entry explains how the role of Japanese engineers differs considerably from that of engineers elsewhere. Specifically, it discusses how Japan closes the gap between graduate engineers and frontline operators by making engineering graduates spend considerable time on the shopfloor before engaging in any design.

407. Olerup, Agneta, Leslie Schneider, and Elsbeth Monod, eds. *Proceedings of the IFIP First Working Conference on Women, Work and Computerization*. Riva del Sole, Italy: Elsevier Science Publishers, 1985.

Keywords: women, automation, computers, workplace democracy

The conference papers published in this volume are directed exclusively toward issues concerning the impacts of computers and new technology on women and their work. Two fundamental goals are noted: "The study and evaluation of women's work and computers, with a view toward promoting research and work on the impacts of new technology in offices, and on women's work in particular. Another aim is to encourage work on strategies for influencing and controlling the introduction and usages of new technology in offices and the impacts on women's jobs."

Part 1 provides the background and design of the conference and discusses the highlights and major outcomes. In part 2 on "Office Automation, Work, and Skill" the focus centers on skills in general, skills in women's work and the impact of computers and new technology on skills. It is argued that women's skills are largely nonvisible and therefore tend to be ignored. The papers in part 3 address "Remote Work" or telecommuting. The organization, division and place of work, as well as the probable impacts on women's and men's work are explored. The degree to which remote work confers flexibility in work routines is examined and it is suggested that real flexibility may only come about through legal guarantees. Part 4 on "Manufacturing" deals with the issues of women and computers in industrial work. The obstacles preventing women from entering skilled jobs are considered. Part 5 on "Practice and Participation in Systems Design" looks at some of the inadequacies of traditional approaches in systems design and offers a women's perspective with an emphasis on workplace democracy. The role of trade unions and formal rights is also explored. Part 6 on "Education and Training" is directed toward the education of female computer professionals and engineers. A longitudinal study of female computer experts is reported, and the work-related attitudes and values of female engineering students are examined.

408. Olsen, Margrethe H., ed. *Technological Support for Work Group Collaboration*. Hillsdale, NJ: Lawrence Erlbaum Associates, 1989.

Keywords: work groups, teams, computers

This volume examines a range of approaches to using computers in the work environment to support work teams. The term "technological support for work group collaboration" is a label for an emerging trend in research on the relationship between computer systems and social systems. "Part of the research is concerned with assessing the ways in which people use computer-based tools to work together and understanding how the tools and the work relationship affect each other. Some of the research focuses on tools that have been around for a while—electronic mail, computer conferencing, project management, etc. Some of it focuses on brand new tools emphasizing 'work group productivity' rather than individual productivity."

The underlying theme common to all the contributions in the book is "a new way of thinking about work—in particular, knowledge work—and the ways it can be made more effective and personally satisfying through information technology." The collaboration of computer scientists with social scientists is stressed throughout the work as a necessary prerequisite for designing effective computer-supported work teams.

Chapter titles include the following: "Assumptions Underlying Systems that Support Work Group Collaboration"; "The Information Lens: An Intelligent System for Information Sharing and Coordination"; "Flexible Interactive Technologies for Multi-Person Tasks"; and "Organizational Architecture for Distributed Computing: The Next Frontier in System Design."

409. O'Reilly, Jacqueline, Inmaculada Cebrian, and Michel Lallement, eds. *Working-Time Changes: Social Integration through Transitional Labor Markets*. Labor Markets and Employment Policy. Northampton, MA: Edward Elgar Publishing, 2000.

Keywords: hours of labor, flexible, full employment policies, labor market, employment contracts, company practices

To begin, the theoretical context and the way in which society has operationalized the concept of transitional labor markets are outlined. This is followed by the implications for working-time changes for the type of transitions that are possible both within the employment relationship and in terms of social integration for those outside paid work. Also, the issue of cross-national comparative and interdisciplinary research is touched upon. And finally, the main results are examined, as are their implications for both policy makers and future research agendas.

410. O'Reilly, Jacqueline, and Colette Fagan, eds. *Part-Time Prospects: An International Comparison of Part-Time Work in Europe, North America and the Pacific Rim*. New York: Routledge, 1998.

Keywords: part-time work, men, women, ethnic minorities, labor standards, low pension income, international perspective

One of the most striking features of industrialized economies over the past forty years has been the growth in part-time employment. By asking questions such as Is part-time work better than unemployment, or is social welfare a disincentive to taking up a part-time job? Is this kind of work becoming an increasingly normal part of most people's working lives, or does it remain a female ghetto of low pay, low pensions and low labor standards?, this book provides a comparative analysis of the common and divergent patterns in the use of part-time work in Europe, North America, and the Pacific Rim. A wide variety of issues are tackled including those related to gender, ethnicity, and the differences between societies.

411. Orr, Julian E. *Talking about Machines: An Ethnography of a Modern Job.* Ithaca, NY: ILR Press/Cornell University Press, 1996.

Keywords: case study, knowledge embedded in experience

Within all of the literature on work, there is very little focus on the actual practice of work. To remedy this situation and to gain insight into the work that technicians do, Julian Orr presents here an ethnography of Xerox photocopier field service technicians. A better understanding of technicians and their work is important because this emerging occupational group is going to be of great significance in the workforce. This new group consists of neither professionals nor craftworkers, wears white collars but does "blue collar" work, uses their hands yet requires education and a high level of skill. As more and more jobs become infused with a technical component, more technicians are required.

Orr discovered that "technical knowledge is best viewed as a socially distributed resource that is diffused and stored primarily through an oral culture." By sharing vignettes from workers' daily lives, Orr reveals that their talk is an essential part of how they do their jobs. Diagnoses are made by verbally creating a description of the malfunctioning machine. The exchange of stories among technicians is the principal method of gaining new knowledge and keeping up to date. By accompanying workers to different service sites, Orr also observed that the triangular relationship of technicians, customers and machines must always be considered when analyzing the work practice of technicians. He maintains that although he studied only photocopier repair people, his general conclusions apply to all technicians.

412. Osterman, Paul, ed. *Broken Ladders: Managerial Careers in the New Economy.* New York: Oxford University Press, 1996.

Keywords: management, quality management, office work, restructuring

Making customer satisfaction and quality management the cornerstone of corporate management, industry has dramatically restructured itself such that the increasing demands of different skills have successfully created a diverse range of job activities. However, contemporary managerial positions have come under great risk, due in part to much of the same constant reorganization and reinvention of corporate structuring. This book examines how and why managerial positions are becoming increasingly insecure, reconceptualized, and displaced within a new era of office work.

A collection of discussions by various authors, the book is the documentation of a Sloan Foundation sponsored conference held on human resource and managerial employment, covering issues of corporate restructuring, organizational deskilling and rising pay inequity, managerial roles in networked organizations, the demographic transformation of labor markets, among others. Edited by Paul Osterman, the book includes essays by Stephen R. Barley, Rosemary Batt, Sara L. Beckman, Peter Cappelli, Renee M. Landers, John Paul MacDuffie, K. C. O'Shaughnessy, Paul Osterman, James B. Rebitzer, Elizabeth D. Scott, Lowell J. Taylor, Michael Useem, and Stacia E. Zabusky.

413. Osterman, Paul. *Securing Prosperity: The American Labor Market: How It Has Changed and What to Do about It.* Princeton, NJ: Princeton University Press, 1999.

Keywords: labor market, trade unions, industrial relations, economic conditions, United States, economic policy

The central thesis of the book is determining what happened in the American labor market over the past two decades and what we should do about it. The premise of the book is that the beginning of the twenty-first century is a transitional period from one form of labor market to another with choices that are much more open. This makes the topic at hand that much more relevant, and in turn presents many new uncertainties about what is happening and what the possibilities may be. Thus, the author tries to operate the book on two levels: a scholarly analysis of the past and a programmatic prescription of the future.

414. Owen, John D. *Reduced Working Hours: Cure for Unemployment or Economic Burden?* Baltimore: Johns Hopkins University Press, 1989.

Keywords: unemployment, work time, comparative

This volume examines the social and economic implications of a reduction in work time for Americans and Europeans. The author introduces the book by noting that "European unions have asked for sharp reductions in work time in order to 'share the work'. . . . Considerable progress has been made, and the struggle for work sharing continues, often with government support." In the United States, however, Owen indicates that this issue is only beginning to be discussed seriously, most probably because of continued economic growth and low unemployment.

The book is divided into three parts. "Part 1 sets out the basic facts about work time, presenting data on weekly hours and on vacations and holidays since 1945 in four countries: the United States and the three largest economies in Western Europe—Germany, France, and the United Kingdom. The analysis shows how the Europeans in this period were consistently more aggressive in demanding and obtaining shorter work time. . . . Part 2 sets out in a systematic form the basic arguments used in the current debate over work sharing and summarizes the principal empirical findings used in that debate. . . . Part 3 considers the long-term consequences for the United States if a major, permanent reduction in work time does take place. This subject has received only a little attention in the work-sharing debate." A discussion of possible effects on leisure time, recreation spending, and metropolitan area development is also included. The analyses presented make clear the quite significant costs, as well as the benefits, of reduced work time.

415. Pahl, R. E., ed. *On Work: Historical, Comparative and Theoretical Approaches*. Oxford: Basil Blackwell, 1988.

Keywords: general, history, sociology

This massive sociological and historical study of work brings together a wealth of information from many well-known contributors on the subject of the relationship between work and society. Part 1 of the book examines the historical experience of work—"the emergence of the male breadwinner and collective mass worker, and the whole concept of unemployment and the unemployed" (i.e., patterns of work and attitudes that lasted around 200 years). Part 2 considers "the receding dominance of such patterns under the stress of new divisions in labor markets and new strategies among employees, workers, and households." Topics discussed here include the following: "Taylorism, Responsible Autonomy, and Management Strategy"; "New Technology and the Labor Process"; "The Decline of the Mass-Collective Worker?", etc. Part 4 looks at work outside employment, collective work and pooling of labor. Part 5 explores "the new processes of disaggregated capitalism—from homeworking to office automation and the new factories in the third world." Finally, part 6 examines fundamental questions about the need to work, in both social science and philosophical terms.

416. Palokangas, Tapio. *Labor Unions, Public Policy and Economic Growth*. Cambridge: Cambridge University Press, 2000.

Keywords: collective bargaining, credibility in collective bargaining, taxation and production efficiency, unions, economic growth

Collective bargaining remains to this day the main vehicle for labor worldwide to negotiate benefits, wages, training, retirement policies, and other terms of working with management in both the public and private sectors. For many years, labor economists have been modeling the relations among collective bargaining agreements, social welfare conditions and labor markets. A new theoretical framework for unions that offers a unified treatment of the centralization of bargaining, the unionization of labor markets, the credibility of labor contracts, and the relative bargaining power of the union are presented in this book. It also assesses the foundations of bargaining, as well as examines collective bargaining interacting with investment and growth, public policy, and international trade and specialization. The author concludes by challenging the commonly held view that collective bargaining has a negative impact on economic welfare and argues that, with the existence of market failure, collective bargaining can be welfare-enhancing.

417. Pardo, Olga, Oliver Strohm, Christina Kirsch, Julia K. Kuark, Loni Leder, Eric Louis, Axel Schilling, and Eberhard Ulich. "Computer-Aided Manufacturing Systems: Work-Psychological Aspects and Empirical Findings from Case Studies." *International Journal of Industrial Ergonomics* 16, no. 4-6 (1995): 327-38.

Keywords: CAM, anthropocentric, automation

The design of computer-aided manufacturing systems should consider not only the technical but also the organizational aspects as well as worker skills. These holistic approaches are more profitable according to the study presented in this paper. Swiss companies in the capital-goods industry were studied in terms of how common the more human-centered approaches such as decentralization, functional integration, work group autonomy and challenging tasks are. The results show that very few companies use these approaches, so the authors outline specific requirements to design more humane CIM systems: (1) organizational design prior to automation, (2) education and training, (3) functional integration and (4) local self-regulation to increase employees' control over their work.

418. Parker, Christopher P., Boris B. Baltes, Scott A. Young, Joseph W. Huff, Robert A. Altmann, Heather A. LaCost, and Joanne E. Roberts. "Relationships between Psychological Climate Perceptions and Work Outcomes: A Meta-analytic Review." *Journal of Organizational Behavior* 24, no. 4 (June 2003): 389-416.

Keywords: psychological well-being, employee motivation, employee performance

In this study, meta-analytic procedures were used to examine the relationships between individual-level (psychological) climate perceptions and work outcomes such as employee attitudes, psychological well-being, motivation, and performance. The authors' review of the literature generated 121 independent samples in which climate perceptions were measured and analyzed at the individual level. These studies document considerable confusion regarding the constructs of psychological climate, organizational climate, and organizational culture and reveal a need for researchers to use terminology that is consistent with their level of measurement, theory, and analysis. The meta-analytic findings indicate that psychological climate, operationalized as individuals' perceptions of their work environment, does have significant relationships with individuals' work attitudes, motivation, and performance. Structural equation modeling analyses of the meta-analytic correlation matrix indicated that the relationships of psychological climate with employee motivation and performance are fully mediated by employees' work attitudes. The article also found that the James and James PCg model could be extended to predict the impact of work environment perceptions on employee attitudes, motivation, and performance. Despite the number of published individual-level climate studies that the authors found, there is a need for more research using standardized measures so as to enable analyses of the organizational and contextual factors that might moderate the effects of psychological climate perceptions. Finally, the authors argue for a molar theory of psychological climate that is rooted in the psychological processes by which individuals make meaning of their work experiences.

419. Parker, Martin. *Organizational Culture and Identity: Unity and Division at Work.* London: Sage Publications, 2000.

Keywords: history and theories of organizational culture, cultures and identification

Hidden by the rise of interest in organizational culture was the assumption that a hard scientific management of institutions could be replaced by an approach that relied on a more humane understanding of people's values and culture. The author suggests that there are in fact more important insights to be gained from applying the term "culture" to organizations. Thus, he explores the history of ideas about culture in organizations and explains why the term has been invoked with such enthusiasm. Further ways of thinking about organizations and culture are presented that suggest that organizational cultures should be seen as "fragmented unities" in which members identify themselves as collective at some times and divided at others.

420. Parker, Mike, and Jane Slaughter. *Working Smart: A Union Guide to Participation Programs and Reengineering.* Detroit: A Labor Notes Book, 1994.

Keywords: management and stress, participation programs, union strategies

Jobs in today's workforce are becoming increasingly insecure and less flexible. The main focus of this book is to warn union members of these issues. The authors claim that the administration is seeking ways in which to encourage labor-management cooperation, however, such an institution already exists in the form of collective bargaining. The issues surrounding how the trade union movement must respond to these circumstances are outlined. First, the authors insist, the starting point must be grounded in the commitment to unionism and workers' welfare. They distill lessons from dozens of workplaces to learn from their successes and mistakes. It is emphasized that concerns for unions, the voice of the workers, must remain paramount and thus all programs should ask the question: How does this affect the union?

421. Parsons, Nick. *Employee Participation in Europe: A Case Study in the British and French Gas Industries*. Aldershot, UK: Avebury, 1997.

Keywords: participation, comparative, Great Britain, France

The research presented in this book examines, through case studies in the gas industry, the workings of employee participation systems in Britain and France. This particular study focuses on trade union based employee participation arrangements at the shop-floor level. The author notes that Britain and France have very different industrial relations systems and practices, "which can therefore be expected to lead to differences in the functioning of participation arrangements in the two countries."

The study examines "the variables affecting these differences, as well as their effects on the attitudes and strategies of trade unions, employers, and employees." In particular, "the effects of the differences in the role and attitudes of the state, and in trade union organization" are emphasized.

The introduction to the book sets out the rationale for conducting the study, and chapter 2 "gives an overview of EU initiatives aimed at increasing the participation of employees in company decision making." Chapter 3 develops the concepts adopted in the research. Chapter 4 looks more closely at "the environment in which participation structures operate in Britain and France and develops hypotheses for the outcomes of trade union based participation in the two countries based on the concepts elaborated in the previous chapter." See also chapter 9 for a discussion of the conclusions that can be drawn from this study.

422. Pascarelli, Emil, and Deborah Quilter. *Repetitive Strain Injury: A Computer User's Guide*. New York: John Wiley and Sons, 1994.

Keywords: computers, repetitive strain injury

This volume offers a detailed examination of the ways in which "the great speed, ease, and efficiency of personal computers can lead to severe physical and emotional pain." The problem is called repetitive strain injury or RSI and includes a wide range of conditions including Carpal Tunnel Syndrome. This "epidemic of the '90s," that damages the muscles, nerves and tendons of the hands, wrists and arms, is a potential concern for every computer user, according to the authors. The book is well-researched, expertly illustrated, and filled with numerous commonsense explanations and practical suggestions for those suffering from all types of repetitive strain injuries, as well as those who wish to prevent such injuries.

Topics explored in the text include the following: the causes of RSI; prevention (a seven-point plan); warning signs of RSI; typing style; posture; the role of stress; personality and attitudes; getting an accurate diagnosis; classifications of various repetitive strain injuries; the role of rest, splinting, and surgery; computer-related eye problems; rehabilitation and the healing process; self-care (eye, neck, arm, hand exercises); the emotional impact of RSI; ergonomic workstations; legal issues; etc.

423. Pasmore, William A., and John J. Sherwood, eds. *Sociotechnical Systems: A Sourcebook*. La Jolla: University Associates, 1978.

Keywords: sociotechnical systems, organizational change, work design, alienation, participation, management, general, policy, organizational design

The goal of sociotechnical systems design is to optimize the relationship between the social/human systems and the technological systems of an organization. This classic sourcebook on sociotechnical systems presents a clear explanation and debate over relevant aspects of sociotechnical systems. Following the introductory section is part 2 "Working with the Organization as an Open System." Here the underlying theme is that sociotechnical organizations are open and living systems that interact with the environment much like biological cells. Part 3 contains classic articles by Trist and by Cherns that outline what the sociotechnical system theory is. Among other things, it studies and describes the relationships between people, tasks and technologies and how they can be optimized, for example, by creating self-directing autonomous work groups that are responsible for their own task performance. Once sociotechnical system theory is understood, managers or consultants can diagnose and change an existing organization system. This is the subject of part 4 that includes, among others, the articles "How to Counter Alienation in the Plant" and "Innovative Restructuring of Work" by Walton. Participation and management strategies are also discussed. The technical systems can be effective, given the right conditions and techniques. But which conditions and techniques? To begin to answer this question, part 5 "Sociotechnical System Studies: What Do We Really Know?" contains case studies of sociotechnical and other interventions. The most notable contributions to part 6 "Perspectives on Sociotechnical Systems" are "Perspectives on Work Restructuring" by Walton and "Sociotechnical Systems: The Design of Work and Quality of Working Life" by Davis.

424. Pelfrene, Edwin, Peter Vlerick, Rudolf P. Mak, Patrick De Smet, Marcel Kornitzer, and Guy De Backer. "Scale Reliability and Validity of the Karasek 'Job Demand-Control-Support' Model in the Belstress Study." *Work and Stress* 15, no. 4 (2001): 297-313.

Keywords: job demand-control-support model, job strain, scale reliability, validity

In studies of occupational stress, a leading theoretical model is the "Job Demand-Control-Support" model (Karasek and Theorell, 1990). This states that the most adverse job-related strain reactions are to be expected in jobs characterized by high job demands, low control and low worksite support. The reliability and validity of the scales was evaluated in a sample of 21,419 employees out of twenty-five large companies across Belgium. Participants completed items from the Job Content Questionnaire (Karasek, 1985) in either French or Dutch translation. Data were handled by a French-speaking and a Dutch-speaking center, respectively. Occupational groups were identified according to the International Standard of Classification (ISCO). Basically, the data support the assumptions of the model. The internal consistency was adequate: Cronbach's alpha varied between 0.77 and 0.83 for psychological demands (9-item version), decision latitude, supervisor social support and coworker social support. These four common factors were clearly distinguished in a factor analysis. A confirmatory factor analysis pointed to the correlation among these factors and illustrated similar loading structures within subgroups according to age, gender and education. Lower occupational grades tended to display lower mean values of psychological demands and decision latitude than those observed in higher grades. Blue-collar workers, at least men, were found to be less exposed to high strain working conditions (high demand and low control) than clerks and service workers. "Feeling stressed" was found to be more strongly associated with psychological demands than with decision latitude or social support; the reverse held true for "job satisfaction."

425. Pelletier, Kenneth R. *Healthy People in Unhealthy Places: Stress and Fitness at Work.* New York: Delacorte Press/Seymour Lawrence, 1984.

Keywords: job stress, psychology, industrial, occupational health services

As workplaces become increasingly unsafe, millions of men and women are taking greater precautions and taking greater measures to improve and maintain their fitness and health. Inescapably for most people, work consumes most of an individual's life on a daily basis, second only to sleep, and is recently coming under close scrutiny as a threat to good health. Physical ailments such as back pain are common among all branches of labor and office workers, as well as the psychologically debilitating illnesses of depression and anxiety. There has also been an increase in recent years of alcoholism, drug abuse, and suicide. The book covers sources of stress, "type A" behavior, stress management, toxic hazards of the workplace, and health promotion programs. It concludes with an overview of possible measures to be taken to create a healthier workplace.

426. Penzias, Arno. *Ideas and Information: Managing in a High-Tech World.* New York: W. W. Norton and Company, 1989.

Keywords: computers

This book, written by a researcher and educator at AT&T Bell Laboratories, aims to provide a straightforward, nontechnical explanation of computerized information processing by penetrating "beneath the slick surface layer that computers often present to their potential users." As well as satisfying the curiosity many people have about the computer technology that surrounds us, the author hopes to reduce the anxiety and confusion these people have abut the impact of technology on their lives.

The book discusses how, "with the steady increase in human knowledge, our employment of technology continues to enhance human specialization and increases the interdependency between communities of specialized knowledge." The author speculates that "many large organizations may therefore grow even larger in order to bring diverse knowledge to bear on complex tasks . . . but this trend needn't dehumanize our lives." The author further argues that "properly directed technology can enhance the role of the individual by giving each of us needed access to heretofore inaccessible information sources."

Topics discussed include the following: information processing as symbol manipulation; the "rules" of logic and grammar; computers and the programming process; computer "languages" and linguistics; the evolution of "thinking" machines; microprocessors; and human qualities and knowledge versus artificial intelligence.

427. Perrolle, J. A. "Expert Enhancement and Replacement in Computerized Mental Labor." *Science, Technology, & Human Values* 16, no. 2 (1991): 195-207.

Keywords: expert systems, skill, professional work, deskilling

What happens to professional and technical work when it is computerized? Exploratory analysis of case studies indicates that when expert systems are used to enhance the work of professionals, some tasks of medium- and low-skilled support personnel are integrated into the work of highly skilled experts. Technical workers are thus at risk of having their jobs automated as part of the computer enhancement of professionals. When computerization replaces expertise, job opportunities for medium-skilled personnel shrink and barriers to upward mobility through on-the-job expertise are reduced. Entry-level professionals or even technicians with computers can perform tasks formerly done by experienced professionals. But working conditions do not promote the development of expertise and professional judgment among these workers. Thus it appears that routinization, deskilling, and automation are not only the problems of manual laborers in the information age; professional workers are also at risk, in complex ways.

428. Perrow, Charles. "The Organizational Context of Human Factors Engineering." *Administrative Science Quarterly* 28 (1983): 521-41.

Keywords: complex systems, human factors, accidents

This article begins by noting that "recent disasters and near disasters in high tech systems have generated increased concern about the interaction of operators and equipment in complex military and industrial systems." The author explores an unaddressed aspect of the operator-machine problem by "analyzing the organizational context that structures the relationship between the two; that is, how organizational structure affects the design of equipment and how new equipment reproduces the organizational structure."

The discussion of organizational context in this paper explains why top management personnel are often "indifferent to good human factors design and shows how the social structure favors the choice of technologies that centralize authority and deskill operators."

In addition, "the role of equipment and system design in shaping cognitive maps and mental models is explored." The author concludes that "rather than technology determining organizational structure, it would appear that machines and equipment are designed so that they reinforce existing structures." The implications of this for potential accidents are also examined.

429. Perry, Martin, Carl Davidson, and Roberta Hill. *Reform at Work: Workplace Change and the New Industrial Order*. Auckland, NZ: Longman Paul, 1995.

Keywords: work design, human resources, sociology, politics

This book adopts a multidisciplinary perspective to explore workplace reorganization and the quality of working life in the context of global economic restructuring, technological change, and increasing economic competitiveness. The text focuses on workplaces in New Zealand and uses the findings drawn from many fields of study: economics, human resource arrangement, industrial sociology, management, and political studies.

The authors begin with the premise that "the successful introduction of new technology depends on an understanding of the cultural and organizational factors in production." Chapter 2 provides the theoretical foundation for the case studies that follow. The studies themselves are well-documented, offer a good cross-section of different workplace reform experiences, and are written in straightforward, nontechnical language. They "document change and reflect conditions and perspectives in individual workplaces up to a particular moment of time," given the inevitability of their continued tendency to change.

While the precise focus of each case study varies, the questions considered in their assessment remain the same. In summary, these questions explore the following concerns: "1. whether there is a blueprint of best practice in workplace reform; 2. the influences determining whether organizations are able to make progress with new workplace methods; 3. the extent to which there is anything progressive in the new practices, in the sense of improvements in the quality of working life experienced by employees and their impact on the distribution of job opportunities; 4. the implications of workplace changes for managers, unions and public policy."

The case studies are presented in chapters 4 through 11 and deal with the meat processing industry, dairy processing, automobile manufacturing, the steel industry, the chemical industry, the service industry, and several other areas. See also chapter 2 "Workplace Reform and the New Industrial Order" for material on JIT and flexible specialization and chapter 12 "Lessons from the Workplace" for preventive practice and healthy work implications. This chapter discusses QWL, specifically union involvement in work design, the role of management, and public policy issues.

430. Petersen, Dan. *Human Error Reduction and Safety Management.* New York: Van Nostrand Reinhold, 1996.

Keywords: accidents, safety, ergonomics, psychology

The author of this text, a consultant in safety management and organizational behavior, describes "how managers, by controlling the physical and psychological situations under which workers operate, can modify employees' behavior in such a way as to reduce error, accidents, and consequently on-the-job injuries and illnesses." The book offers a multidisciplinary approach to workplace safety that integrates findings from psychology, ergonomics, business management, and safety management.

Major contributions to the volume include the following: "a model of accident causation that exemplifies the processes of today's safety technology; a treatment of the managerial sources of error; a chapter on the ways in which the 'culture' of an organization determines what methods will and will not succeed; a discussion of ergonomics—how design causes error; . . . insight into how to reduce psychological overload on the job; . . . and material on risk assessment techniques." See especially part 3 of the book on overload.

431. Petersen, Dan. *Safety by Objectives: What Gets Measured and Rewarded Gets Done.* New York: Van Nostrand Reinhold, 1996.

Keywords: total quality management, safety

This book explores the philosophy and practice of safety management in the workplace. The author shows "how to devise, install, operate and maintain tailor-made accountability systems that will foster a sense of safety responsibility, first in upper and middle managers and finally throughout the entire organization, thereby reducing on-the-job injuries and illnesses."

The book advances the position that measuring accident prevention efforts and rewarding effective safety performance are the foundation of any successful safety system. Drawing from modern management concepts, including Total Quality Management and Management by Objectives, it provides essential guidance on how to understand the corporation's individual culture; assess current safety systems using audits and perception surveys; identify the hazards that cause injuries and illnesses; set safety objectives and evaluate whether they have been met; and establish rewards for meeting safety performance goals.

This text is intended primarily for safety managers, safety engineers, industrial hygienists, and environmental professionals.

432. Piore, Michael J., and Charles F. Sabel. *The Second Industrial Divide: Possibilities for Prosperity*. New York: Basic Books, 1984.

Keywords: political economy, sociology, mass production, flexible production, general, technology

This now-classic work of industrial sociology/political economy argues that "we are living through the second industrial divide"—a historical period that offers an opportunity for a significant shift in the direction of technological development, away from the dominant principles of mass-production and toward the craft methods of production (using flexible equipment) that lost out at the first industrial divide. The authors suggest that the first industrial divide came in the nineteenth century when the emergence of mass-production technologies limited the growth of less rigid (i.e., more flexible) manufacturing technologies. It is further argued that "under somewhat different historical conditions, firms using a combination of craft skill and flexible equipment might have played a central role in modern economic life—instead of giving way, in almost all sectors of manufacturing, to corporations based on mass production. Had this line of mechanized craft production prevailed, we might today think of manufacturing firms as linked to particular communities, rather than as the independent organizations—barely involved with their neighbors—that, through mass production, seem omnipresent." The authors look at the history of industrial capitalism with a focus on the way in which technologies and organizations have been organized. They examine how a particular technology came to dominate industrial production and reopen the debate about the alternative possibilities of technological advance. "This reexamination of the past—together with a survey of the contradictory changes now in progress—illuminates the preconditions for the survival of any of the emerging economic alternatives." See especially chapter 2 "Mass Production as Destiny and Blind Decision," chapter 4 "Stabilizing the Economy," chapter 6 "Mass and Craft Production Abroad," chapter 7 "The Mass-Production Economy in Crisis," chapter 10 "Possibilities for Prosperity: International Keynesianism and Flexible Specialization," and chapter 11 "The United States and Flexible Specialization."

433. Poynter, Gavin. *Restructuring in the Service Industries: Management Reform and Workplace Relations in the UK Service Sector*. Employment and Work Relations in Context Series. New York: Mansell, 2000.

Keywords: service industries workers, Great Britain, service industries, management, personnel management, industrial relations, financial services industry, employees, insurance companies, health facilities, National Health Service

By focusing on industrial restructuring and workplace relations in the UK service sector, this book examines the complex processes of transformation in technology, labor, work organizations, and product markets that have occurred in recent years. This analysis also entails an in-depth study of the enterprise and the workplace and a broad appreciation of structural developments within the economies of the advanced industrial nations.

434. Pratt, Joanne, and Karen Jacobs, ed. *Work Practice: International Perspectives*. Oxford: Butterworth-Heinemann, 1997.

Keywords: health, occupational therapy, comparative

This volume uses a "person-environment framework" to provide evidence that "occupational therapy has broad and unique capabilities related to improving individuals' work performance." Section 1 of the text offers an introduction to the diversity of work patterns given cultural, gender, and historical factors. This section also discusses current models and trends in work practice service delivery (issues considered here include workers' compensation, health insurance, community resources, health maintenance organizations, health and wellness promotion programs, etc.).

Section 2 attempts to deepen the readers' understanding of the broad concept of "environment" by providing "a framework for the utilization of occupational therapy concepts in response to the breadth of environmental demands." (Topics covered include the following: the healthy community model; barriers to satisfactory work; adapting the work environment to facilitate work performance; and the person-environment model of occupational health.)

Section 3 focuses on specific areas of work performance enhancement. For example, "Work Programs to Enhance Psychosocial Performance Components." This section also examines cognitive and motor/neuromuscular performance.

Section 4 discusses "outcome measures in work practice" and some of the challenges to be faced by those employed in this area of practice, from an international perspective.

435. Prietula, M. J., and H. A. Simon. "The Experts in Your Midst." *Harvard Business Review*, January-February 1989: 120-24.

Keywords: skill, expertise, intuition, knowledge embedded in experience

The article examines the nature of skill and expertise among workers in corporations. It implicitly identifies expertise as related to knowledge embedded in experience (KEE). This is important, for misunderstanding this point can lead to not recognizing who the real experts are.

436. Pulat, Babur Mustafa, and David C. Alexander, eds. *Industrial Ergonomics: Case Studies*. New York: McGraw-Hill, 1991.

Keywords: ergonomics, stress, human factors

This book highlights recent innovative efforts in the growing field of industrial ergonomics. Case studies are presented that focus on the qualitative relationship between workers and their tools, workplace, work space, equipment, and environment. A human integrated design approach is used throughout the text—one that considers the human's role from the beginning of the design process and emphasizes human interaction with other systems.

The authors indicate that ergonomists are capable of playing a significant role in improving working conditions and the quality of working life for industrial workers. Other benefits of ergonomic designs for the workplace include the following: "higher production output; decreased lost time; lower medical and material costs; decreased absenteeism; high-quality work; fewer injuries and strains; decreased probability of accidents and errors; and decreased labor turnover."

See especially section 1 "An Overview of Industrial Ergonomics" and section 4 "Design of Work Space and Work Methods." In particular, see chapter 13 "Work Center Redesign Combines Tasks to Improve Productivity and Reduce Job Stress," chapter 17 "A Perspective on Solving Ergonomic Problems," and chapter 19 "Implementation of Human Factors Principles in the Design of a Manufacturing Process."

437. Puryear Keita, Gwendolyn, and Joseph J. Hurrell Jr., eds. *Job Stress in a Changing Workforce: Investigating Gender, Diversity and Family Issues*. Washington, DC: American Psychological Association, 1994.

Keywords: stress, family, coping, corporate culture, women

This book presents new research on occupational stress and "workplace wellness" in the context of recent social, economic, technological, and demographic trends. Some of these fundamental trends discussed include the increasing number of workers employed in service industries; the technological and organizational restructuring of corporations; the growing participation of women, ethnic minorities and older workers in the labor force; and the increasing pressures resulting from working adults attempting to balance the demands of work and family.

All of the essays are grouped into two broad stress-related themes: "workplace diversity and the interface between work and nonwork life." The first section of the book focuses on gender, culture, ethnicity and aging. "The second section includes two parts, exploring work and family functioning and work and family conflict, respectively."

Part 1 deals with the additional stress that women face as a result of their entry into male-dominated and patriarchal organizations as well as how to develop stress management programs to deal with this stress. Part 2 focuses on issues especially relevant to ethnic minorities and dealing with coping with workplace stress. Part 3 concentrates on issues of aging, including the effects of anxiety and depression. In part 4, the effect of work on family is investigated, along with specific problems related to two working parents, violence, self-esteem and unemployment. Part 5 focuses on work and nonwork conflict. Questions examined include the following: "How do the conditions of work thwart or further the developmental tasks of adulthood? How do individuals resolve conflicts between the demands of work and the needs of self, spouse, and children?"

438. Puryear Keita, Gwendolyn, and Steven L. Sauter, eds. *Work and Well-Being: An Agenda for the 1990s*. Washington DC: American Psychological Association, 1992.

Keywords: stress, health, coping, work design

Improved training, better job design, and reduction of stress in the workplace can contribute to health, well-being, and the prevention of work-related psychological disorders. This is the basis on which these papers from the conference of the same title as the book are based. The conference, a joint effort between the American Psychological Association (APA) and the National Institute of Occupational Safety and Health (NIOSH), aimed to develop additional strategies to protect workers from psychological disorders. The original document that the paper seeks to expand on, "Prevention of Work-Related Psychological Disorders: A National Strategy Proposed by the National Institute of Occupational Health and Safety," is also included. The aforementioned aim is approached from three different perspectives: health promotion, education, and treatment; surveillance of psychological disorders in the workplace; and work design and stress (the only one with a preventive inclination).

In the paper by this last panel, a variety of possible stressors in the workplace are studied. Section 1 considers stressors related to the psychological architecture of work. Section 2 considers ones related to the social aspects of that architecture. Sections 3 and 4 deal with control and the nature of work and task demands, respectively. Following this is an analysis of the exogenous versus endogenous nature of the stress debate. In other words, are stressors products of the environment or the individual's reaction to it? The authors conclude that exogenous and endogenous variables interact to produce strain. The paper concludes with recommendations for intervention and for research. The major design variables are identified as control, uncertainty, conflict and task/job demands.

Aside from the papers from the three panels, the book also contains an invited presentation entitled "Psychosocial, Occupational, Environmental, and Health Concepts; Research Results; and Applications."

439. Quick, James C., Debra L. Nelson, and Jonathan D. Quick. *Stress and Challenge at the Top: The Paradox of the Successful Executive.* Wiley Series on Studies in Occupational Stress. Chichester: John Wiley and Sons, 1990.

Keywords: stress, executives

As the title suggests, this book explores occupational stress from the perspective of the corporate executive. See chapter 2 "Executive Stress: The Risks of Success," which outlines the dynamics of stress; the stress response (physiological reactions to stress); the behavioral, psychological and medical consequences of stress; the health benefits of stress; and modifying the stress response. Also noted is the fact that "individual moderating factors" influence the body's response to stress. Factors suggested by Seyle include "internal conditioning factors" such as personality, family illness patterns, age and sex, as well as "external conditional factors" such as diet, drugs and social setting. See also chapter 3 "Preventive Stress Management: What Works and What Doesn't" and chapters 4 and 5 for case studies on the varied responses of different executives to stressors in the work environment.

440. Rain, Jeffrey S., Irving M. Lane, and Dirk D. Steiner. "A Current Look at the Job Satisfaction/Life Satisfaction Relationship: Review and Future Considerations." *Human Relations* 44, no. 3 (1991).

Keywords: job satisfaction, sociology, psychology

Sociological and psychological research studies have for many years postulated a correlation between job satisfaction and life satisfaction (JSLS). This paper reviews the literature on this relationship (usually referred to as the "spillover effect") and considers the theoretical, empirical, and methodological grounds for such a claim. The authors argue that "recent theoretical work is too often characterized by repeatedly confirming the spillover hypothesis to the exclusion of advancing further theoretical developments." Specific attention is given to the theoretical and methodological requirements for more insightful future research.

The authors report that support for the spillover hypothesis is strong in many studies to date. "A consistent positive relationship between global measures of job satisfaction and life satisfaction can be found." However, given the consistency of empirical results, the researchers wonder why "greater attention has not been paid to provide a consistent theoretical basis for the spillover hypothesis." The authors also suggest that intervening variables, such as how successfully people cope with work stress, "could moderate the impact of this stress on life satisfaction." In addition, this paper contends that "life stage, as operationalized by relative importance of work and nonwork, and the roles considered as salient in either job or life domain appear to be potentially important moderators."

441. Ransome, Paul. *The Work Paradigm: A Theoretical Investigation of Concepts of Work*. Brookfield: Avebury, 1996.

Keywords: work ethics, work history, economic rationality, Protestantism, Weber

Historically, cultures of each period have created work paradigms by conflating the concept of productive means with a specific idea of work, or a work ethic. This balance has, as the book explains, been the pervasive theoretical model of work in society from antiquity onwards until the industrial revolution. As a new technological paradigm, or concept of productive means, has radically shifted the work ethic, job security is put at risk alongside expectations of formal paid employment.

As advancing technologies have rapidly revolutionized our concepts of what work is and how it is carried out in our day-to-day lives, constantly changing concepts of work—in regards to issues of income, security, creativity, and social contact—demand that a new theoretical model is provided. Members of contemporary, advanced, post-industrial society face a growing endemic of joblessness due to technological advancement.

Divided into three major areas of study, the book begins with an overview of Marxian ideas of work with additional discussion of Lucien Seve and Andre Gorz in order to establish the theory of a contemporary work paradigm. It then progresses into stage two, discussing the work paradigms of classical, pre-Christian and early medieval society, as well as extensive discussion of Max Weber's Protestant Ethic Thesis, drawing an association between Protestant ethics and acquisitive capitalism. Upon establishing the relationships between belief systems and practice of work, the book moves into its third and final stage, discussing the developments of the late-twentieth century. Turning our attention to the changes brought by the "technological paradigm" onto the fundamental organization of work, the dislocated relationship between the concept and practice of work will be discussed, as well as how a new concept of work may work to reestablish a much-needed equilibrium.

442. Ransome, Paul. *Sociology and the Future of Work: Contemporary Discourses and Debates*. Brookfield: Ashgate, 1999.

Keywords: Marx, Durkheim, industrialism, feminism, Weber

The new world of work is fragmentary and insecure, demanding flexible and diverse skills. Focusing upon fundamental changes in today's workforce and job market, Ransome proposes an analysis from which some idea of what the future holds can be theorized. In doing this, the book criticizes some currently held debates on the future of the workplace and job market.

The future of the job market and of work is, in fact, a matter of perspective. From the old to the young, from the less educated to college and university graduates, such projections carry different weight and meanings, and in theorizing the future of work, it is of greater use to specify underlying patterns of work itself and not the individual experience. Likewise, there is no single analytical framework from which to create a solid model, and so discourse is more situated on key trends and dimensions, such as the decrease of employment in manufacturing with technological advancement, and the increase of employment for women across different fields with the breakage of gender roles.

Taking into account that in sociology, knowledge is more provisional than absolute, Ransome looks to the combination of continuity and change in industry, in several major parts. Beginning with the narrative theorists of industrialism, predominantly Karl Marx, Max Weber, and Emile Durkheim, as well as post-Ford industrialism, the book goes on to discuss how work paradigms are renovated by newer technology. Further study is made from a feminist perspective, specifically with regards to the engendering of specific occupations. The contradicting identities of production and consumption are also addressed, as well as questions of social divisions between the unemployed and employed, and contemporary notions of individuality, or "new individuality." Ransome concludes with a discourse of economic globalization and the sociological impact of a "Network Society" on the future of work.

443. Rasmussen, Bente, and Tove Håpnes. "Excluding Women from the Technologies of the Future? A Case Study of the Culture of Computer Science." *Futures*, December 1991: 1107.

Keywords: women, computers

The case study reported in this article was undertaken because of the authors' concern over the low level of representation of women in computer science. "The authors show how the culture and ideas of a small male minority of students, the computer hackers, come to dominate computer science in the eyes of the female students. This minority culture is reinforced by the values and interests of the most powerful (male) groups in computer science, the male professors and teachers and their disciples, the dedicated students. In this way, a male-dominated and machine-fixated culture works to marginalize women."

In order to analyze the culture of a computer science education, the researchers "deconstructed the cultural images and representations of the different groups in the Department of Computer Science at the Norwegian Institute of Technology." Both teachers and students were interviewed for the study—on the curricula and the cultural conditions, their experiences and ideas, and their values and interests. Throughout the article the authors' perspective is the viewpoint of the female students.

444. Rasmussen, Jens. "Human Error and the Problem of Causality in Analysis of Accidents." *Transactions of the Royal Philosophical Society, London. Part B.* 32 (1989): 449.

Keywords: human factors, accidents, complex systems

This paper explores the changing nature of human factors problems faced in industrial safety as technological systems become larger and more complex. The author argues that "in previous periods, the analysis of industrial systems could be treated separately by different professions . . . human factors specialists were primarily involved in attempts to match the interface between people and equipment to human characteristics." However, in the modern context, "human factors problems of industrial safety have become a true cross-disciplinary issue."

Current human factors concerns "not only include the classical interface problems, but also problems such as the ability of the designers to predict and supply the means to control the relevant disturbances to an acceptable degree of completeness, the ability of the organization . . . to maintain an acceptable quality of risk management."

Topics examined in the paper include the following: the nature of causal explanations for accidents; accident analysis; allocation of responsibility; suggestions for system improvements; error in sociotechnical systems; the problem of human adaptation; system safety and error-recovery; and the control of safety in high hazard systems. The fundamental conclusion of the paper is that "some of the deficiencies presently attributed to operator of management deficiencies may very well be structural problems that have to be considered at a much more fundamental level than efforts to improve human reliability."

445. Rasmussen, Jens. "Perspectives on the Concept of Human Error." Paper presented at the First Danish Conference on Cognitive Science Research, Roskilde University: 1992.

Keywords: human error, cognitive science, complex systems

This fascinating paper, written with a cognitive science frame of reference, explores the concept of human error in the context of industrial/technological environments. The implications for accident prevention and the design of safe and reliable systems are also considered. The author argues that the notion of human error is very elusive, and that many accidents attributed to human behavior are often due to problems inherent in complex, nonlinearly structured technological systems.

The paper examines the definition and identification of human error from the perspective of psychology, engineering, risk analysis and law. "From here, the cognitive aspects of errors and the close relationship with human learning and adaptation are discussed." The author contends that "the theme of research should be the cognitive control of activities in complex work systems, not human error in a laboratory setting."

This paper also provides some suggestions for the "design of error tolerant systems." The role of systems design in improving safety is seen to be the responsibility of many different specialists, including law makers, company authorities, engineering designers, and operations planners.

Conclusions are summarized as follows: "In a modern dynamic environment, where discretionary decision-making to a large degree is replacing routine tasks, definition of a correct or normal way of doing things is difficult, and the focus of research should be on the understanding of the way in which features of the work environment shape human behavior and the conditions under which normal psychological mechanisms result in unsuccessful performance." The author also states that "the aim . . . is to design work systems that support the actors in coping with the effects of their actions." This requires "a better understanding of the relationship between human adaptation to a dynamic environment and human errors."

446. Rasmussen, Jens, Berndt Brehmer, and Jaques Leplat, eds. *Distributed Decision Making: Cognitive Models for Cooperative Work*. New Technologies and Work. Chichester: John Wiley and Sons, 1991.

Keywords: complex systems, cognitive science, decision making

This rather technical volume explores "the basis for design of decision support systems in different kinds of complex, collective modern work environments." The authors contend that decision making in work settings has all too often been analyzed "in terms of isolated 'decisions' made by one person," whereas in reality, "decision making is a continuous interpersonal process." Rather than approaching the subject from a management or sociological perspective, the writers in this collection advance a "cognitive approach."

The book can be argued to be overburdened by excessive statistical data, complex methodological schema, and modeling jargon that detract from this important field of investigation. In summary, this is a very specialized analysis of a difficult subject. Any possible implications of this work for (direct) application to healthy work strategies are obscure and implicit.

447. Rasmussen, Jens, Annelise Mark Pejtersen, and L. P. Goodstein. *Cognitive Systems Engineering*. Wiley Series in Systems Engineering. New York: John Wiley and Sons, 1994.

Keywords: cognitive science, human factors, expert systems

The human conditions of work are being rapidly transformed by new information technologies. As the authors point out, "levels of mechanization and automation are steadily increasing and computers are used in planning and control within most work domains." The consequence of this is that "computer-based interfaces are being inserted between humans and their work."

The central thesis of this book is that "a new approach to the analysis of work is needed together with the development of a new frame of reference that can serve the strategic planning, design, and evaluation of sociotechnical systems based on advanced technology."

The authors emphasize that for the design of information systems and user interfaces, expertise is needed not only in the work domain for which the system is going to be used—but is also crucial with respect to "human cognition." Therefore, it becomes increasingly important that "human factors considerations should be an integral part of the basic design process, and not merely an add-on polish to the interface." Here is where the preventive component of cognitive systems engineering is clearly evident.

The introduction to the text also discusses the present change toward flexible manufacturing systems in order to illustrate "the conceptual issues caused by the introduction of information technology in a complex, modern work domain." Topics covered in the book include "basic modelling problems, functional abstraction versus structural decomposition, relational and causal representations, control strategies in work systems (open-loop control, closed-loop control, control by trial-and-error, adaptive control), the design of adaptive systems, and cognitive systems analysis." To a great extent this is a technical volume for specialists. Nevertheless, the application potential for the area of healthy work is substantial.

448. Ray, Darrel, and Howard Bronstein. *Teaming Up: Making the Transition to a Self-Directed, Team-Based Organization*. New York: McGraw-Hill, 1995.

Keywords: teams, management, self-directed work groups

This book examines the advantages of self-directed work teams in company organizations—both for the benefit to employees themselves and for the employer—in the form of productivity and efficiency gains. The authors make the assumption that the "art of managing is in empowering individuals and groups to do what they already do for themselves in their private lives." The strategies suggested here for "opening up corporate life to *all* so that workers can fully participate" are regarded as a whole ensemble, a new management "technology" rather than a number of individual, self-contained techniques. Essentially, the book is about "changing the patterns of communication in organizations" so that all parties involved can take greater control of their workplace destiny.

See especially part 2 "Designing for Self-Direction." Topics include key considerations; size, structure and consensus; assessing the work environment; employee perceptions; the design team: techniques and strategies; and the role of the team developer and interpersonal processes in teams. Also see part 3 "A System for Self-Directed Work Teams." This section explores topics such as organizing the self-directed work team, training the self-directed work team, modeling and communication, and techniques for receiving feedback.

449. Rayman, Paula M. *Beyond the Bottom Line: The Search for Dignity at Work*. New York: Palgrave for St. Martin's Press, 2001.

Keywords: work ethic, psychological aspects, dignity

The book is concerned with "having work that provides dignity and a family life that provides unrushed time for caring." The author argues that externalities must be included in calculating the costs and benefits of our current economy. What is productive for our economy, the well-being of families, and the viability of society need to be considered in this equation. The author challenges current skepticism and cynicism by arguing that a change in how we live and work is not only possible but that there are undeniable signs that it is beginning to take place.

450. Raynauld, Andre, and Jean-Pierre Vidal. *Labor Standards and International Competitiveness: A Comparative Analysis of Developing and Industrialized Countries*. Cheltenham, UK: Edward Elgar Publishing, 1998.

Keywords: labor policy, labor laws and legislation, employee rights, comparative industrial relations, labor economies, wages, developing countries, labor productivity, competition, international

The central purpose of this book is to study the impact of labor standards on the competitiveness of firms in the context of a comparison between developed and developing countries. Generally speaking, labor standards include government regulations concerning working conditions as well as rules arising from collective agreements—for example, minimum wages, the freedom to form labor unions, restrictions on the number of working hours, and other similar examples of considerable importance. In developing countries, the lack of a strict code of labor standards has been seen in the more advanced countries as fostering unfair competition and, rightly or wrongly, as justifying the adoption of protectionist measures. On the whole, developing countries have been opposed to the adoption of labor standards because they view such measures as likely to interfere with their competitiveness in world markets.

451. Rayner, Bruce. "Trial-by-Fire Transformation." *Harvard Business Review*, May-June 1992: 117-29.

Keywords: work design, labor-management relations, case study

This interview with the CEO of an innovative metallurgical company revolves around the changes that he has made over the past eight years. He talks about implementing flexible, cross-functional work teams and a quality program. The company also gained a strong emphasis on research and development and a niche marketing strategy. Many of the changes that the CEO implemented are the results of lessons learned during a labor strike that forced managers to run the furnaces themselves.

452. Reckman, Bob. "Carpentry: The Craft and Trade." 73-102 in *Case Studies on the Labor Process*, edited by Andrew Zimbalist. New York: Monthly Review, 1979.

Keywords: skill, knowledge embedded in experience, design, deskilling

The historical evolution of carpentry is not a subject often written about. This paper traces this evolution in the United States, from colonial times to the present. The focus is on the technologies the carpenter used, the network of social relations within which he worked, and the relationship between the two.

Reckman begins by illustrating the importance of building as a human activity through the use of statistics regarding its share of GNP, number of companies, number of employees, etc. The change in the definition of carpentry is discussed next. Anyone who worked with wood used to be called a carpenter. Today, the narrower definition encompasses only the use of wood in buildings and represents a loss in skill embedded in experience. Reckman proposes that the carpenter's activities be thought of as consisting of both the craft and the trade dimension. Craft refers to the "skills, tools, technologies, and logic of the work," while trade refers to "control over the process and products toward which that craft is applied."

After the introductory section, Reckman comments upon "the art of building with wood in the material world of time, weather, and people." This art, he states, can be described in terms of four characteristics. Firstly, carpentry is an *art*—there is no absolute right or wrong way to build. Secondly, the possibility that exists for compromise versus lasting quality must be considered. Thirdly, the integration of the design and layout stages within the sequential building process is important. Finally, all buildings have a lot in common yet contain endless differences.

The next section consists of a historical synopsis. The colonial period, the period between the Revolutionary War and the Civil War, the period between the Civil War and the turn of the century, and the twentieth century are examined in detail. The main pattern that emerges is that the "expanding capitalist/industrialized social relations and forces have destroyed parts of the carpenter's craft skill or trade autonomy."

This deskilling trend and others are described in the final section. The influence of complementary trades with which carpenters must now share the job site is considered. As well, the impact of technologies and trades that displace the carpenter, such as factory-produced parts and even houses prefabricated on an assembly line, is reviewed. The purpose of building used to be to provide a structure for a family or store owner that met their long-term needs. Today, buildings are built for their value on the market. The far-reaching implications of this key change are analyzed.

453. Reich, Robert B. *The Work of Nations: Preparing Ourselves for 21st Century Capitalism*. New York: Alfred A. Knopf, 1991.

Keywords: capitalism, political economy, policy, forecasting

This highly-regarded book by one of America's foremost political economists examines the transformation of work in the context of the emerging global economy. The increasing irrelevance of the concept of a national economy (and corporate nationality) is analyzed. Conventional indicators of economic prosperity, such as the gross national product, national economic growth, and national competitiveness are criticized for their serious limitations in explaining the new economic realities of the twenty-first century.

In an era in which "almost every factor of production—money, technology, factories, and equipment—moves effortlessly across borders," the author argues that there is only one aspect of a national economy "that is relatively immobile internationally: the American workforce, the American people." Consequently, the author contends that "the real economic challenge facing the United States in the years ahead . . . is to increase the potential value of what its citizens can add to the global economy by enhancing their skills and capacities and by improving their means of linking those skills and capabilities to the world market."

This book also focuses on "the future of American *society* as distinct from the American economy, and the fate of the majority of Americans who are losing out in global competition." The author clearly recognizes the critical importance of full participation by the majority of workers in the new global economy if the well-being of society is to be preserved. See especially part 1 "The Economic Nation," part 2 "The Global Web," and part 3 "The Rise of the Symbolic Analyst."

454. Reid, Donald G. *Work and Leisure in the 21st Century: From Production to Citizenship*. Toronto: Wall & Emerson, 1995.

Keywords: leisure, forecasting, Canada

This book, written from a Canadian perspective, "examines the balance between work and leisure, and the resulting alternative social organization strategies available to society." The fundamental premise of the author is that "work must not be seen as the only venue for gaining a sense of self-worth and identity. Given the present trends in the economy and workplace, people may come to rely more on non-work and leisure activities to enhance individual well-being and the health of the communities in which they live than on the work they do."

The author discusses the importance of citizenship and community, arguing that society faces a greater problem of citizenship than production. "We tend to assess the worth of individuals more by their contribution to the production process rather than by their involvement in and contribution to society."

The chief aim of the book is to describe and promote a more positive "post-capitalist social formation, a system based on a lifestyle which transcends our present understanding of the concepts of work and leisure . . . emphasis moves from production to citizenship, cultivated through leisure and education."

The author also endorses the movement toward, first, a guaranteed annual wage and, then, a guaranteed annual income as a means of promoting more meaningful civic participation by everyone in society. Other topics discussed include the following: the globalization of the economy and its effect on work; the effect of technology in the work environment; the post-materialist society; radical planning and community development; and leisure as a liberating concept.

455. Reilly, Peter. *Flexibility at Work: Balancing the Interests of Employer and Employee*. Hampshire, UK: Gower Publishing, 2001.

Keywords: hours of labor, flexible, manpower planning, industrial relations

The key to success lies in balancing the needs of employers to be efficient and competitive with the needs of employees to protect their incomes and to lead the lifestyle that suits them. It is commonplace to find that flexible work arrangements are not developed with consideration given to the individual circumstances of employees. The argument of this book is that it is becoming increasingly difficult to achieve success in developing flexible work arrangements due to the rhetoric of flexibility, the elasticity of the term, and the different mental models held by those responsible for defining employment relationships. To overcome these difficulties, organizations should attempt to get beyond the rhetoric and discover mutually beneficial approaches that cater to the needs of their increasingly diverse work force. Organizations must also take into account the changing demography of the workforce, the changing external environment, the social context within which it operates, and the political environment, in order for a real solution to take place.

456. Reynolds, Shirley, and David A. Shapiro. "Stress Reduction in Transition: Conceptual Problems in the Design, Implementation and Evaluation of Worksite Stress Management Interventions." *Human Relations* 44, no. 7 (1991).

Keywords: stress, medicine, psychology, organizational change

This article discusses the impact of the medical model in occupational stress research and "explores the extent to which it has constrained the design, implementation, and evaluation of stress management interventions." The authors contend that two basic problems have been found in existing evaluation studies. The first is that many of these studies "share common methodological problems which include the use of inadequate controls . . . and lack of follow-up." The second problem, which relates most directly to the issue of developing preventive/healthy work strategies, "concerns the limited range of intervention strategies which have been chosen" and "the extent to which these strategies attempt to change attributes of the individual rather than characteristics of their working environments."

The study examines conceptual issues in stress research, the challenges of reducing occupational stress, the design and implementation of stress management intervention strategies, and future directions and recommendations for occupational stress research. The authors conclude that "psychologically compatible models such as systems theory may provide a more fruitful basis for development and research and a focus for collaboration between occupational and clinical psychologists."

457. Rifkin, Jeremy. *The End of Work: The Decline of the Global Labor Force and the Dawn of the Post-Market Era*. New York: G. P. Putnam's Sons, 1995.

Keywords: technology, unemployment

This volume examines "the technological innovations and market-directed forces that are moving us to the edge of a near workerless world." Section 1 "The Two Faces of Technology" presents an overview of the current technology revolution with an eye toward understanding its effect on employment and the global economy. The author discusses the "two competing visions of technological progress that have spurred the drive to an automated society," in order to better assess the impacts and potential outcomes of the Third Industrial Revolution.

Section 2 "The Third Industrial Revolution" looks at how early innovations in automation affected the livelihoods of American workers and trade unionists, and how "their experience could be a harbinger of what lies ahead for millions of service and white collar workers as well as a growing number of middle-class management and professional employees around the world." The section ends with an analysis of "the revolutionary changes being made in corporate organizational structures and management practices to accommodate the new high technologies of the twenty-first century."

In section 3 "The Decline of the Global Labor Force," Rifkin explores in depth "the vast technological and organizational changes taking place in the agricultural, manufacturing, and service sectors that are greatly reducing the number of workers needed to produce the world's goods and services."

Section 4 "The Price of Progress" considers the human consequences of the restructuring of production practices and the permanent replacement of machines for human laborers. The author argues that "information and communications technologies and global market forces are fast polarizing the world's population into two irreconcilable and potentially warring forces—a new cosmopolitan elite of 'symbolic analysts' who control the technologies and the forces of production, and the growing numbers of permanently displaced workers who have little hope . . . for meaningful employment in the new high-tech global economy."

458. Rijnsdorp, J. E., ed. *Proceedings of the IFAC Workshop*. Pergamon Press, 1977.

Keywords: automation, work design, participation

These proceedings of the International Federation of Automatic Control workshop contain papers presented under the subject headings of "general," "supervision of processes and systems," "numerical control, assembly, and robots," "other subjects," and "late papers." A "discussion report" and list of participants are also included. Although dated and not the most comprehensive collection of papers in this bibliography, it is nonetheless a good resource for studying automated systems.

The main conclusion reached is that a complete redesign of work is necessary for its humanization. This new design is characterized by two-way communication, cooperation among different functional units, flexibility, and transparency to the outside world. As well, the humane organization must promote worker participation through familiarization with various processes, autonomy for groups, vertical job enrichment, and ergonomics. Discussions also revolve around the dangers of extreme automation. The impossibility of jobs that require monitoring of VDTs in the case of calamities is affirmed. The computer should be a partner, not a master or an adversary, the editor declares. Concern is also raised regarding the social needs of isolated workers.

As well, it is acknowleged that problems with implementing radical changes in work organization exist. Firstly, lower management may feel threatened when vertical job enrichment is provided to workers below them. Secondly, economic limitations come into play.

459. Rinehart, James. "Improving the Quality of Working Life through Job Redesign: Work Humanization or Work Rationalization?" *Canadian Review of Sociology and Anthropology* 23, no. 4 (1986): 507-30.

Keywords: QWL, work design, participation

Quality of Working Life (QWL) programs claim to benefit both capital and labor: managers gain a more cooperative and productive workforce and workers gain job satisfaction. This assertion faces two lines of criticism in this article. Rinehart begins by describing two types of QWL programs: participative management and job redesign. He shows that the latter does not follow the resistance-integration explanation of productivity increase. That is, he postulates that productivity gains are due to work rationalization and not due to workers' improved attitudes toward the employer and resulting lowered resistance. The second line of criticism theorizes that employees' gains are overestimated due to two factors: (1) overestimation of QWL's effect on organizational hierarchy and job content and the resulting psychological gratifications, and (2) underestimation or outright denial of workers' possible decrease in job security, bargaining power and power of workers' organizations.

460. Rinehart, J. W. *The Tyranny of Work*. 2nd ed. Toronto: Harcourt Brace Jovanovich, 1987.

Keywords: QWL, participation, work design

This book provides a skeptical treatment of QWL's claims and the claims of job redesign in general. In whatever form it is packaged, QWL is used by the corporation insofar as it is compatible with cost reducing and profit maximizing objectives. Job redesign is implemented not to humanize work but to intensify labor, lessen labor costs, or to meet production exigencies that a highly specialized division of labor cannot handle economically. Participatory mechanisms are introduced to appropriate workers' knowledge and to turn resistant workers and adversarial unions into willing collaborators with management policies.

461. Robbins, Stephen P. *Organizational Behavior: Concepts, Controversies, and Applications*. Englewood Cliffs, NJ: Prentice Hall, 1993.

Keywords: organizational behavior, work design, job enrichment

This textbook tries overly hard to be fun and readable, and it contains a brief mention of job redesign. The self-managed team concept is introduced through the example of the Volvo plant in Uddevalla, Sweden. Other types of job design such as job rotation, job enlargement, and job enrichment are given. The author, however, seems to be somewhat critical of job enrichment and self-managed work teams. In the chapter on work stress, job redesign is listed as an organizational stress management strategy. After stating that "Redesigning jobs to give employees more responsibility, more meaningful work, more autonomy, and increased feedback can reduce stress" and mentioning the demand-control model, the author curiously makes the following statements: not everybody wants an enriched job, and for some workers less responsibility and increased division of labor are beneficial. Also contained in this chapter are explanations of stress, its consequences, its sources, individual differences in dealing with stress, and implications for performance and satisfaction.

Other than this, the book is a standard textbook on organizational behavior, divided into sections examining the individual, the group, and the organization. Appendix A contains a valuable discussion of the history of organizational behavior. Early influences of Adam Smith, Charles Babbage, and Robert Owen are recounted. Taylor's scientific management, Fayol's administrative theory, Weber's structural theory and the "social man" theory are explained and put into perspective. Discussions of the behavioral era and "OB today" conclude the section.

462. Rodrigue, John C. *Reconstruction in the Cane Fields: From Slavery to Free Labor in Louisiana's Sugar Parishes, 1862-1880*. Baton Rouge: Louisiana State University Press, 2001.

Keywords: sugar workers, Louisiana, history, plantation workers, slavery, slaves, emancipation, sugarcane industry

By using the sugar plantations as a basis for his study, the author displays the intense political struggles that followed the American Civil War, with insights into the evolution of labor relations after slavery. Sugar plantations, unlike cotton or tobacco, functioned much like factories in the fields where the laborers worked for their wage. It is in this light that the strategies planters and free people devised, respectively, to produce a valuable product in a fiercely competitive international market and to earn a living in an atmosphere of security and dignity are explored.

463. Rogers, Jackie Krasas. *Temps: The Many Faces of the Changing Workplace*. Ithaca, NY: Cornell University Press, 2000.

Keywords: temporary employment, part-time employment, lawyers

Temporary employees constitute a much-discussed but poorly understood segment of the labor force, even though it is now an established fixture of the American workplace. The realities of temporary work are explored from the points of view of workers, agencies, and clients, concentrating on issues of race, gender, power, and identity.

464. Rolfe, Heather. "In the Name of Progress? Skill and Attitudes toward Change." *New Technology, Work and Employment* 5, no. 2 (1990): 107-21.

Keywords: skill

This article uses case study data to explore the relationship between skill and workers' attitudes to technological change. A detailed model of skill is constructed to examine whether and how jobs are deskilled. The influence of a range of skill-based and other factors on attitudes is then assessed.

465. Ronco, William, and Lisa Peattie. *Making Work: Self-Created Jobs in Participatory Organizations*. New York: Plenum Press, 1983.

Keywords: participation, egalitarian work

This volume looks at small participatory and egalitarian work organizations where workers have maximum autonomy and control. The researchers seek to "know both the organizational conditions for satisfying work and the conditions under which collaborative work organizations can keep functioning." Among the organizations studied are a teacher-controlled public school, a fishermen's cooperative, a potter's studio, a public-interest advocacy group, and an architectural firm.

Essentially, the book explores the question of work satisfaction by focusing on three aspects of the organizations' experience: (1) the extent to which the organizations contribute to members' work experience, (2) members' ability to control and govern the organizations, and (3) the organizations' effectiveness and ability to learn. The book also examines how different individuals exhibit work accomplishment and the question of what it means for work satisfaction or dissatisfaction to have to define a chosen and satisfying activity as "work."

See especially chapter 1 "Making Work" on "The Social Construction of Work" and the "Inherent Dilemmas of 'Good Work.'" Also see chapter 8 on "Participatory Organizations." The case studies are found in chapters 2 through 6.

466. Roney, Alex, and Cary Cooper, eds. *Professionals on Workplace Stress: The Essential Facts*. Essential Facts Series. Chichester: John Wiley and Sons, 1997.

Keywords: stress, coping

This volume seeks to develop an acceptable definition of stress and how it relates to the workplace. It also gives practical advice on preventive and coping strategies. The contributors, consisting of a psychologist, human resource manager, business adviser, occupational physician, lawyer, and victim, link their combined skills and knowledge to offer an overall strategy to manage stress at work. The book details the devastating impact stress can have at both a personal and financial level. But once the reality of the problem is recognized, say the authors, "it is possible to implement effective tactics to identify and limit the negative aspects of stress."

Chapter 1 provides an "Introduction to Workplace Stress." Topics discussed here include the following: changing work patterns; temporary work and stress; debt as a stressor; stress and the self-employed; stress management techniques; general observations; etc. Chapter 2 identifies sources of stress in the workplace and gives a strategy to deal with them. Chapter 3 provides a "Human Resource Perspective on Managing Stress," which considers the symptoms, root causes, employers' responsibilities, and preventive strategies. Chapter 4 outlines "An Occupational Physician's Experience of Workplace Stress." The author gives an example of a stress audit and discusses stress awareness seminars and employment assistance programs. See chapter 5 on "The Legal Implications for Employers and Employees of Workplace Stress." Chapter 6 gives "A Victim's Tale of Stress" and presents a detailed overview of the stress-related hazards of self-employment.

467. Roobeck, Annemieke J. M. "The Crisis in Fordism and the Rise of a New Technological Paradigm." *Futures*, April 1987: 129-54.

Keywords: Fordism, mass production

The sometimes contradictory general tendencies in social and institutional structures spring partly from control problems and partly from the application of new technology. In contrast to the mass-production concept that was so characteristic of Fordism, now other features are appearing: flexibility, deregulation, dualization and polarization, and segmentation. As a result, existing labor and social relations, as well as interindustrial relations, will be drastically changed. In nearly all economic and social areas there appears to be a tendency toward flexibility. Greatest flexibility is found in the size of the workforce and tasks demanded of employees (so-called internal flexibility).

468. Rose, H., I. McLoughlin, R. King, and J. Clark. "Opening the Black Box: The Relation between Technology and Work." *New Technology, Work and Employment* 1, no. 1 (1986): 18-26.

Keywords: technology, case study

This article argues that social scientists need to develop a detailed understanding of technology and its relationship to social variables if the full implication of new technologies is to be adequately investigated. Material from research on telephone exchange modernization in British Telecom is used to develop such an approach.

469. Rosen, Ned. *Teamwork and the Bottom Line: Groups Make a Difference.* Series in Applied Psychology. Hillsdale, NJ: Lawrence Erlbaum, 1989.

Keywords: teams, work groups, stress

A group can work synergistically as a team under certain conditions. Ned Rosen investigates why and how from a social psychology/organizational behavior perspective. Topics covered include the group life cycle, the manager's role, the impact of office automation, group development, how groups affect their members, job satisfaction, communication, group status, motivation, recognition, rewards, group tasks and participation in decision making. The section most relevant to healthy work is chapter 6 "Stress, Strain, and Conflict: By-Products of Group Processes." However, it is not truly preventive, for the focus is on increased productivity for its own sake. The chapter outlines three categories of sources of employee frustration: (1) stress encountered while performing one's job, (2) stress due to balancing work and home life, and (3) stress due to employer's system of rules and policies and their administration. Consequences of stress, factors affecting reactions to stress, as well as conflict within the group round out the chapter.

470. Rosenberg, Richard S. *The Social Impact of Computers*. San Diego: Academic Press, 1992.

Keywords: computers, general

This volume offers a good introduction to "the social implications of current and future applications of computers." Appropriate as a textbook for students, the book makes use of research findings from sociology, economics, history, political science, and philosophy.

Seven basic themes are explored: "1. The changing nature of work in response to technological innovation as well as the threat to jobs. 2. Personal freedom in the machine age as manifested by challenges to privacy, dignity and work. 3. The relationship between advances in computer and communications technology and the possibility of increased centralization of authority. 4. The emergence and influence of artificial intelligence and its role in decision-making, especially in military applications. 5. The growing importance of information as both a means to improve productivity and as a commodity in its own right. 6. The hidden influence of computers as microprocessors embedded in a myriad of products. 7. The diffusion of the personal computers at work, at home, in schools, and elsewhere."

More specifically, this book also addresses the following issues: privacy and freedom of information; computer crime; information technology in the political process; women and computing; Videotext systems; military applications of computers; medicine and computers; popular attitudes toward computers; robotics and industrial automation; and ethics and professionalism in computing.

471. Rosenberg, Richard S. *The Social Impact of Computers*. 2nd ed. San Diego: Academic Press, 1997.

Keywords: computers, general

This volume is a substantially revised and updated version of the 1992 edition. In response to a number of major technological innovations, the author has made significant additions to the text, especially in regard to issues such as the Internet, the Information (Super) Highway, the National Information Infrastructure, Virtual Communities, MUDs, the Clipper Chip, the Communications Decency Act, etc. A wider view and more extended analysis has also been given to social/ethical concerns such as privacy, free speech, security, risks, access to information, personal responsibility, and national interests. Special emphasis has been paid in this edition to new computer technologies and problems including: industry regulation, electronic financial systems, electronic stock markets, international competition, and productivity. See especially chapter 2 "Computers and the Human Imagination" (computers as a creative medium, artificial intelligence, etc.); chapter 4 "The Business World" (information technology, the office of the future); chapter 5 "Medicine and Computers" (medical information systems, computers and the disabled, medicine and the Internet, etc.); chapter 6 "Computers and Education" (computer-assisted instruction, computer literacy); chapter 8 "Computers and the Law" (computer crime, legal issues on the Internet, etc.); chapter 10 "Employment and Unemployment" (telecommuting, women and computers, the union response, etc.); chapter 12 "The Information Society" (virtual communities, access, risk and security); and chapter 13 "Ethics and Professionalism" (pedagogy and ethics, professional organizations and ethics). See also the appendix for a long list of organizations that are concerned with many of the social issues addressed in the book.

472. Rosenbrock, H. H., ed. *Designing Human-Centered Technology: A Cross-Disciplinary Project in Computer-Aided Manufacturing*. Springer Series on Artificial Intelligence and Society. London: Springer-Verlag, 1989.

Keywords: CAM, anthropocentric, participation, collaborative work

This second volume in a series on Artificial Intelligence (AI) and Society "explores the issues involved in the design and application of human-centered systems in the manufacturing area, with particular reference to the introduction of AI systems." The book provides a participatory design approach that focuses on collaborative learning and enhancement and creation of new skills. The concern for a human-centered perspective is reflected in the text's emphasis on the role of intuition, subjective judgement, and tacit knowledge in the human expert.

This book clarifies the debate on the tacit dimension of skills and practice and "lays a foundation for the design of practical systems in working life environments where the fundamental issues of collaborative design will be common." The authors suggest that the "design challenge" may be seen as dealing with such issues as: "sharing of knowledge space; . . . distribution and diffusion of knowledge; open and distance learning; tacit knowledge; social and cultural determinants; human factors; information flows; internationalization of knowledge." The book also includes an outline of a human-centered CIM project carried out by the University of Manchester Institute of Science and Technology (UMIST).

In the foreword, Mike Cooley and Karamjit Gill state that "a great strength of the book is that it raises at a practical and a philosophical level sets of alternatives to the given orthodoxy."

See especially chapter 6 "On the Collaboration between Social Scientists and Engineers," chapter 7 "How Can Technology Be Redirected? A Scandinavian Perspective," and chapter 10 "Human-Centered Systems" by Mike Cooley.

473. Rossler, Paul E. "Challenging Mainstream IE Thinking: The Human Element." *Industrial Engineering*, September 1991: 53-8, 73.

Keywords: engineering, Taylorism

This article examines the Tayloristic paradigm in industrial engineering that is imported into management strategies. The author finds this paradigm of scientific management short-sighted and suggests a more humanistic approach to industrial engineering.

474. Rouse, William. *Design for Success: A Human-Centered Approach to Designing Successful Products and Systems*. Wiley Series in Systems Engineering, Wiley Interscience Series. New York: John Wiley and Sons, 1991.

Keywords: anthropocentric, engineering, design

This volume argues that engineers and designers "need to understand users' needs and preferences in order to design products and systems that are user-friendly in the broadest sense of the phrase." The author attempts to meet this objective by presenting "a comprehensive methodological framework for human-centered design of complex systems." This new approach to system design includes four phases that cover the entire product life cycle. A wide variety of methods and tools are discussed in the context of this methodological framework, and the use of these techniques is illustrated by several case histories.

The design philosophy presented in the book "focuses on the roles of humans in complex systems . . . and the design objectives are elaborated in terms of roles of humans." These features distinguish the human-centered design philosophy from more conventional approaches. The author's perspective of design is one that does not focus primarily on performance, productivity or economics. While these are seen as very important, "they subserve human-centered design issues because achieving, for example, performance goals is the consequence of good design rather than the means for creating the design."

This text follows through in its application of a human-centered method of design for all phases of product or system development: design and measurement, marketing, engineering, sales and service, system evaluation, etc.

475. Rousseau, Denise M., and Rene Schalk, eds. *Psychological Contracts in Employment: Cross-National Perspectives*. Thousand Oaks, CA: Sage Publications, 2000.

Keywords: organizational behavior, cross-cultural studies, contracts, psychological aspects, commitment, industrial relations

There is an ever-changing relationship worldwide between workers and firms, and nowhere is this more evident than in the psychological contracts of employment, that is, the obligations workers owe to their employer and vice versa. This book examines how societies differ in the nature of psychological contracts in employment and how global business initiatives are bridging these differences. International knowledge is given to the topic at hand as scholars from thirteen countries delve into the issue, thus involving both local and global psychological contract phenomena.

476. Rowe, Christopher. *People and Chips: The Human Implications of Information Technology*. 2nd ed. Oxford: Blackwell Scientific Publications, 1990.

Keywords: video display terminal, information technology, industrial relations, deskilling, skills

This updated version of a 1986 edition considers the human implications of the introduction of information technology (IT), with particular reference to employment, industrial relations, citizenship and leisure. The book does not focus on the technology itself but on people, "first as consumers, and how IT affects patterns of expenditure, changes in lifestyle and developments in leisure patterns; secondly as citizens, and the impact on democracy and privacy; and finally as workers, and the effects on employment, industrial relations, and occupational skills." The author considers these issues by drawing on sociology, economics, law, and politics to explore the central question of the human effects of new technology.

Particular emphasis is given to the influence of information technology in the workplace. Topics explored here include the following: the deskilling and reskilling arguments; computer-aided design; robotics; flexible manufacturing systems; automated factories; health and safety concerns; the information office (i.e., new office technology); VDTs; and the role of management and unions in the introduction of new computer technology. See also chapter 8 on citizenship and chapter 10 "A New Work Ethic?"

477. Rubin, Marcus, and Ray Richardson. *The Microeconomics of the Shorter Working Week*. Aldershot, UK: Avebury, 1997.

Keywords: work time, policy

In the United Kingdom, the number of working hours has been decreasing for almost 200 years. Why is this the case? Do people really want to work fewer hours? Would they prefer a pay raise to a shortened work week? Does a shorter work week mean more efficient use of time? What is the relationship between the shorter working week, unemployment and productivity? These and other interesting questions are probed with a UK focus. The central question asks how the shorter working week affects economics. The micro-, rather than macro-, economic approach is taken. Past research shows that a reduction in hours stimulates productivity but does not decrease unemployment. These studies are the focus of chapter 2. The research undertaken by the authors is described in chapters 3 and 4 and suggests that reduced hours are not related to changes in productivity. While this study focuses on engineering work, chapter 5 studies factory reports of the result of reduced hours. Conclusions and policy implications are presented in the final chapter.

478. Rudolph, Barbara. *Disconnected: How Six People from AT&T Discovered the New Meaning of Work in a Downsized Corporate America*. New York: Free Press, 1998.

Keywords: corporate America, downsizing, corporations

While the world of work rapidly changes, job instability has come with the territory, even among high ranking executives of corporate America. Following the lives of six laid-off employees of AT&T, Rudolph discusses the disregard of perceived old workplace concepts of loyalty, security, and community for the contemporary attitude of blunt individualism and emotional detachment. Emphasizing the connection between sense of self and sense of career, the book considers the personal as well as social implications of corporate downsizing.

The book covers issues of job security from a historical perspective, as well as providing an overview of the technicalities of corporate downsizing and statistics. Told narratively from the personal aspect of each real-life case study, the book charts the failure and recovery of self and identity through the loss and regaining of corporate work.

479. Sagie, Abraham, and Zeynep Aycan. "A Cross-Cultural Analysis of Participative Decision-Making in Organizations." *Human Relations* 56, no. 4 (April 2003): 453-73.

Keywords: organizational behavior, cross-cultural studies, employee involvement

Despite considerable awareness about various forms and meanings of participative decision-making (PDM) in different parts of the world, there is less agreement on the causes of variation in PDM. This article argues that among other exogenous (e.g., sociopolitical, legal, historical) forces, the sociocultural context plays an important role in the observed differences among PDM approaches and practices across nations. Similarly, subcultures and organizational cultures may influence PDM within nations. Two cultural dimensions, individual-collectivism and power distance, are linked with four widespread employee participation approaches: face-to-face PDM, collective PDM, pseudo-PDM, and paternalistic PDM. The attributes of each PDM form, including the cultural determinants, underlying beliefs, the types of decisions made, and the relationship between a specified form and other PDM meanings (e.g., self-managing teams) are elaborated.

480. Sale, Kirkpatrick. *Rebels against the Future: The Luddites and Their War on the Industrial Revolution: Lessons for the Computer Age*. Reading, MA: Addison-Wesley, 1995.

Keywords: history, computers, Luddites, politics, technology

This book documents the struggles of the Luddites at the end of the eighteenth century and the beginning of the nineteenth century in their efforts to "preserve their jobs and way of life" in the wake of the Industrial Revolution. Sale presents the Luddite movement of machine-breaking as a passionate expression of resistance against the personal and cultural impact of industrialism and technological change. The author notes that this form of English industrial protest had existed as job grievance activity since the late seventeenth century, but that by the 1790s and into the early 1800s, the destruction of textile factory equipment and other industrial machinery had become a symbolic attack on "a feared technological revolution."

The book also contains an account of contemporary "neo-Luddites who challenge the current Industrial Revolution" being heralded by computerization. Sale argues that "this time around the technology is even more complex and extensive, and its impact even more pervasive and dislocating, touching greater populations with greater speed and at greater scales." Sale examines the many ways in which computer technology has "deskilled and often dehumanized" its operators, subjecting them to constant monitoring and machine-discipline, etc. This volume is well-researched and rich in historical detail, with extensive references and a good bibliography.

See especially chapters 8, 9, and 10 for information on "The Second Industrial Revolution" and the sociocultural consequences of computerization.

481. Salvendy, Gavriel, and Waldemar Karwowski, eds. *Design of Work and Development of Personnel in Advanced Manufacturing*. Wiley Interscience Series. New York: John Wiley and Sons, 1994.

Keywords: automation, personnel management

There has been a real shift in traditional thinking about manufacturing technology, and this is illustrated here through people's central roles in automated production environments. Successes of manufacturing enterprises became largely dependent on the symbiotic relationship among social, technical, organizational, management, and ecological design efforts, due to an increasing use of computers. The goal of this book is to present a framework of problems, issues, and solutions relevant to the design of work and development of personnel in the advanced manufacturing area. Within the range of articles written by various experts in the field, the issues covered are the following: job design; taxonomy for work analysis; human supervisory control; technical choice and work design; alternatives for the factory of the future; design of work and technology; skills and education requirements; personnel selection and training; meeting the training needs of employees; decision support systems for computer-integrated manufacturing; uses and benefits for flexible assembly systems design; sources of performance variability; human planner and scheduler; human factors in test and inspection; human factors in AMT maintenance; managing human reliability in advanced manufacturing systems; worker attention and fatigue; human aspects of industrial robotics; operational model for increasing quality, productivity, and profitability in maintenance; and future trends in computer-integrated manufacturing. Although all the articles in this book are quite good, the ones on design of work and technology (chapter 5) and worker attention and fatigue (chapter 16) are particularly relevant to healthy work.

482. Salvendy, Gavriel, and M. J. Smith, eds. *First International Conference on Machine Pacing and Occupational Stress*. London: Taylor and Francis, 1981.

Keywords: machine-paced work, stress, disease

When this book was published in 1981, over fifty million people worldwide were working on machine-paced jobs. Because of the suspected correlation between these jobs and ill-health and social unrest at work, the First International Conference on Machine Pacing and Occupational Stress was held. The papers presented at this conference were collected and printed in this book. According to the preface, the contributors are interested in enhancing the paced-work environment without hindering productivity.

Section 1 offers various perspectives on working pace and stress. Section 2 studies models of human stress and the related fields of organizational stress, cognitive load and performance. Karasek has also contributed a chapter, entitled "Job Decision Latitude, Job Design, and Coronary Heart Disease." Variables relating to stress, such as job satisfaction, mental fatigue, noise and physical illness, are examined in section 3. The measurement of stress is the topic of section 4. "Select Issues" in machine-paced research, for example work repetition, short-cycle repetitive work and working patterns and the relation to stress, are investigated in section 5. The sixth section, entitled "Impact of Machine-Paced Work on Stress," deals with symptoms such as psychoneuroendocrine correlated strain and discomfort. The next section contemplates the impact of computer-paced work on stress using examples of railroad control centers, clerical VDT operators, CRT display terminal workers and information-processing jobs. Finally, section 8 consists of a single paper that considers the difficulty of determining the relationship between machine-paced work and stress as well as research needs. The book is an excellent resource on the relationship between stress and machine pacing.

483. Sandberg, Åke, ed. *Enriching Production: Perspectives on Volvo's Uddevalla Plant as an Alternative to Lean Production*. Aldershot, UK: Avebury, 1995.

Keywords: automotive industry, case study, job enrichment

This volume, a product of the Swedish Institute for Work Life Research, focuses on the human-centered production methods of Volvo's car assembly plant in Uddevalla, Sweden. The experiences of the plant that closed down after four years of operation are gathered here in a book with an international and comparative perspective.

The authors do not support the view of many proponents of "lean production" that there is one single best work organization model. Rather, the concept of enriching production is promoted—"production that is enriching to work and workers and to investors and owners." This book thus helps shape the contours of a necessary alternative to the lean production concept—one which can make the workplace a decent place for human activity. The innovative techniques of Volvo's Uddevalla car assembly plant are described and debated. Special attention is given to the abandonment of assembly-line methods, the adoption of work groups acting in parallel independently of each other, and the use of advanced computer technology to support skilled workers.

Part 1 describes the development of the Uddevalla plant from the first ideas of conventional line assembly to qualified workers building whole cars in a completely parallelized production. Production system design strategies are outlined. Part 2 explores the performance of the Uddevalla plant in a comparative perspective, focusing on the plant's impressive performance regarding customized cars with very short delivery times. Criticism of Volvo's decision to close the plant is also discussed. Part 3 examines Volvo car plants internationally and the alliance with Renault. Part 4 "Beyond Lean Production" criticizes social aspects of Japanese production concepts; humanization of the production system and work at Toyota; and social preconditions for post-lean management strategies.

484. Sandberg, Åke, et al., eds. *Technological Change and Co-Determination in Sweden*. Labor and Social Change. Philadelphia: Temple University Press, 1992.

Keywords: QWL, case study, democracy

"This book describes efforts to meet the strategic problems that labor unions in Sweden face in improving the quality of working life" in the context of rapid technological change. The authors note the pivotal role of the Swedish labor movement in improving the quality of work for both Swedish workers and workers abroad. "Good work" is envisioned by the authors and the Swedish Quality of Working Life (QWL) movement as "work that enables people to develop, grow, and expand their capabilities . . . it is safe, and provides scope for increasing responsibility, autonomy, variety, and social interaction." Moreover, "the democratization of decision making about work is deemed crucial, both for the process of replacing bad work with good and for the content of good work. Through national policy and local action, management need to be induced and constrained to incorporate the requirements of good work into job design. The devolution of responsibility for production to autonomous groups of workers and their participation in the choice of technology and work organization are themselves among the key attributes of good work."

See especially chapters 5, 6, and 7 for excellent case study material, along with a discussion of their implications for industrial democracy. Also, see chapter 2 "Industrial Relations and Co-Determination" and chapter 3 "Innovations in Production and Work Organization."

485. Sanne, C. "How Much Work?" *Futures*, January-February 1992: 23-36.

Keywords: forecasting

The future of work is a constant topic of discussion. This article approaches it with the deceptively simple notion of demand and supply: How much work is required to yield a reasonable standard of living? And how much work would people prefer to put in? Answers are given from two studies of a mature welfare state: Sweden. The answers also point to the following underlying questions: What are the driving forces behind the present pattern of work? Is there a lagging self-understanding about needs, risks, and possibilities in our type of society?

486. Satchell, Paul. *Innovation and Automation*. Aldershot, UK: Ashgate, 1998.

Keywords: automation, case study, human factors, anthropocentric

This volume develops a framework for understanding the interactions between innovation and automation in organizations. After noting that both innovation and automation are key to organizational competitiveness, the author adds that their compatibility has been little considered. Moreover, "current approaches to blending innovation and automation are failing to comprehend the consequences for humans or machines." The central proposition of this book is that "organizational success will depend upon optimization of the interaction between the organization's ability to innovate and the manner in which organizational functions are automated." The author considers innovation first by looking at its importance and its current place in organizations. In addition, "the process underlying innovation is considered at the level of human creativity, as this is the key element." The book views creativity in an environmental context. "The environmental view is particularly apt, because creativity in organizations is not the creativity of a particular individual in isolation, but reflects a mixing of the creativity of many people in social networks, faced with challenges specific to their workplace."

The book next addresses current approaches to the process of automation. The author points out that while automation has undoubtedly had many beneficial effects, "it has frequently proved disappointing, even impinging harmfully on creativity." Satchell further adds that "harmful effects are contained within the current technology-centered approach and its propensity to control without providing feedback." The book discusses how the unwanted effects from automation have been unexpected, costly and have reduced usefulness. These negative consequences issuing from automation, suggests the author, "reflect the underlying values that the technology-centered approach has ascribed to humans, which manifests as humans and machines being seen as comparable." Much of the remaining part of the book discusses a new approach called human-centered automation, which has tried to break free from viewing human-machine sharing in terms of compatibility. The book uses many case studies and examples to illustrate various creative, human-centered methods of involving people and technology in organizational contexts.

487. Sauter, Steven, Marvin Dainoff, and Michael Smith, eds. *Promoting Health and Productivity in the Computerized Office: Models of Successful Ergonomic Interventions*. London: Taylor and Francis, 1990.

Keywords: ergonomics, occupational health and safety, computerized offices

The majority of papers contained within this book were prepared for a workshop with the same title as the book and sponsored by the National Institute of Occupational Safety and Health. The research presented ranges from controlled laboratory experiments to field studies. The settings for all of the research are VDT workstations and workplaces, that is, computerized offices. The papers in the first section report the effects of ergonomic and job/task redesign on worker well-being and organizational performance. The management approaches' effects are studied in the second section. In both cases, the conclusion of all the papers taken together is that these factors can improve worker satisfaction, health, and productivity and can decrease complaints, absenteeism, turnover rates, sick leaves, and compensation claims. The third section reports on clinical techniques for assessing and managing health complaints due to VDTs, such as visual problems and neck and arm pain.

488. Sauter, Steven L., Joseph J. Hurrell Jr., and Cary L. Cooper, eds. *Job Control and Worker Health*. Wiley Series on Studies in Occupational Stress. Chichester: John Wiley and Sons, 1989.

Keywords: stress, health

This book begins with the premise—widely subscribed to in the occupational health field—that worker control over working conditions is integral to health and well-being. The contributors (scientists well-known for their research in the arena of worker control and occupational stress/health) examine the methods and theory of research linking job control to health. The book is one of the first major efforts to systematically review and assess this expanding research field. Specifically, "the book documents what is currently known about the influence of job (i.e., worker) control on worker well-being." The implications of modern work practices for worker control/health are considered in detail—with an emphasis on both theory and application. The book is directed toward researchers and educators alike in occupational health and safety, management/business, industrial engineering, and psychology.

It contains excellent chapters by Robert Karasek, Stanislav V. Kasl, Steven Sauter and others. Part 1 considers the "Effect of Job Control on Worker Health: A Look at the Evidence." Part 2 explores "Theoretical and Methodological Issues" and part 3 considers "Control Problems and Solutions in Modern Work."

489. Sauter, Steven L., and Lawrence R. Murphy, eds. *Organizational Risk Factors for Job Stress*. Washington, DC: American Psychological Association, 1995.

Keywords: stress, health, organizational culture, productivity

That there is a connection between job stress and health problems is becoming common knowledge, but exactly what is the relation? What are the health problems? What factors contribute to job stress? These are the questions that this book addresses. The editors criticize American organizations for treating their employees poorly—as depreciating costs, not appreciating assets. The authors show that changing this attitude will not only improve the health of all involved but will result in improved worker performance and economic success.

Part 1 "Organizational Culture and Climate" explores this relatively new area of study within job stress research. The macroscopic aspects of jobs defined by organizational culture and climate are studied. Different researchers dimensionalize these aspects differently and theorize different mechanisms linking them to stress. This shows that it is indeed a new area of study. However, all three research groups found a link between culture-climate factors and well-being. One of the papers in this section also deals with measuring hostile workplace climate.

Part 2 "The Job Demand-Job Control Model" seeks to challenge, evaluate and expand on Karasek and Theorell's model of stress. One paper in this section expresses the need for validation studies of health problems other than cardiovascular disease. It also considers broadening the demand and control dimensions in order to better predict health outcomes. Other papers use other dimensions to predict job stress and come to the same conclusions as Karasek and Theorell. One study finds that some health effects are more reliably associated with job demands than with control. The final paper in this section echoes this thought, adding that decision latitude, perceived locus of control and coping style can intervene with the effect of demand on health.

"A Risky Management Practice: Electronic Performance Monitoring" is the title of part 3. It begins with a paper summarizing current practices and suspected health and performance effects. The next paper describes an empirical study that asks "whether it is close monitoring of performance per se that is stressful or whether the presumed stress effect is specific to the use of computers . . . for performance monitoring." The third and final paper concludes that electronic performance monitoring is stressful because it affects perceived workload or job control.

Suicide rates among health professionals are higher than those of the general public. This thirty-year old finding is the basis for a closer look at job stress felt by those working in the emergency/crisis health and helping professions. In this fourth part, the chapters discuss various themes such as the need for intensive psychoeducational interventions, the importance of social support, the negative effects of high technology on nurses and how mental health care providers can protect themselves from patient violence, stress risks among musicians, and the attraction some people feel to dangerous, exhilarating jobs.

"Methodological Developments" in job stress studies is the focus of part 5, which criticizes the common self-report method of data gathering. Some suggestions for improvements and alternative methods are given. The notion of emotional labor and the lack of data regarding chronic effects are also discussed.

490. Scalet, Elizabeth A. *VDT Health and Safety: Issues and Solutions*. Lawrence, KS: Ergosyst Associates, 1987.

Keywords: video display terminal, health

This volume focuses on the health implications of video display terminals (VDTs). The various complaints that are common among VDT operators are examined and the causes of these complaints (as they are currently understood) are discussed. In many cases, there are specific suggestions about what can be done to improve the situation. But "the most important 'finding' of this report may be the appreciation of the human system as a complex, highly sensitive mechanism, which deserves at least as much consideration in its use at work as the highly complicated and sensitive computer systems that are the tools of today's office worker."

The author notes that "although the VDT is just a piece of equipment, it is only one component of a wider system or series of systems. These systems include the computer system itself, the business system and procedures it is used to support, and the organizational system to which the user belongs. VDT health problems may occur in any or all of these systems." The book goes on to argue that it is often the interaction between these systems that are most problematic—that is, the interaction between the VDT, its environment, and how it is used. In other words, "some of the health problems are VDT specific, some are VDT work related, and some are more to do with the nature of modern office work."

The author notes in conclusion: "one lesson that has emerged most clearly in the VDT health debate is that it never does any harm to improve the ergonomics of the workplace. It may solve the health problem completely. Even if it does not, it is probably good for productivity. It is certainly good for morale and that helps staff and management."

Contents include chapters on VDTs and radiation, eyes and vision, strain and injury, stress, pregnancy and reproduction, and policy and regulatory issues. See also "References and Further Readings."

491. Schabracq, Marc J., and Cary L. Cooper. "Toward a Phenomenological Framework for the Study of Work and Organizational Stress." *Human Relations* 51, no. 5 (1998).

Keywords: stress, sociology

In this article, "elements from different stress models are embedded in a phenomenological framework for work and organization stress based on practical insights on the one hand and ideas and methods from ethology, microsociology, and cultural anthropology on the other. The framework is compatible with most of the existing research and theoretical views, and pays attention to some lacunas in these views. The central concept is integrity, i.e. the ways in that the process of situated individual functioning is organized in a niche, consisting of a limited set of situations. Integrity refers to the interval integration of individual functioning and the integration of the individual in his or her niche (and thereby in an organization and society at large). . . . Situations are cultural spaces, that provide their actors with a shared reality in which they can attain recurrent goals by following the situated roles, that is, the standardized lines of morally acceptable action inherent in the situation. Integrity in a situation and its disturbances can be described and analyzed in terms of individual options for action, that is, what one can (is able), will (wants to), may (is allowed to), and must (ought to, has to) do. Analysis in these terms can generate insights in ways to improve both integration processes of integrity." The authors suggest that adequate integrity provides the individual with a number of gains: "it enables one to develop skills for coping with the recurrent problems of life, ensuing from the necessity of meeting one's cyclical vital needs; it provides the individual with meaningful and morally acceptable ways of living, such as working, in a reality that one can share with other individuals; it provides someone with a morally acceptable identity; it positions and anchors an individual life and identity in society; it allows room for exploration, learning, and further development; it is conducive to individual well-being and health."

492. Schabracq, Marc J., Jacques A. M. Winnubst, and Cary L. Cooper, eds. *Handbook of Work and Health Psychology*. Chichester: John Wiley and Sons, 1996.

Keywords: stress, psychology

This volume examines the contributions of various branches of psychology to the domain of work stress and well-being. The authors note that despite the considerable interaction between the different approaches, "there is no such thing as a generally accepted 'unifying' theory of stress."

The book's chapters reflect the subdisciplinary interest areas within the field of psychology. For data on the (psycho)physiology of stress and the "ecology" of stress, see chapter 7. The contributions of clinical psychology in the areas of anxiety and trauma (chapter 14), burnout (chapter 15), coping and personality factors (chapters 3, 7, and 18), quality of life, general stress, and psychotherapy (chapters 21 and 22) are presented. The tradition of industrial, organizational, and work psychology (which overlaps with general experimental psychology) explores such research areas as work stressors, fatigue and job characteristics (see chapters 2, 6, 8, and 16). Studies from social psychology on person-environment fit, social support and role theory can be seen in chapters 4, 5 and 15. Finally, there is the developmental psychological tradition, which studies subjects such as career-related issues (chapters 14 and 15) and management development (chapter 17).

Of special relevance to the context of preventive strategies and healthy work models are chapter 1 "Work and Health Psychology: Toward a Theoretical Framework," chapter 2 "Job Control and Health," chapter 4 "Social Support, Stress, and Organization," and chapter 6 "Assessment of the Psychosocial Hazards at Work." Also see part 6 of the text (especially chapter 21) for data on "interventions for the improvement of occupational health and well-being that affect organizational culture in a positive way."

493. Schellenberg, Kathryn, ed. *Computers in Society*. 4th ed. The Annual Edition Series (Computer Studies). Guilford, CT: Dushkin Publishing Group, 1992.

Keywords: computers, general, deskilling

This collection of readings is designed to familiarize students with the philosophical, economic, political, social, and psychological dimensions of the so-called computer revolution. Contributors come from a variety of disciplinary backgrounds and offer diverse, sometimes contradictory points of view. The major themes of the book are economy, community, and conflict—discussed in both a national and international context. The final section looks at some of the philosophical challenges posed by emerging information technologies.

Section 1 deals with "The Changing Economy" and touches on issues such as robotization, office automation, the question of corporate nationality and the myth of a post-industrial economy. Section 2 examines "Employment and the Workplace" and considers deskilling, telecommuting, the growing service sector, etc. Section 3 discusses "Social Interaction and Participation in the Information Age." Topics explored here include computers and disabilities, effects of computerization on human interaction, virtual reality, education, and computer literacy. Section 4 explores ethical and legal issues and section 5 considers "Individual Privacy in the Information Age." Section 6 looks at "Computer System Reliability and Safety" and section 7 discusses computerization in an international context. See also section 8 for a discussion of philosophical concerns in the field of computers and society (the mind/machine debate, computers and "thought," etc.).

494. Schenk, Christopher, and John Anderson, eds. *Re-shaping Work: Union Responses to Technological Change*. Don Mills, ON: Federation of Labour, 1995.

Keywords: human resources, unions, technology

From the work of union researchers and members of the Technology Adjustment Research Program (TARP) comes this compilation of papers on technology and how the decision makers use new technologies to transform the world of work and thus the lives of those involved. It is meant to serve as an example to others of ways in which technology can be used for the greater good of society, but also as a warning as to its abused use by corporations seeking increasing profits at the expense of workers who lose their jobs, are used as guinea pigs, or suffer mental or physical stress. The introduction "Technology on Trial: Lessons from the Labor Frontiers" looks at what technological change is, whether this is a new economy or a new phase of an old system, whether there will be worse periods of technological change ahead of us, government action or technology, workplace reorganization committees, new laws on adjustment, research capacities, collective bargaining, new ownership and nailing down technology, and a look at the future. Following articles address such issues as the confrontation of work reorganization by unions and the rise of precarious employment in terms of home-based work in the garment industry and federal public service, the impact of technological change on the building trades, a case study at Walker Exhaust of the impact of work reorganization on employee attitudes toward work, the company and the union, the theory and practice of free trade and its implications for unions, a summary of a study on Labor Adjustment Programming, lean production to agile manufacturing, and the long struggle of postal workers and technological change. There is also a very good article on knowledge at work: human-centered machinery technology.

495. Schlenning, Nila. *Idle Hands and Empty Hearts: Work and Freedom in the United States*. New York: Bergin and Garvey, 1990.

Keywords: ethics, work ethic

This book's general philosophical/sociological perspective on the meaning and ethics of work emphasizes the personal and sociocultural dimensions of work. The author poses many of the central questions having to do with work in our time: "Why do human beings work? What can we learn about work from history? What is the impact of technology on work? How does work affect our political lives? Do women have a different perspective on work? And finally, what is good work and how do we create a future in which good work can be realized?" In addition, commonly-held assumptions are examined and critiqued: the idea that machines will improve the quality of life, the notion that assembly-line and automated production techniques create efficiency in work, and the belief that unions can substantially change the way work is conducted in capitalist society. The author connects the subject of work with issues of ethics, community, and environment in an effort to develop strategies for change that will promote healthy and meaningful work in vital and sustainable communities.

496. Schonberger, R. J. *World Class Manufacturing: The Lessons of Simplicity Applied*. New York: Free Press, 1986.

Keywords: manufacturing, case study

This is a comprehensive treatment of techniques that constitute world class manufacturing (WCM). The fundamental goal of WCM is continual and rapid improvement in quality, cost, lead time, customer service and flexibility (i.e., "faster, higher, stronger"). Elements of production affected include the following: management of quality; job classification; labor relations; training; staff support; souring; supplier and customer relations; product design; plant organization; scheduling; inventory management; transport handling; equipment selection; product line accounting system; role of computers; and automation. All of this material emerges from an in=depth look at how the Harley-Davidson Motorcycle Company turned itself around to become a world competitor.

497. Schor, Juliet, and Jong-Il You, eds. *Capital, the State and Labor*. Brookfield, VT: Edward Elgar Publishing Company, 1995.

Keywords: comparative industrial relations, labor policy, capitalism, labor economics, industrial policy, economic policy

Throughout the twentieth century issues such as the relations between capital, state, and labor have had a significant influence on economic development and political stability. However, these are changing again as the dismantling of the welfare state, technological progress, economic difficulties and new industrial and occupational patterns are having an impact on all countries. This raises fundamental questions for the future: Can capital-labor relations be better synchronized, and can the state play a meaningful role in this process? This book, which studies the development of capital-labor relations, demonstrates that a discontinuity has become especially apparent in the last ten to fifteen years that coincided, perhaps by accident, with the end of the Cold War period. One of the main points of this book is that even in capital-labor relations, the world has arrived at a point where old practices and approaches have lost much of their appeal and potential for success. The main conclusion of the book is that predictions regarding the future development of capital-labor relations are uncertain at the best of times, thus more research is needed because it is one of the most fundamental issues in the economy.

498. Schor, Juliet B. *The Overworked American: The Unexpected Decline of Leisure*. New York: Basic Books, 1991.

Keywords: work time, leisure, unemployment

This remarkable book documents and explains the trend in the United States toward increasing worktime by both men and women. While the growing participation of women in the workplace is widely acknowledged, the author notes that the fact "that both women and men are working longer hours has still not been recognized." The second component of the book concerns the decline of leisure time for workers as productivity and prosperity have increased.

The author begins her analysis by noting the rise of a new view of the labor market—one that "emphasizes asymmetries between workers and their employers." She goes on to state: (1) "A key asymmetry is the existence of a chronic shortage of jobs, which puts workers at a disadvantage in their dealings with employers," and (2) "a second asymmetry is the preference of employers for long hours, which makes it difficult to translate productivity increases into free time."

This book scrutinizes the consensus view that capitalism has delivered increases in leisure. The author's research indicates that "far from raising leisure time, the development of capitalism involved a tremendous expansion of human effort . . . people began to work longer and harder."

The author's fundamental argument is that "key incentive structures of capitalist economies contain biases toward long working hours. As a result of these incentives, the development of capitalism led to the growth of . . . long hour jobs."

See especially section 2 "Time Squeeze," chapter 3 "A Life of Hard Labor: Capitalism and Working Hours," and chapter 5 "The Insidious Cycle of Work-and-Spend."

499. Schuler, Douglas, and Aki Namioka, eds. *Participatory Design: Principles and Practices*. Hillsdale, NJ: Lawrence Erlbaum, 1993.

Keywords: participation, design, computers

This volume is about participatory computer systems design. It takes up "the problem of how to establish meaningful and productive interactions" among people who are involved in processes of technology design and use. The book stresses the importance of humane and creative relationships between computers and human activities and "makes explicit the critical . . . presence of values in the system development process. To predominant values of product quality and work productivity are added broadened participation and skill development. The premise is that these values are closely related; that the productiveness of our work is tied to the extent of our involvement, and that product quality is a matter of a technology's support for the continually expanding work practices of skilled practitioners."

The contributors to this collection make clear the difference between European, Scandinavian, and American environments for system development. See especially part 3 "Approaches to Participatory Design" and the case studies of part 4.

500. Schuller, Tom. *Democracy at Work*. OPUS. Oxford: Oxford University Press, 1985.

Keywords: democracy, participation, politics

This book reviews a variety of conceptual approaches to industrial democracy and offers a simple framework for its analysis. The book's basic premise is that "we should be actively exploring ways of achieving a more equitable distribution of power at the workplace" while recognizing that "conflict is an inherent if uneven feature of society." Rather than providing the usual descriptive accounts of participation systems, the author focuses on presenting "a relatively straightforward way of looking both at the general theme of worker participation and at specific issues which have contemporary significance." Some of the issues discussed include the following: pension scheme management; health and safety; industrial democracy within public services; worker directors; and the relationship between knowledge, power and the division of labor.

The author does not believe that power-sharing at work will "dissolve tensions," nor does he believe that it is "necessarily the case that greater democracy inspires greater efficiency." Nevertheless, he contends that "it is inconceivable that current patterns of authority and power will—or should—remain as they are." This book explores one important method (i.e., industrial democracy) through which these current patterns of authority can be challenged.

See especially chapter 6 "Determining the Work Environment" and chapter 7 "Political and Industrial Democracy."

501. Schultz-Wild, Rainer. "CIM and Future Factory Structures in Germany." *Futures*, December 1991: 1032-46.

Keywords: computer integrated manufacturing

The author summarizes his findings as follows: "Recent debates on the 'factory of the future' refer almost exclusively to computer integrated manufacturing (CIM); but there is still a long way to go toward the realization of fully automated and computer integrated production. The current dynamic diffusion of CIM components creates new problems for the organization of future factory and work structures. Our findings from the German capital goods industry illustrate that there is presently no uniform structural paradigm emerging from these computer-based innovation processes. Efforts to make traditional Tayloristic forms of work organization more efficient is the path still taken by many companies, while others are seeking ways of maintaining or revitalizing forms of skilled production work on the shopfloor. The restructuring of industrial labor seems more than ever a political question. Concepts of technology, the system of education and vocational training, as well as the management of innovation on the company level, have important influences in determining the direction of further development."

502. Schumacher, E. F. *Good Work.* New York: Harper & Row, 1979.

Keywords: technology, self-development, philosophy, economics

This is a classic, philosophical, and eco-sensitive treatment of the subject of work by one of the innovators of "intermediate" or appropriate technology. Schumacher begins by asking the question, "How does work relate to the end and purpose of man's being?" He regards human work as having three fundamental purposes: "First, to provide necessary and useful goods and services. Second, to enable every one of us to use and thereby perfect our gifts like good stewards. Third, to do so in service to, and in cooperation with, others, so as to liberate ourselves from our inborn egocentricity."

The first essay examines the social and ecological consequences of large-scale production and technological giantism. The author makes the case for a return to viable systems of technology that have an appropriate human scale. Chapter 2 identifies the major problematic characteristics of modern industrial society and considers the ethical and intellectual resources required to create a technology and social system that responds directly to real human needs. Chapter 3 explores the issues of responsible corporate management and just systems of organizational life. Chapter 4 considers "Appropriate Forms of Ownership and Action" and chapter 5 looks at the role of education in a humane society.

503. Schwalbe, Michael. *The Psychosocial Consequences of Natural and Alienated Labor*. SUNY Series in the Sociology of Work. Albany: State University of New York Press, 1986.

Keywords: alienation, psychology, capitalism

The author makes his political/sociological orientation very clear in the opening preface, in which he states that the capitalist form of labor is one that "generally denies freedom, aesthetic pleasure, and moral responsibility, thereby undermining human well-being and development." This book "offers a new perspective on how the capitalist labor process shapes the character of its participants." Schwalbe argues that "with appropriate social psychological elaboration, Marx's original analysis of alienated labor can provide a powerful theoretical framework for understanding the psychological consequences of working for capitalism." The author uses the social psychological perspective of G. H. Mead "to specify the processes whereby alienated labor produces particular psychological outcomes."

Case study material from five capitalist firms provides the empirical foundation for the author's study of work experiences. Particular topics discussed in the context of the labor process include the following: constraints on intellectual and moral development; self-objectification in work; and limits on the opportunities for problem-solving.

504. Scott, Ronald M. *Introduction to Industrial Hygiene*. Boca Raton: CRC Press, 1995.

Keywords: industrial hygiene, occupational health and safety

A clear and concise introduction to workplace hazards and workplace safety issues is presented in this textbook. Section 1 "Chemical Hazards in the Workplace" first discusses different types of toxic effects. Then the reader is introduced to measuring and reporting toxicity, how toxins enter and leave the body, and government regulations. Following this, toxic exposure through skin contact and through inhalation are discussed. Protecting the worker by monitoring the plant atmosphere and by providing clean air are the next topics. A chapter on fires and explosions concludes section 1.

Section 2 "Physical Hazards in the Workplace" deals with hearing loss, radiation and heat stress. These chapters contain information regarding the nature of the hazards, different types of hazards, how they harm the body and protective measures. The chapter on workstation design informs the reader on ergonomics, vibrations, cumulative trauma and designing for prevention of accidents.

Section 3 "Specific Hazards" deals with different types of metals, their uses and their potential to harm. Different types of operations involving metals are also examined in terms of how they can pose a threat to workers' health. Polymers are the last group of specific hazards to be considered. Plastics, textiles, adhesives and their hazards during synthesis and processing are examined. Each chapter concludes with a very useful "Key Points" segment that summarizes the chapter, a problem set, and bibliography.

505. Senker, Peter, and Mark Beesley. "The Need for Skills in the Factory of the Future." *New Technology, Work and Employment* 1, no. 1 (1986): 9-17.

Keywords: automation, skill, forecasting, deskilling

The "automated factory" as the culmination of ingenuity has fascinated engineers and social visionaries (albeit for different reasons) for a considerable period. This article discusses the skill requirements of advanced automated production. The authors of this paper attempt to challenge the rhetoric that often surrounds discussions of the automatic factory. Firstly, they question the assumption that the automatic factory inevitably implies the total deskilling of the workforce, and secondly, that automation is as far advanced as is sometimes assumed. These two assumptions tend to color the debate about automation and distract attention from the very real problems associated with automation. In this paper, the authors consider a number of case studies on various aspects of automation in factories. In this context, they conclude that managers will have to give workers broader training if they wish to gain benefits from automation in its most extreme forms: inevitably, this will cause particular difficulties in countries such as Britain and America, where there is a long tradition of controlling the labor force through deskilling.

506. Seppälä, Pentti. "Semi-Autonomous Work Groups and Worker Control." 291-306 in *Job Control and Worker Health*, edited by S. L. Sauter, J. J. Hurrell, and C. L. Cooper. Chichester: John Wiley and Sons, 1989.

Keywords: work groups, work design

The organization of work and the design of jobs are related to the product, the production technologies, and the production phase as well as the type of employee. This chapter analyzes the experience of work groups in different industries and the varying degrees of achievement of autonomy and thus decision latitude for the worker. The analysis is based on studies of work organization in Finnish automobile, electrical, and sawmill industries in the 1970s. The remainder of the article discusses production philosophies, such as cellular manufacturing, that were created in the early 1970s in engineering companies. In cellular manufacturing, whose underlying technical principle is group technology ("parts or products which can be processed or manufactured by similar machines or tools are coded and grouped together"), promoting healthy work is secondary to cutting costs and shortening throughput times. The chapter continues to describe production cells in operation in the 1970s as well as the production philosophies of the 1980s, such as flexible manufacturing systems. The chapter is realistic in its documentation of the different attempts to create healthy work in the specific industries mentioned.

507. Shaiken, Harley. *Work Transformed: Automation and Labor in the Computer Age*. New York: Holt, Rinehart and Winston, 1985.

Keywords: labor process, rationalization, automation, unemployment, Taylorism, deskilling, numerical control

This book begins with the promise that "the technical potential is there for new productions systems to be designed in a way that both enriches life on the job and benefits society." The author examines the growing gap between the promise and the reality of more humane work designs by uncovering "the mystery that surrounds the process of technological development, exploring the managerial strategies that govern its use, and analyzing the experiences of workers and managers in the workplace." Emphasis is given to the social decisions (rather than just the technical requirements) necessary for the creation of new forms of automation. Special consideration is also given to the issues of deskilling, flexible computer technology, the monitoring and control of workers, and the political implications of modern reorganized production systems.

Chapter 2 looks at the case of the machine shop to illustrate the problems of "scientific management" and the rationalization of the labor process. Chapter 3 examines "managerial control as a criterion of design, minimizing human input as a pervasive engineering philosophy." The author also "questions the extent to which the current direction of technological change blocks other paths of development." Chapter 4 offers a case study of numerical control (NC) and considers its ramifications for the skill acquisition of workers. Chapter 5 analyzes the operation of the computerized factor as a whole by looking at the overall changes in the organization of production, including flexible manufacturing systems. Chapter 8 provides a good summary of the challenges automation poses for society in general and labor in particular.

508. Shain, Martin. "Returning to Work after Illness or Injury: The Role of Fairness." *Bulletin of Science, Technology & Society* 21, no. 5 (October 2001): 361-8.

Keywords: accidents, coping, illness

The author's abstract summarizes the article as follows: "Research has confirmed the existence of a robust relationship between certain conditions of work (high demand/low control, high effort/low reward) and a variety of adverse health outcomes including cardiovascular disease, mental disorders, and immune system dysfunctions. Recently, these same conditions have been implicated in the defeat of certain capacities, such as adaptability, coping, ability, memory, and creativity. Such conditions appear also to influence the likelihood of making successful recovery from illness or injury and of returning to productive employment. The dynamic processes linking these conditions and outcomes nonetheless remains somewhat unclear. In this article, the role of fairness as a mediator of these connections is explored. In particular, the psychoneuroimmunological significance of promises explicit or implicit in the employment relationship is identified as being crucial to our understanding of how stress affects health and capacities. Practical implications are explored."

509. Shallis, Michael. *The Silicon Idol: The Micro Revolution and Its Social Implications*. Oxford: Oxford University Press, 1984.

Keywords: computers, general

This volume, written fairly early on in the so-called computer revolution, examines the social aspects of computerization from a number of different perspectives. The first half of the book deals with the workings, applications, and projected futures of computers. Topics here include "intelligent" machines, the anthropomorphizing of computers, fundamental differences between humans and machines, the internal components of computer technology (i.e., hardware and software), how computers function, automation and the computerization of the office, and artificial intelligence in the future.

The second half of the text is concerned with the historical and social origins of computers and the effects they are having on employment and the structure of society. Topics discussed here include the development of modern science and technology; the myth of technological neutrality; the origins of microtechnology; industrial mechanization and the computerization of work; and computers and security/privacy issues.

The book ends with a discussion of the information technology revolution and its ethical and philosophical implications.

Considering this book's early date of publication, it offers many surprisingly keen insights and makes good use of first-rate reference material from leading scholars in the field of technology and society studies.

510. Sheil, Beau. "Thinking about Artificial Intelligence." *Harvard Business Review*, July-August 1987: 90.

Keywords: computers, artificial intelligence

This article examines the unique problems of deploying artificial intelligence (AI) in a large organization and attempts to reveal the keys to understanding the real potential of this new technology. The author notes that although AI is indeed moving from the research lab into business, industrial, and professional applications, it is still a long way from delivering on the more extravagant claims that some have made for it. Moreover, the subtlety required to integrate such complex technology into the daily operations of a large organization is often overlooked. The author further contends that "although many seemingly 'obvious' applications of AI are unlikely ever to happen, there are some very effective and near-term ones that are so subtle they're apt to be missed." One of the aims of this article is to differentiate these applications. After discussing some of the more philosophical and abstract aspects of AI (such as our unconscious beliefs about "intelligence," the inherent limitations of AI, rule-based systems, knowledge-based accounts of intelligence, and common-sense "intelligence") the author explores their very real and practical implications for the senior manager who is considering using AI technology. "What that person wants to know is whether the AI system is reliable. Will it perform to specifications? Will its answers always be right, or, at the very least, defensible?" The article stresses that if AI applications are to achieve widespread commercial use, a wide range of operational issues must be addressed. One approach, the author suggests, is simply to give AI a low profile—"to call the technology by a different name that removes the notion of intelligence with all its implicit problems . . . a second approach is to concentrate on low-responsibility applications in which the consequences for errors are nil . . . a third approach is to package AI technology as an assistant rather than as the primary decision maker."

511. Sheridan, T. B., T. Vamos, and S. Aida. "Adapting Automation to Man, Culture and Society." *Automatica* 19, no. 6 (1983): 605-12.

Keywords: automation

Anxiety about the effects of automation on workers and society is at least 150 years old. The recent explosion of microelectronics and robotic applications has sharpened our understanding of both the gains and the risks: mismatch to human physiological, psychological and cultural characteristics; alienation from fulfillment and dignity in work; widening of the gap between skilled and unskilled workers and between technologically developed and underdeveloped communities; and decrement in individual security. Attention to these problems can ensure that automation results in a better society. The control engineer, who is responsible for enlarging the scale of automation, should also play a role in adapting it to people. For the time being, technology should be individually designed to each culture.

512. Shipper, F., and C. C. Manz. "Employee Self-Management Without Formally Designated Teams: An Alternative Road to Empowerment." *Organizational Dynamics*, Winter 1992: 48-61.

Keywords: QWL, participation, productivity

The managerial practices of W. L. Gore and Associates are examined as a viable method of worker empowerment leading to competitive advantage. The advantages and disadvantages of various forms of decentralization and self-management are discussed. It is found that worker empowerment is strongly correlated with increased productivity, better attendance, less turnover, better product quality, and improved quality of working life.

513. Shorris, Earl. *A Nation of Salesmen: The Tyranny of the Market and the Subversion of Culture*. New York: W. W. Norton and Company, 1994.

Keywords: capitalism, democracy, marketing/selling, culture studies, culture of capitalism

The role of the salesman has come to subvert the role of the human being. For all its commonality, the act of selling draws an opaque veil of human complexity, begging the question: Is the dominance of selling in our time a result of modern capitalism, or is it closer to the base of human nature, who we are?

What is selling? Who is hurt in the process, and what are the qualifications for innocence in the life of a salesman? Only through answering these questions and more can one gain an understanding of the salesman's place and the role of capitalism in our cultural, social, political, and moral life.

Writing a series of case studies and narratives to discuss the nature of the capitalist world, Shorris covers historical perspectives, issues of democracy, and concludes with a discussion of the moral and social life of human beings, in the context of a pervasive salesman's culture.

514. Siegrist, Johannes. "Adverse Health Effects of High-Effort/Low-Reward Conditions." *Journal of Occupational Health Psychology* 1, no. 1 (1996): 27-41.

Keywords: health, stress, reward imbalance model

The author summarizes his article as follows: "In addition to the person-environment fit model (J. R. French, R. D. Caplan & R. V. Harrison, 1982) and the demand-control model (R. A. Karasek & T. Theorell, 1990), a third theoretical concept is proposed to assess adverse health effects of stressful experience at work: the effort-reward imbalance model. The focus of this model is on reciprocity of exchange in occupational life where high-cost/low-gain conditions are considered particularly stressful. Variables measuring low reward in terms of low status control (e.g., lack of promotion prospects, job insecurity) in association with high extrinsic (e.g., work pressure) or intrinsic (personal coping pattern, e.g., high need for control) effort independently predict new cardiovascular events in a prospective study on blue-collar men. Furthermore, these variables partly explain prevalence of cardiovascular risk factors (hypertension, atherogenic lipids) in 2 independent studies. Studying adverse health effects of high-effort/low-reward conditions seems well justified, especially in view of recent developments of the labor market."

515. Singleton, W. T. *The Mind at Work: Psychological Ergonomics*. Cambridge: Cambridge University Press, 1989.

Keywords: ergonomics, psychology, organizational design

This textbook concerns itself with making work more effective and safer by applying the principles of psychological ergonomics. It emphasizes the changes that need to take place in ergonomics as a result of the changes in technology, particularly the computer. The book consists of seven chapters: "Human Resources and System Design," "Skill and Training," "Needs and Organizations," "Performance and Job Design," "Information Processing," "Risk and Reliability," and "The Citizen and the Environment." Each of these chapters clearly sets out the concepts, knowledge, principles, methods, and procedures and applications involved, but does not provide strong preventive insights.

516. Singleton, W. T. and J. Dirkx, eds. *Ergonomics, Health and Safety: Perspectives for the '90's*. Leuven, Belgium: Leuven University Press, 1991.

Keywords: ergonomics, occupational health

The chapters included in this volume "represent a cross-section of current thinking and action in the related fields of Ergonomics, Health, and Safety." In the context of this book, health refers largely to occupational health.

Section 1 deals with "Ergonomics and the Developing Countries." The problem of servicing advanced equipment is emphasized in relation to the general problems involved in technology transfer.

Section 2 explores current topics of interest in ergonomics. Topics include the following: night work for women; workload and dirty work; and the concerns associated with workers using visual display terminals.

Section 3 looks at application studies, with case study material pertaining to health issues in dental offices and banks. An integrated approach to "overload risks" is also given.

Section 4 considers health in the organizational context. Topics include the following: the social construction of work and organizational problems; stress at work; and the organization of occupational medicine.

Section 5 is on occupational safety. Topics dealt with include the following: the role of the individual; technological innovation and occupational accidents; the development of safety law; and prospects for improving road safety.

517. Skorstad, Egil. "Mass Production, Flexible Specialization and Just-in-Time." *Futures*, December 1991: 1075-84.

Keywords: flexible specialization, just-in-time production

For many years, industrial mass production has been criticized for its consequences on conditions of work. Today, this mode of production is facing another crisis caused by its inability to respond to changing market demands. According to some observers, a new mode of production—flexible specialization—is seen as an answer to both of these crises. Moreover, it is also seen as a dominant paradigm of industrial production for the years to come. One can question such a claim. Another mode of production—often labeled just-in-time—seems to represent a competing paradigm. This mode of production represents a probable solution to the required responsiveness of the firm. It does not, however, automatically mean an end to Taylorized conditions of work.

518. Smith, George E. "The Dangers of CAD." *Mechanical Engineering* 108, no. 2 (1986): 58-64.

Keywords: CAD, deskilling

This article argues that computer-aided design (CAD) methods, for all their advantages, "also pose certain dangers, primarily in the form of unintended side effects." The author illustrates these dangers "by drawing on examples from the area of turbomachinery design, where computers have been in use since the mid 1950s."

The article first outlines the problem of undetected program errors, and then notes that "much worse problems have come from incorrect modeling of physical phenomenon in computer solutions. . . . Even the most sophisticated computer-aided design programs invariably use idealized models of phenomena." The author details the two ways in which mismodeling can occur, and then discusses another problem with CAD—"systematically misleading outputs." It is noted that "inexperienced users have always been inclined to draw unwarranted inferences from the form in which outputs are presented."

Possibly the most important of the side-effects of automated design systems is the loss of the intellectual skills of workers. The author notes that "before computers, the critical skill turbomachinery designers had was an ability to devise simple, but often ingenious, models of pertinent phenomena. . . . This skill went hand in hand with what are sometimes called *physical intuitions*. As computers have come to have an increasing role in turbomachinery design, however, this skill has been atrophying."

The final section of the article offers suggestions concerning what can be done to counteract the dangers of computer-aided design.

519. Solow, Robert M., and Alan B. Kruger, eds. *The Roaring Nineties: Can Full Employment Be Sustained?* New York: Century Foundation Press, 2001.

Keywords: employment forecasting, labor market, full employment policies, United States, economic conditions

All of the papers in this book attempt to explain the success of the roaring '90s. No overriding explanation was discovered. However, there were a number of likely explanations; for example, an unsustainable demand for dollar-dominated wealth, a plunge in energy prices, and a temporary surge in productivity growth might account for a period of low unemployment with stable and low inflation. The economy could be given a more sustained boost by a steady surge in productivity growth if perhaps advances in information technology were made. But, several of the authors warn that unemployment cannot remain as low as it was in the late 1990s, even if productivity remains high, due to the fact that people will begin to act with this in mind. The contributors to this volume note that much depends on healthy capital investment and the continued growth of a skilled workforce, which could be in future jeopardy in the United States, thus urgency must take place in order to search for explanations for the variability of productivity growth.

520. Sproull, Lee, and Sara Kiesler. *Connections: New Ways of Working in the Networked Organization*. Cambridge, MA: MIT Press, 1991.

Keywords: electronic mail, organizational behavior

This volume examines computer-based communication technology in organizations, electronic mail in particular, and how such technology influences and changes organizational behavior and structure. The social science research reported here explores the following questions: "Does a computer network make work groups more effective? How do people treat one another when their only connection is a computer message? What kinds of procedures best suit long-distance management using a computer network? What problems do these technologies alleviate—and what problems do they create?"

The authors seek to demonstrate "how computer-based communication can alleviate barriers and distortions in organizational communication and can create opportunities for new connections among people. . . . Ours is a social and organizational view of computer-based communication."

Chapter 1 "draws on the social history of nineteenth century technologies . . . to introduce a two-level framework for thinking about technology changes in organizations." That framework is then used to explain the early history of networked computer communication. Chapters 2 and 3 discuss the first social effects people are likely to notice with these new technologies ("electronic etiquette" is also described). Chapters 4, 5, and 6 focus on specific kinds of changes that are likely to occur in three areas: meetings, connections among peripheral workers, and patterns of control. Chapters 7 and 8 discuss longer-range changes that can be expected in organizational procedures and structures, respectively, as networked communication becomes more ubiquitous.

521. Stacey, Neill H., ed. *Occupational Toxicology*. London: Taylor and Francis, 1993.

Keywords: occupational health and safety, chemicals

Since many occupational health and safety professionals do not have a strong background in toxicology, this book intends to provide an accessible overview (but not a reference manual) of toxicology to them. The contributors hope to introduce these people to the basis of toxicology and how toxicological information can be used in dealing with workplace health issues. The first section provides this overview. The second section explains the effects of chemicals on various target tissues such as those of the respiratory system, the skin, and reproductive systems and fetuses. A chapter is devoted to genotoxicity, and another one to the prevention of cancer. The toxicity of different groups of chemicals such as metals, pesticides, solvents, plastics, gases and particulate matter is the topic of section 3. The subject of toxicology is of importance to many different fields of study. Thus, "Fields Interfacing with Toxicology" is the title of the fourth section. These fields, explored one at a time in separate chapters, are occupational hygiene, occupational medicine and occupational epidemiology. Finally, section 5 contains three chapters entitled, "Managing Workplace Chemical Safety," "Working Examples in Occupational Toxicology" and "Chemicals, Workplaces and the Law."

522. Standing, Guy. *Global Labor Flexibility: Seeking Distributive Justice.* New York: St. Martin's Press, 1999.

Keywords: quality of working life, industrial relations, foreign trade and employment, labor, distributive justice

The twentieth century has been the century of the laboring man. It has been dominated by the competition between two laborist models of society, state socialism and welfare state capitalism, both of which reached their peak in the 1970s and promoted forms of labor security. Also, since the 1970s, globalization, flexible labor markets, and supply-side economics have added to the feelings of insecurity and inequalities. This means that politicians and social thinkers must now find ways of promoting distributive justice based on new forms of voice representation and regulation. This book presents a vision combining security of income and representation without moralistic state control, where the right to occupational security is given pride of place.

523. Star, Susan Leigh, ed. *Ecologies of Knowledge: Work and Politics in Science and Technology.* Albany: State University of New York Press, 1995.

Keywords: computers, general, science, technology

The essays in this collection examine the following questions: "Whose side are we on in social studies of science and technology? What hierarchies of credibility are we tacitly or explicitly assigning? And what language can we invent to investigate these questions honestly?" These questions are designed to assist in reminding sociologists that pretensions to value neutrality are themselves value laden. It is suggested that "we must choose to recognize that all perceptions are located in a hierarchy of credibility. In other words, people consider the source of any statement or perception, and discount those produced by lower-status people." These essays all attempt to frame the question of whose side we are on "by examining science as a radically contextual, problematic venture with a very complicated social mandate, if any." The authors take an ecological view of work and politics. To quote from the editor's introduction: "Our work challenges the moral order of science and technology making—and in turn places us in a complex, often tense moral position."

Ecologies of knowledge here means trying to understand the systematic properties of science by analogy with an ecosystem and, equally important, all the components that constitute the system. The editor hastens to add that "this is not a functional (or functionalist) approach, with a closed-system organic metaphor at its core. . . . We want to approach science as a set of linked interdependencies inseparable from 'personal troubles, public issues, and social change agendas,' not a social structure with one or more dysfunctional parts." See especially "Computerization Movements and the Mobilization of Support for Computerization," by Rob Kling and C. Suzanne Iacono. In this chapter, the authors examine "how specialized 'computerization movements' advance computerization in ways that go beyond the effect of promotion by the industries that produce and sell computer-based technologies and services." The main thesis here is that "computerization movements (i.e., as social movements) communicate key ideological beliefs about the favorable links between computerization and a preferred social order, which helps legitimate relatively high levels of computing investment for many potential adopters. These ideologies also set adopters' expectations about what they should use computing for and how they should organize access to it." In this chapter attention is focused primarily upon the character of the computerization movements and their organizing ideologies.

Also see the two essays in part 3 dealing with "Workplace Ecologies."

524. Stark, Andrew. "What's the Matter with Business Ethics?" *Harvard Business Review*, May-June 1993: 38-48.

Keywords: ethics, management, business ethics, corporate ethics

The author of this article asks, "What is the matter with business ethics? And more important, what can be done to make it right?" Texts in the field are reviewed in order to shed light on both questions. They point to the gulf that exists between academic business ethics and professional management and suggest that business ethicists themselves may be largely responsible for this gap. "Far too many business ethicists have occupied a rarified moral high ground, removed from the real concerns and real-world problems of the vast majority of managers. They have been too preoccupied with absolutist notions of what it means for managers to be ethical, with overly general criticisms of capitalism as an economic system, with dense and abstract theorizing, and with prescriptions that apply only remotely to managerial practice." In this article, the author reports on recent efforts by a number of prominent business ethicists to take stock of their field and to introduce fundamental changes in the way the enterprise of business ethics is conducted. A guide is offered to business ethics for perplexed managers: "why it seems so irrelevant to their problems and how it can be made more useful in the future." Considerable attention is given to the dominant approach to the moral dimension of business in the 1960s and 1970s, known as corporate social responsibility, before turning to more recent attempts to inculcate responsible business behavior. See especially the subsections of "The Myopia of Moral Philosophy," "Mistakes and Missed Opportunities," and "Toward a New Business Ethics?" The article ends with a few new key words that are intended to represent the essence of contemporary business ethics: moderation, pragmatism, and minimalism.

525. Starrin, Bengt, Per-Gunnar Svensson, and Helmut Wintersberger, eds. *Unemployment, Poverty and Quality of Working Life: Some European Experiences.* Berlin: Edition Sigma (on behalf of the WHO), 1989.

Keywords: unemployment, comparative, health, coping

This volume of essays examines the fundamental relationship between work, quality of life, and human health. The basic premise of the book is that "health for all means guaranteeing for every citizen an economically and socially productive life." The authors further contend that "the right to work is a basic human right" and that poor-quality work and unemployment are associated with "health-related behavior, the suicide rate, higher mortality rates, diet, and even physiological changes in the neuroendocrine and immune systems."

The book offers suggestions for "participatory approaches in intervention programs to lessen the impact of unemployment on the health of individuals and families." Research on coping mechanisms is also provided. Contents include a World Health Organization perspective on unemployment, poverty and quality of working life. Additional chapter titles include the following: "Unemployment, Social Support, Psychological Well-Being, and Psychosomatic Symptoms"; "Stress Reactions to Unemployment"; "Unemployment, Overtime Work, and Work Intensity"; and "Continuity and Change in the Submerged Economy." See especially part 3 of the book on "Interventions and Mobilizations" and part 4 on "Policy Implications."

526. Statham, Anne, Eleanor M. Miller, and Hans O. Mauksch, eds. *The Worth of Women's Work: A Qualitative Synthesis*. SUNY Series on Women and Work. Albany: State University of New York Press, 1988.

Keywords: women, unemployment, health

Improving working conditions for women is an important part of the move toward healthier work. This book contains many suggestions on how to improve these conditions. It draws upon qualitative research through participant observation, unstructured interviews, analysis of diaries, and review of historical documents to describe the lives of working women. After the introductory section, a series of articles focus on women in traditionally female-dominated jobs such as nursing assistants, domestic workers, janitors, and street hustlers. Next, the focus is shifted to higher status women in the traditionally female professions of nursing, counseling and teaching. Part 4 "Making It in the Male World" features the stories of women in jobs such as police officer, manager, salesperson and factory worker. Collectively, the essays challenge various entrenched assumptions regarding women's work. For example, the notion that feelings of self-esteem are determined by the status of one's job is discredited by showing that workers devise methods for maintaining dignity even in the face of oppression.

527. Statt, David A. *Psychology and the World of Work.* London: Macmillan Press, 1994.

Keywords: general, psychology

This highly readable yet rigorous study of the psychology of work would make a very good introductory textbook. An overview of historical trends in the field of work is provided with interesting reviews of work during the Industrial Revolution, Taylorism and scientific management, the impact of behaviorism and psychoanalysis, Henry Ford and the assembly line, and the emergence of automated technology.

Chapter 5 offers a solid summary treatment of "Work and Mental Health." Topics discussed include the following: the physiological experience of stress; causes of stress at work; issues of control; overload and underload; emotional labor and role conflict; burnout; personality factors and stress; and the fit between person and job.

See chapter 16 for "The Effects of New Technology." Topics explored here include the following: the idea of progress; control of the workplace; job redesign (ergonomics, sociotechnical systems, QWL); and the new technology.

Also, see the "Key Studies" appended to the text for a review of fifteen select studies that have contributed significantly "to our understanding of psychology and the world of work in the twentieth century."

528. Stebbins, Leslie F. *Work and Family in America: A Reference Handbook.* Contemporary World Issues. Santa Barbara: ABC-Clio, 2001.

Keywords: family, research, statistics

The role of the parent in relation to the family and their job has changed over the past few decades, and it is these changes that are explored. A historical overview is given in which the Industrial Revolution and other factors are used to explain the separation of work and home, leading to two separate worlds of work and family, as well as men and women. These two worlds collided once women began to enter the workforce in greater numbers during the 1970s. The effect that work was having on women, both mentally and physically, became more prevalent in research fields, as well as concerns such as inequality, employment discrimination and pay equity that came to the foreground. These concerns also meant that the role of men became included in the work-family equation, broadening their ideas about what role men should play in child rearing and household duties. Recent research has shown that men, as they become more involved in their family life, have become more stressed all the while the workplace remains largely unresponsive. These roles become that much more difficult as the income level decreases as parents cannot afford caregivers for their children or time off to care for them themselves. The final topics deal with social scientists and activists calling for a greater role to be played by the government and the community, as well as alternate ways in which work can be restructured and the roles of family members, community members, and employees can be more evenly balanced for both men and women.

529. Steele, Fritz. *Making and Managing High-Quality Workplaces: An Organizational Ecology*. New York: Teachers College Press, 1986.

Keywords: workplace design, work design

Not only does the physical setting of the workplace affect workers and how they work, but settings are designed and altered by users. These reciprocal processes that the author calls organizational ecology should be understood by managers and other decision makers in order to provide high-quality work environments. Focusing on office environments, the author seeks to provide the knowledge regarding organizational ecology that is required for this understanding as well as to provide guidelines on how to actually design high-quality offices.

Part 1 consists of four chapters that describe the ecological point of view for dealing with offices, the most prevalent patterns and problems in the management of workplaces, how social dynamics of organizations influence the workplace design process, and the impact of the social system on the way workplaces are used. Part 2 "Processes for Making Workplaces" provides suggestions regarding how to influence and manage the ecological relationships in order to enhance the health and well-being of individuals, groups and organizations. Part 3 "The Ecological Impact of Work Settings" consists of detailed discussions on different ways that work settings affect the users and the organizations. The most important areas that are affected are identified as the sense of identity and ownership, social interactions, energy levels and excitement, task effectiveness and efficiency, power and influence, boundary relations, organizational climate and quality of work life experiences. Various office designs are assessed in terms of advantages and disadvantages. Finally, part 4 delves into future applications of organizational ecology.

530. Steptoe, Andrew, Olga Evans, and George Fieldman. "Perceptions of Control over Work: Psychophysiological Responses to Self-Paced and Externally-paced Tasks in an Adult Population Sample." *International Journal of Psychophysiology* 25 (1997): 211-20.

Keywords: stress, work pace

This article reports the results from an experiment that tested the hypothesis that externally-paced task administration would produce greater blood pressure and heart rate responses than self-paced tasks. The study uses the demand-control model of job strain formulated by Karasek and Theorell (1990) as its theoretical foundation. As the authors point out, "recent studies indicate that the control dimension may be particularly important for cardiovascular risk."

"One hundred and thirty-two adults aged 30-65 years (64 men and 68 women) were randomized to self-paced and externally-paced task conditions." The hypothesis was only partly supported. For some of the tasks given to the two groups, "systolic blood pressure responses were heightened in the externally-paced condition, but for other tasks, differences in blood pressure readings and heart rates were not significant for the two groups."

The authors conclude that "further psychophysiological investigations" are required but that "the modelling of job control or decision latitude in the laboratory is an important step toward understanding the processes through which job stress may increase cardiovascular disease risk."

531. Stigliani, Joan. *The Computer User's Survival Guide*. Sebastopol, CA: O'Reilly and Associates, 1995.

Keywords: computers, health, work design, radiation, repetitive strain injury, stress, ergonomics

Written as a practical guidebook, the health issues faced by workers using modern computer systems are examined. The author begins by noting that computers have drastically altered the way office work is done and that this has brought about new working conditions that pose health risks to a large number of people. "The terminal at your desk changes the surface you read from, how you sit, how you move (or don't move), how much light you need, how much radiation you're exposed to, and how fast you have to work." The book gives background about how bodily systems work, how computer work affects those systems, and what you can do about it. "Risks to your health will vary with the kind of equipment you use, how long, and intensely you use a computer, the physical layout of your office, your work habits, your general health, and so on." While the text is written for computer users themselves, primarily, it is also directed at members of safety committees, those working in human resources or personnel, managers who need an overview of the risks faced by computer users, occupational health specialists, ergonomics consultants, and occupational and physical therapists.

Part 1 offers a holistic overview of the subject of computers and human health, with information on proper posture, body awareness, and work-station design. Part 2 looks at all aspects of repetitive strain injury. Part 3 considers eyestrain and part 4 examines the subject of computer-related stress. Part 5 explores the potential risks of electromagnetic fields. Part 6 offers suggestions on office computer equipment purchases in light of ergonomic principles and the psychosocial effects on users. An excellent resource guide and a suggested reading section are also appended to the text.

532. Stinglhamber, Florencea, and Christian B. Vandenberghe. "Organizations and Supervisors as Sources of Support and Targets of Commitment: A Longitudinal Study." *Journal of Organizational Behavior* 24, no. 3 (May 2003): 251-70.

Keywords: organizational support, job conditions

The main objective of this study was to examine the relationship between perceived support and affective commitment, and the linkages between these constructs and some of their common antecedents and consequences. Using a sample of 238 employees, the authors conducted a longitudinal study to examine the linkages between the favorableness of intrinsically and extrinsically satisfying job conditions, perceived organizational support, perceived supervisor support, affective commitment to the organization and supervisor, and turnover. Affective commitment to the supervisor was found to completely mediate the effect of perceived supervisor support on turnover, whereas neither perceived organizational support nor organizational affective commitment were significantly related to turnover. Perceived organizational support partially mediated the effect of favorable intrinsically satisfying job conditions on organizational affective commitment and fully mediated the effect of extrinsically satisfying job conditions on organizational affective commitment. Finally, perceived supervisor support totally mediated the effect of favorable intrinsically satisfying job conditions on affective commitment to the supervisor. As a whole, findings suggest that exchange relationships between employees and their supervisors should be further investigated in future turnover research.

533. Stover, Ronald G., Melodie L. Lichty, and Penny W. Stover. *Industrial Societies: An Evolutionary Perspective*. Upper Saddle River, NJ: Simon & Schuster, 1999.

Keywords: industrial sociology, industrialization, economic development

The workplace is changing and this is having an effect on people's lives. People's work and lives are affected by government policies, international trade, dangers in the workplace, sexual harassment, environmental degradation resulting from industrial production, and the negative impact that long hours at work have on marital relationships and on child rearing. These are the central themes of the book as they relate to everyday working life, as well as the experience of working in an industrial society.

534. Sullivan, William M. *Work and Integrity: The Crisis and Promise of Professionalism in America*. New York: HarperCollins, 1995.

Keywords: professional ethics, integrity, expertise, professional culture

This book examines the long-term prospects and integrity of the professional/managerial class in the American workforce. The author, an associate of Robert Bellah and coauthor of *Habits of the Heart*, expresses deep concern over the (questionable) role of professionals in the emerging global order. He argues that this group of workers "embodies enormous human capital in the form of knowledge, skill, and organizational abilities" and that "these are a key resource, not only for the growth of the world economy, but for any conceivable solutions to the problems of global population growth, social conflict, and environmental degradation."

This book makes the case that professional life can and needs to be restructured in ways that suffuse technical competence with civic awareness and purpose.

The author explores the relationship between professionalism and integrity, both in terms of individual responsibility and from a social/institutional perspective. He suggests that "integrity and responsibility need knowledge and orientation. These depend upon institutions that are organized to recognize and promote the application of expertise toward those socially and environmentally conserving functions that are needed to rescue competitive striving from its self-induced narrowness of sympathy."

This volume also considers the profoundly divergent outcomes of professionalism. "At its worst, professionalism can lock individuals in a narrow focus upon technical competence . . . to the exclusion of all other considerations. At its best . . . by taking responsibility through one's work for ends of social importance, an individual's skills and aspirations acquire a value for all. Professionalism thereby forms a crucial link between the modern individual's struggle for a fulfilling existence and the needs of the larger society."

See especially chapter 4 "The Era of Expertise," chapter 5 "Reinventing 'Professionalism,'" and chapter 6 "What Is Professional Knowledge? Expertise and Professional Education."

535. Sumanth, David J., Johnson A. Edosomwan, D. Scott Sink, and William B. Werther Jr., eds. *Third International Conference on Productivity and Quality Research*. Miami: Industrial Engineering and Management Press, 1991.

Keywords: total quality management, quality circles, productivity, teams, participation

This book contains 148 papers presented at the Third International Conference on Productivity and Quality Research in 1991. The editors describe this collection as a mixture of papers containing new models, innovations and applications for a wide range of topics. They also note that the two topics of productivity and quality are becoming increasingly interrelated in research. The section headings are as follows: measurement, evaluation and planning; improvement; TQM and productivity management; applications and case studies; and education and training. Some preventive content is provided in articles dealing with team work, employee participation, quality circles, and total quality management.

536. Sumanth, David J., Johnson A. Edosomwan, Robert Poupart, and D. Scott Sink, eds. *Fourth International Conference on Productivity and Quality Research*. Miami: Industrial Engineering and Management Press, 1993.

Keywords: productivity, quality, total quality management

This volume and the second volume combined contains over two hundred papers presented at the Fourth International Conference on Productivity and Quality Research in 1993. The editors describe this collection as a mixture of papers containing new models, innovations, and applications for a wide range of topics. They also note that the two topics of productivity and quality are becoming increasingly interrelated in research. The section headings are as follows: productivity measurement; productivity evaluation and planning; productivity, quality, and technology linkages; productivity and quality management process; transfer of knowledge in productivity and quality research; formal productivity and quality education; and awards for productivity and/or quality excellence.

The book, unfortunately, has low preventive potential. For example, the paper entitled "Resolving the Quality-Productivity Dilemma" presents a conceptual framework for studying the link between total productivity and quality. It provides a very technical, scientific approach to the link that does not consider human aspects.

On the other hand, the Danish article "Corporate Excellence through Technology, Environmental, and Quality Management" calls for a new managerial philosophy that incorporates technological, environmental and quality considerations. They call this approach Total Corporate Excellence (TCE). Total quality management will not be enough to remain competitive, the authors state. Rather, environmental aspects of industry must be sensitively handled.

537. Sundstrom, Eric. *Work Places: The Psychology of the Physical Environment in Offices and Factories*. Environment and Behavior Series. Cambridge: Cambridge University Press, 1986.

Keywords: work environment, psychology

When considering how the physical work environment affects the worker, it is important to remember that the worker affects the environment as well. This mutually influential and interactive perspective is the one forwarded by this book. The author also espouses the importance of distinguishing between various levels of analysis. He considers the relationship between the workplace and (1) the individual, (2) interpersonal relations, and (3) organizations separately, while recognizing that they are interrelated. The respective processes that mediate the influences of the environment are psychological, social-psychological and organizational.

Sundstrom's three-unit model thus calls for an analysis of different aspects of the physical environment at different levels. At the individual level, the workstation, ambient conditions and surrounding areas are considered. The chapters focus on lighting and windows, temperature and air, noise, music, color and psychological processes related to job performance and satisfaction. At the interpersonal level, the field of view must be broadened to include the layout of rooms, the layout of buildings and symbolic qualities of workspaces. In this section, the chapters investigate topics such as communication, privacy, small groups and symbols of status and self-identity. An even broader view of the environment encompassing the entire building must be adopted for the organizational level of analysis.

Two themes emerge from this work. Firstly, factories and offices have been shaped by their history. Thus two chapters on historical evolution are included. Secondly, the influences of the workplace affect different people differently.

538. Susman, Gerald I. *Autonomy at Work: A Sociotechnical Analysis of Participative Management*. New York: Praeger, 1976.

Keywords: work design, sociotechnical systems, health, mental health

This volume deals with the quality of working life in advanced industrial societies. Though written over twenty-five years ago, the book presents outstanding and fundamental research on the subject of work redesign in the context of worker autonomy. The author makes clear the close relationship between the quality of work and mental and physical health, adjustment to leisure and retirement, and the ability to retrain for new jobs.

The book "presents an analysis of current conditions and the forces for improving the quality of work in advanced industrial societies, as well as a framework for designing new work forms to improve the quality of work."

The author "assumes that the reader is acquainted with basic psychological and sociological concepts related to work and motivation, organizations, and industrial society." The concepts related to general systems theory that are used in this volume are explained by the author.

The book is intended for industrial psychologists, sociologists and industrial engineers, as well as for "members of managerial and technical staff in public and private organizations who are concerned with the problems of quality of work and wish to redesign the work places of their employees so as to improve productivity and create more meaningful work experiences."

"Part 1 discusses the reasons for developing a new framework for the design of work and introduces a model of motivation that assumes that human behavior is purposeful and future-oriented. Part 2 presents a framework for understanding work groups as systems in dynamic interaction with their environment. It is proposed that work groups be designed as autonomous, self-regulating systems." Part 3 discusses principles of sociotechnical design that are based on achieving a "best match" between a social and a technical system. The author concludes, "Work-group members perform best when achievement of desired outcomes leads them to experience self-enhancement."

539. Swearingen, Michael H. *Participative Management: An Analysis of Its Effect on Productivity*. New York: Garland Publishing, 1997.

Keywords: QWL, participation, organizational change, productivity

Although participative management is a highly touted tool, what kind of results does it actually yield? Does it lead to increased productivity as claimed? This book presents an empirical study that seeks to answer this question. It is based on the analysis of questionnaires to determine the style of management and the financial rating of the organization. Swearingen proposes the following five hypotheses that—except for number four—were not rejected by the research results: "1) The higher the education level of the organization's manager is, the more likely they are to use a participative management style of management. 2) The older an organization is, the less likely they are to use a participative style of management. 3) The older the organization's managers are, the less likely they are to use a participative style of management. 4) Organizations that use a participative style of management are more likely to be smaller in size than organizations that use a more rigid style of management. 5) Organizations that use a participative style of management will have increased productivity that will result in increased financial stability."

The book does not take a preventive approach. Its usefulness lies in the second chapter that provides a literature review of what the author deems the essential components of participative management: increased communication, quality circles, quality of working life, joint decision making, conflict resolution, increased job satisfaction and increased cooperation. The literature on the relationship between participative management and productivity is also reviewed.

540. Széll, György. *Concise Encyclopaedia of Participation and Co-Management*. Berlin: Walter de Gruyter, 1992.

Keywords: participation

This volume provides an overview of the international debate on workers' participation and employee involvement schemes in more than one hundred contributions by more than fifty specialists in the field. Each entry gives a historical presentation of the concept in theory and praxis, the main theories and debates, a critical evaluation, and references and further readings. This text is intended as a basic reference manual for practitioners, students, and teachers in the fields of industrial sociology, organization studies, management and business.

541. Tan, Joseph L. H., ed. *Human Capital Formation as an Engine of Growth: The East Asian Experience*. Pasir Panjang, Singapore: Institute of Southeast Asian Studies, 1999.

Keywords: East Asia, human capital formation, economic growth, developing countries

On the whole, the East Asian countries have been more advanced than other developing countries in the field of human capital development. This was proven to be true as far back as the 1960s, when they managed to attain higher levels of human capital compared with other low- and mid-level economies in the developing world. This book examines the role of human capital formation in the rapid growth of the East Asian economies. Aside from the formal education variable, other factors such as nutritional status of the population, on-the-job training, and better health care of the labor force are important concerns, but they were not given much attention in the 1993 World Bank study *The East Asian Miracle*. The authors seek to offer many insights of interest to policy makers and specialists with regard to developing (and transitional) economies.

542. Taris, Toon W., Raija Kalimo, and Wilmar B. Schaufeli. "Inequity at Work: Its Measurement and Association with Worker Health." *Work & Stress* 16, no. 4 (2002): 287–301.

Keywords: health, burnout, equity theory, inequity measurement

The equity theory of Adams (1963, 1965) predicts that people pursue a balance between their investments in and the rewards gained from their work, such that their own investment/reward ratio is the same as that of similar others. Disturbance of this balance is expected to result in a range of negative outcomes, even if people are comparatively well off. The current study among a representative sample of 1,297 Finnish workers examined two assumptions of this theory more closely, namely: (1) whether the relationship between inequity and selected health-related outcome variables is U-shaped (is receiving too much as detrimental as receiving too little?) and (2) whether the reference to "similar others" should be included in the measure tapping inequity. Multivariate analysis of variance only partly confirmed the hypothesis that the relationship between inequity and selected outcome variables is U-shaped. The reference to "similar others" in the measurement of inequity seems to be superfluous.

543. Teich, Albert, ed. *Technology and the Future*. 7th ed. New York: St. Martin's Press, 1997.

Keywords: general, technology, forecasting, gender, anthropocentric, ethics

In this well-known collection of essays by specialists in the field of technology and society studies, the theme is how technological change affects the individual and all aspects of society. Twenty-six readings are presented, with a number of them focusing on various aspects of computer technology. In "Computer Ethics," Tom Forester and Perry Morrison survey the social problems and the range of ethical issues raised by developments in information technology—issues that face computer users as well as computer professionals. Sherry Turkle's selection from "Identity in the Age of the Internet" takes a different approach to related issues, examining the impacts of computer-mediated communication on individual identity as well as the cultural implications of life in cyberspace. See also "An Unforeseen Revolution: Computers and Expectations, 1935-1985" by Paul Ceruzzi. In this essay, Ceruzzi, a historian, conducts a kind of retrospective technology assessment, looking at early expectations of the utilization and impact of computers and finding them remarkably short-sighted. A number of essays also deal with the subject of technology, work and employment trends. For example, in "Less Work for Mother," Ruth Schwartz Cowan examines the relatively low technology of the American household and explains why "labor saving" technology has not resulted in less household work for women. In an excerpt from *In the Age of the Smart Machine*, Shoshana Zuboff reports on a major study of how information technology ("the smart machine") is influencing the working lives of men and women and the nature of work itself. Also see "Toward Human-Centered Design" by Donald A. Norman, "Buddhist Economics" by E. F. Schumacher, and "Feminist Perspectives on Technology" by Judy Wajeman.

544. Tenner, Edward. *Why Things Bite Back: Technology and the Revenge of Unintended Consequences*. New York: Alfred A. Knopf, 1996.

Keywords: computerized offices, technology, general

This immensely interesting book gives dozens, perhaps hundreds, of examples of what Tenner calls the revenge effects of technology. These are the unintended and unpleasant consequences that counteract the purpose of the technologies surrounding us. For example, the spread of computer use has increased paper use. Power door locks actually decrease safety because it is easy for drivers to lock themselves out and be stranded in unsafe places. Similarly, helmets and other protective gear make football more dangerous than rugby. Filter-tip cigarettes do not reduce nicotine intake. Tenner examines revenge effects in the areas of health and medicine, the environment, the office, and sports. Throughout the book, it is stressed that in many ways, technology *has* improved our lives. However, the vast number of technologies we use require constant and vigilant monitoring. And controlling against catastrophic problems leads to chronic problems that are more difficult to solve or control.

The two chapters regarding the computerized office are valuable additions to this bibliography. One of the chapters examines why there are so many reported and suspected computer-related health problems when white-collar work seems to be clearly less damaging than manual labor. The other chapter asks the important question: Why hasn't computerization dramatically increased productivity as predicted? In fact, productivity has hardly increased at all. Tenner blames not the large scale system breakdowns and virus infections (they are relatively rare), but the smaller, everyday revenge effects of computers. For example, the time needed to learn each new piece of software reduces productive time. The constant upgrading of hardware and software keeps employees in an endless loop of learning new skills. As well, computerization of offices leads to downsizing of staff, just when computer support staff is desperately needed. As a result, certain employees in higher positions unofficially become helpers to computer-using staff, which cuts away at his or her productive time. Throughout the discussion, it is emphasized that new technologies require careful vigilance and may bite back.

545. Terkel, Studs. *Working: People Talk about What They Do All Day and How They Feel about What They Do*. New York: Pantheon Books, 1974.

Keywords: general

This is an excellent collection of firsthand personal accounts of work experience. A vast range of occupational groups are represented: blue- and white-collar workers, cab drivers, bank tellers, car mechanics, dentists, farm workers, janitors, musicians, college professors, teachers, industrial designers, policemen, hair stylists, and others.

Through numerous case study reports, Terkel conveys the subjective/lived experience of workers, their joys and accomplishments on the job, as well as their sorrow, their alienation, and frustration. The author explores the attitude of workers toward the work ethic, changes in technology, conflict with bosses, dreams and aspirations of workers, and the place and meaning of work in the lives of workers.

As a sociological work, this book stands out as a masterful piece of participation research, penetrating into the heart of the world of work. Terkel is able to convey, through his phenomenological approach to work, much of what evades those who apply an academic/theoretical perspective to the subject. Although-written thirty years ago, the book's insights remain valid and revealing.

546. Theobald, Robin. *Understanding Industrial Society: A Sociological Guide*. New York: St. Martin's Press, 1994.

Keywords: history, sociology, general, Taylorism, industrial society

The origin, spread, and impact of industrial capitalism are outlined in this book. It is written for students with little background in the social sciences and is therefore clear and easy to read. The author seeks to reflect upon what it means to live in an industrial society. He stresses that in order to do this, one must first understand the transition from slower paced community life to frantic industrial city life. Of course the problems associated with this transition are also focused upon.

The most useful chapters are those that trace the changes and developments in working life and business enterprises as well as their relation to social changes. In chapter 6 "The Organization of Work," the difficulty farmers and craftsmen experience in adjusting to factory work and the resulting "iron fist" management strategies are addressed. As well, Taylor's view of workers as "Economic Man" is contrasted with the "Social Man" view revealed by the Hawthorne studies. Chapter 7 "Mass Production in Crisis" first describes and comments upon Fordism. It has contributed to the problem of work alienation and deskilling through job fragmentation. These problems are contemplated in the context of first Blauner's and then Braverman's theory. While Blauner foresees a brighter future with reduced alienation once we pass the mass production stage, Braverman's theory hypothesizes a bleaker future. He maintains that deskilling and dehumanization will certainly continue. The author seeks to evaluate these contrasting theories. Firstly, the fact that it is difficult to clearly distinguish between skilled, semi-skilled and unskilled occupations makes the analysis of the situation arduous. Although Theobald does not provide, nor intend to provide, a detailed critique of Blauner's and Braverman's theories, he posits that the generally negative work consequences of the rise of mass production are undeniable. In order to counteract these consequences, restructuring for more participative forms of management and the increase in worker autonomy are necessary. In light of this, various job enrichment and organizational restructuring programs are reviewed.

The post-industrial society has become a popular phrase. Up until now, industrialization has moved through a number of distinct stages. But will the next phase really be a post-industrial one? Chapter 8 outlines Daniel Bell's scenario in favor of this view. He believes that we are moving into a society based on services and knowledge instead of manufacturing and material goods. As a result, the majority of work will be white-collar, in small businesses and involve reskilling. The work situation will thus improve. Theobald criticizes this view by first noting that the "services" sector is ill-defined. Secondly, labor in the services sector is actually cheaper than in manufacturing, and the labor force is more flexible. This generally means poorer working conditions. According to Theobald, the immediate future will still be dominated by large multinational corporations with a small group of privileged workers surrounded by a peripheral work force with a much lower quality of working life.

547. Theorell, Töres. "How Will Future Worklife Influence Health?" *Scandinavian Journal of Work, Environment and Health* 23, supplement 4 (1997): S16-S22.

Keywords: stress, work environment, forecasting

The author introduces this paper by noting, "Before we can discuss psychophysiological mechanisms relevant to our understanding of future worklife and its influence on future health, we need a theoretical model with which to separate stressors from both individual coping mechanisms and physiological reactions." Such a model is presented here and used "to analyze the interaction between work conditions and health. The individual coping patterns are determined partly by genetic factors and partly by life experiences. Since genetic factors determine approximately one-third of the variance in different relevant components of coping patterns, the environment is of considerable importance. Our coping patterns are constantly changing due to our experiences. Our experiences at work are embedded in our social context, and conditions outside work, such as social support from family and friends, are also important in determining the health effects of work conditions. In this review, the emphasis is on the environmental aspects of the total interplay." Theorell also notes that "due to structural developments, with increasing demands on effectiveness and increasing threats of becoming unemployed, employees will be more and more reluctant to report problems at work. Accordingly, the foreseeable development will necessitate increasing emphasis on external ratings of the psychosocial work environment and on physiological monitoring. It will be particularly important to study long-term consequences of the new work environment."

548. Theriault, Reg. *How to Tell When You're Tired: A Brief Examination of Work*. New York: W. W. Norton and Company, 1995.

Keywords: general, working class

This compelling volume, written by a longshoreman of over thirty years, "gives voice to the thoughts and conditions of the laboring classes from the privileged point of view of a man well used to tough manual labor. With a humorous sense of balance—and a refreshing absence of working-class cant—he examines the real world of the workplace: the constant struggle for respect and autonomy, the perennial tendency of management to treat workers as merely one part of the production process, the parallel habit of unions to bargain away precisely the wrong things, the nature of bosses, the sheer grinding tedium and danger of moving heavy objects, and the sense of accomplishment gained from doing a piece of work right."

The author is a keen observer of the workplace and of human nature, and conveys his insights with a moving sense of conviction. He provides "an engaging defense of the working class's right to its portion of credit and dignity for building, job by dirty, demanding job, the civilization we inhabit."

This engaging, firsthand account of the working class world has the same powerful impact as the general experience of work documented in Studs Terkel's book *Working*, in this bibliography.

549. Thomas, Robert J. "Organizational Politics and Technological Change." *Journal of Contemporary Ethnography* 20, no. 4 (1992): 442-77.

Keywords: sociology, politics, technological change

Sociologists tend to pay far greater attention to the "impacts" of technology on work and organizations than they do the process of achieving technological change. This is an unfortunate situation because it invites researchers to ignore the critical choices that organizational members make about what technology should do to organizations. Two detailed case studies of the entire process of change—from the decision to change an established technology to the implementation of a new one—suggest that early choices provided important clues regarding the impacts. Close examination reveals that the process of choice is influenced as much by political considerations as by economic and technical ones.

550. Thomas, Robert J. *What Machines Can't Do: Politics and Technology in the Industrial Enterprise*. Berkeley: University of California Press, 1994.

Keywords: technological innovations, management, organizational change, manufacturers, case study, manufacturing resource planning, organizational change, appropriate technology

The central purpose of this book can be stated rather simply: to explain what new technology does to organizations and what people are trying to do to organizations and, by extension, to themselves by means of new technology. The author argues that smart machines may not hold the key to industrial renaissance, and in so doing uses four successful manufacturing enterprises to reveal the complicated social and political dynamics that surround the design and implementation of new production technology. The author also explores the roles played by organizational power struggles and differences in worldviews in determining the form and the performance of new technologies by advocating a "power-process" perspective.

551. Thompson, Paul. *The Nature of Work: An Introduction to Debates on the Labor Process*. New York: Macmillan Press, 1983.

Keywords: working class, labor process, sociology

This is a comprehensive sociological analysis of work and labor process theory. The author begins by noting that "labor process perspectives are distinguished by their ability to place work activity within the total system of production" (that includes human labor, technology, surplus appropriation and class relations). The author also indicates that one of the problems in mainstream social science is that work is often described in terms of the various structures and tasks connected to levels of economic and technological development, rather than in terms of social relations, skills and machinery. As a result these latter components are usually taken for granted.

Chapter 1 of the text looks at the main features of the treatment of work in the various branches of social science. Chapter 2 places the labor process concepts used throughout the book (such as deskilling, subordination and the division of labor) in the context of Marx's writings. The strengths and limitations of the Marxist approach are outlined. Chapter 3 examines the contemporary labor process debates themselves. The focus is on the fundamental argument forwarded by Braverman. See especially chapters 4 and 5 for research on the degradation of labor, deskilling, the weakening of workers' autonomy, the role of new technology, worker resistance, and modern schemes of job enrichment and work humanization.

552. Tilly, Chris. *Half a Job: Bad and Good Part-Time Jobs in a Changing Labor Market*. Philadelphia: Temple University Press, 1996.

Keywords: part-time employment

At the center of the author's analysis of the study of part-time work lies the organizations that hire part-time workers. In the 1990s, there was at least one person involuntarily working part-time for every person officially counted as unemployed. It is this growing trend, the fact that there is a growing number of people with only half a job, that the author takes issue with and discusses at length.

553. Tilly, Chris, and Charles Tilly. *Work under Capitalism*. New Perspectives in Sociology. Boulder: Westview Press, 1998.

Keywords: labor, labor market, economics, sociological aspects

History plays a very strong role in the structure of labor markets, and the authors demonstrate how attention to the historical and social context of work provides important insights into the employment relationship in contemporary capitalist societies. Many examples of their theoretical approach as applied to hiring, earning distributions, promotions, and similar topics are used to provide a counterpoint to behavioral approaches based on narrowly constructed economic reality. In this study, many worlds of work, such as the household, the prison, the farm, the school, and the family business, are integrated into a theoretically coherent whole. This work also clarifies that compensation—wages and monetary benefits—constitutes only one form of work incentive and that we must be aware of commitment and coercion as other forms.

554. Toomingas, Allan, Töres Theorell, Hans Michélsen, and Rolf Nordemar. "Associations between Self-Rated Psychosocial Work Conditions and Musculoskeletal Symptoms and Signs." *Scandinavian Journal of Work, Environment and Health* 23, no. 2 (1997): 130-9.

Keywords: stress, medicine, support

The authors' abstract summarizes the research reported in their article: "Objectives: The aim was to study the associations between self-rated psychosocial work conditions and the characteristics and location of musculoskeletal symptoms, signs, and syndromes.

"Methods: Perceived psychosocial work conditions were recorded in a cross-sectional study with 358 men and women in various occupations. Symptoms were recorded from the musculoskeletal system with a questionnaire, and signs were detected in a medical examination of all body regions. The analyses of statistical associations between the psychosocial factors and musculoskeletal disorders were performed with control for age, gender, and physical load.

"Results: The most consistent and pronounced associations were mainly seen between poor psychosocial work conditions and coexisting symptoms and signs of the neck and back regions. Poor psychosocial work conditions were more consistently and strongly associated with signs of muscular (soft tissue) tenderness than with signs of tenderness in the joints, tendons, or muscular insertions or signs in nerve compression tests. Mainly low social support at work, but also high psychological demands and high job strain, were associated with such symptoms and signs, whereas decision latitude at work showed few associations with musculoskeletal disorders.

"Conclusions: Perceived poor psychosocial work conditions are statistically associated mainly with symptoms and signs of muscular tenderness in the central body regions. Studies on associations between psychosocial work conditions and musculoskeletal disorders should separate effect measures of different clinical signs and different body regions in order to avoid attenuation of the risk estimates."

555. Trice, Harrison M., and Janice M. Beyer. *The Cultures of Work Organizations*. Englewood Cliffs, NJ: Prentice-Hall, 1993.

Keywords: organizational cultures, cultural forms, organizational passages and cultural continuity, occupational subcultures, subcultures in organizations, leadership and organizational cultures, cultural interchange between organizations and environments

Culture is one of the main underlying processes in much of what happens in modern organizations, as it filters the ways in which people see and understand their worlds. It also encourages some behaviors and forbids others, and thus is responsible for the emotional responses that people have to events. Thus, it is this important and close relationship that culture shares with work that is explored.

556.Troup, Carolyn, and Philip Dewe. "Exploring the Nature of Control and its Role in the Appraisal of Workplace Stress." *Work and Stress* 16, no. 4 (May 2002): 335-55.

Keywords: appraisal of stress, perceptions of control, coping, stress

The concept of control is a prominent component of theories of stress. From a transactional framework, appraisal of control is seen as important in influencing coping behavior. However, little attention has been paid to the measurement of the appraisal of control in a work-related situation. In this paper it is argued that situational control should not be reduced to a simple assessment of whether or not an individual has control over a given situation. Instead it is believed that it is important to identify the factors that an individual strives to have control of, as well as the perceived degree of control over those factors. A major component of the present study was the use of a measure that viewed control in this way and that examined control as a multifaceted construct (task control, predictability, self-control and general control). This paper reports on an analysis that examines the multifaceted nature of perceived control with other situational appraisals in the process of coping with workplace stress. A total of 134 employees from four public sector organizations in New Zealand took part in this research. Having control over work tasks was for this sample considered to be less important in giving a sense of control than either predictability or self-control. When it came to reporting how much control they actually had, respondents reported higher levels of self-control than other aspects of control. However, in general respondents reported lower levels of actual control than what they perceived it was important for them to have. This research emphasizes the importance of having a sense of self-control, particularly when it comes to the use of different coping strategies. Overall these findings point to the need to better understand the nature and type of control and its importance if we are to advance our knowledge of work stress.

557. Tsiganou, Helen A. *Workers' Participative Schemes: The Experience of Capitalist and Plan-Based Societies*. New York: Greenwood Press, 1991.

Keywords: comparative, labor-management relations

This volume attempts to explain "the diversity of workers' participation schemes in broad comparative sociological terms." It offers a comprehensive analysis of worker involvement strategies in both "developed . . . capitalist countries . . . and the centrally-planned socialist countries." Specifically, the author addresses the following critical points: "the conditions under which these plans emerge; and the reasons that account for the similarities or differences among them in the national settings examined. . . . Why, for instance, do countries that face similar problems or have similar political and economic systems differ in regard to the participation schemes they develop? Who are the main initiators of these plans?"

Chapter 1 provides an analytical research framework, and chapter 2 discusses the Scandinavian approach to worker participation. Chapter 3 examines the English, French, and German experiences with worker participation schemes. Chapter 4 elaborates on the American and Japanese experiences in this area. Chapters 5 through 8 discuss worker participation in "some centrally planned socialist societies," and chapter 9 summarizes the findings of the study.

558. Turner, Lowell. *Democracy at Work: Changing World Markets and the Future of Labor Unions*. Ithaca, NY: Cornell University Press, 1991.

Keywords: industrial relations, comparative, unions, automotive industry

"This book examines the comparative political economy of advanced industrial societies, with a focus on comparative industrial relations." The author notes that increasing interest in the field is largely due to "intensified world market competition and industrial restructuring." The central concern of the text is "to cast light on contrasting cross-national outcomes for industrial adjustment, for industrial relations, and above all for the changing role and position of contemporary unions." An accompanying question is explored by the author: "Are unions important and appropriate in early stages of industrial development but necessarily inappropriate and counter-productive later on?" The implications of this question for industrial democracy, successful industrial adjustment, and future social legislation are also considered.

The book's largest empirical content is on United States and West German automobile industries, with a focus on "the politics of new work organization at the plant level." Chapter 2 discusses union-promoted group work concepts in Germany. The greatest emphasis in the volume is given to "core" work forces, a declining segment of the overall work force, rather than part-time, unskilled, largely non-union workers.

To sum up, the author is primarily interested in analyzing "the general driving force of world market changes and new technologies and the particular national institutions that represent workers' interests, shape domestic response, and account for contrasting national outcomes." See especially the conclusion "The Politics of Work Reorganization: Summary and Implications."

559. U.S. Department of Transportation. *Transportation Implications of Telecommuting*. U.S. Department of Transportation, 1993.

Keywords: telecommuting, job satisfaction, gender

This report addresses the potential costs and benefits of telecommuting. It focuses on future impacts of telecommuting on transportation, environment, and energy use. It is noted from the onset that "telecommuting is still in a very early stage, despite the existence of many telecommuters and numerous pilot projects and studies." Chapter 1 provides background to the subject, discusses the purpose and scope of the report, and looks at the historical evolution of telecommuting. This section also considers jobs with telecommuting potential, telecommuter demographics, transportation implications, telecommuting and the public sector, forms of telecommuting (e.g., home-based and regionally centered), and examples of existing telecommuting programs. Chapter 2 explores "Factors Affecting the Future Degree and Impacts of Telecommuting." See especially "Employee Benefits and Concerns" (topics examined here include social isolation, career advancement, job satisfaction, overworking, work/life boundaries, and remote supervision and management). Also see "Health and Safety Concerns," "Legal and Regulatory Issues," and "Estimates of Potential Telecommuters." Chapter 3 focuses on "Potential Transportation-Related Impacts of Telecommuting." In this section, see "Changes in travel behavior, impacts on location, changes in modal choice, congestion mitigation, energy use impacts, air quality impacts, safety implications, time savings, health care effects, economic development, rural area development, job creation, and telecommuting/urban sprawl." And see the final chapter 4 for major conclusions. Here is a sample of the principal conclusions: "Telecommuting is now practiced by approximately 2 million workers and could reach 7.5 to 15 million within a decade. . . . Telecommuting has the potential to provide significant transportation-related public benefits in this decade. . . . The congestion and air quality improvements potentially attainable through telecommuting could be substantially diminished if telecommuters removed from the highways are replaced by the emergence of latent travel demand. . . . Telecommuting could stimulate urban sprawl and have other adverse impacts on land use and public transportation."

560. Upton, David M. "What Really Makes Factories Flexible?" *Harvard Business Review*, July-August 1995: 74-81.

Keywords: computer integrated manufacturing, human resources, flexible production

The author begins this paper by noting that "in the face of fierce, low-cost competition and an army of high-quality suppliers, companies are increasingly focusing on flexibility as a way to achieve new forms of competitive advantage." The article indicates that many managers have collectively invested tens of billions of dollars in hardware and software in the hope that computer integrated manufacturing (CIM) will transform their factories into highly flexible operations. Time and time again, however, the author reports that "mangers have been disappointed and frustrated because they have not understood exactly why enhanced flexibility has eluded them." In an effort to help manufacturing managers understand why the improvement of flexibility has been so elusive, Upton undertook an extensive study of sixty-one factories in North America that produce fine paper. The results are reported here. The findings turn much of the conventional wisdom on its head. In the plants studied, "there was little direct correlation between the degree of computer integration and the degree of operational flexibility. I found that large plants were not inherently less flexible than small plants. Contrary to what many believe, newer, bigger processes were typically better able to perform quick changeovers than older, smaller machines." The biggest revelation for the author was the role of people—both managers and operators. "The flexibility of the plants depended much more on people than on any technical factor. Although high levels of computer integration can provide critically needed advantages in quality and cost competitiveness, all the data in my study point to one conclusion: Operational flexibility is determined primarily by a plant's operators and the extent to which managers cultivate, measure, and communicate with them. Equipment and computer integration are secondary." The author further points out that while managers often embraced computer integration as the "solution," in reality, "computer systems were often a quick fix that helped managers avoid the tremendously difficult task of defining precisely what kind of flexibility they required from a plant . . . and then overhauling work practices in order to achieve that flexibility." The author's case, stated simply, is that "most managers put too much faith in machines and technology, and too little faith in the day-to-day management of people."

561. Vallas, Steven Peter. *Power in the Workplace: The Politics of Production at AT&T.* SUNY Series in the Sociology of Work. Albany: State University of New York Press, 1993.

Keywords: American Telephone and Telegraph Company, employees, telecommunications, case study, industrial relations, industrial sociology, organizational behavior

There are many trends in managerial authority in the workplace that are revealed by the author with the use of a case study of the high-tech communications industry. The mechanism that enabled the advance of capitalist firms to achieve and maintain control over the workers they employ is revealed by the author. How the integration and spread of automated technologies place lower level human labor in positions of declining power is also demonstrated. The author concludes that the new regime does not deskill workers and does not need to fall toward what some have called electronic sweatshops. However, increasing managerial control over production poses a major challenge to those who advocate labor participation in the management of American industries.

562. van Beinum, Hans. "The Kaleidoscope of Workplace Reform." 169-202 in *Constructing the New Industrial Society*, edited by Frieder Naschold, Robert E. Cole, Björn Gustavsen, and Hans van Beinum. Assen, The Netherlands: Van Gorcum, 1993.

Keywords: democracy, participation, sociotechnical systems

This chapter provides a commentary on LOM, a Swedish program for organizational renewal called "Leadership, organization, and co-determination." The aim of LOM is to promote the role of research in workplace development. The author chronicles the development of new forms of work organization starting in the late 1930s. This is a useful summary of various movements such as those by Lewin, Tavistock, sociotechnical systems, and participative design. The subsequent section presents a debate on participative democracy and its relation to the economic effectiveness of enterprises. Finally, the social psychological and relational aspects of research into operating systems in action are explored.

563. Van Den Besselaar, Peter. "The Future of Employment in the Information Society: A Comparative, Longitudinal and Multi-Level Study." *Journal of Information Science* 23, no. 5 (1997): 373.

Keywords: information society, unemployment, forecasting

"This paper aims to analyze the relationship between information technology and employment as a systematic property of societies, in terms of 'per capita' labor demand." The author begins by noting that the everyday experience in the developed information societies is one of rapid technological change and, simultaneously, of a persisting high level of unemployment, suggesting that technology is a net job-killer. On the other hand, it is also noted that most economists and politicians argue that technological change has a positive overall effect on employment. The article makes the point that "despite the abundance of research conducted during the last two decades on the effects of information and communication technology (ICT) on employment, some fundamental disagreement among researchers persists." The author maintains that the complexity of the problem makes it difficult to draw general conclusions about this controversy. "A central problem is that the effects of ICT can be studied at various levels of aggregation, and from different perspectives." In order to solve this problem, the author and a team of researchers conducted several projects, designed to account for the various levels of aggregation at which the effects of technological change on employment can be studied. Long-term trends in employment are also considered here, thus allowing for a more solid foundation for assessing the future impacts of information technology on employment. This is a comprehensive report with detailed information on a number of relevant concerns including: notes on earlier research, theoretical considerations (technological development and structural change; long waves in employment, the shift to services, etc.), design and data, measuring employment, and research results. See especially section 5, "Conclusions and Discussion: The Future of Employment in the Information Society."

One of the fundamental conclusions reported in this research article is that "In the long run, the amount of work available per capita in developed economics decreases. This observation at the macro level is corroborated by the findings on the micro level, where the degree of ICT use was positively correlated to decreasing employment. Not only do advanced process innovations result in rationalization, but product innovations also prove to be a substitution of more labor-intensive products and services by less labor-intensive products and services. . . . Also, the growth of employment in the expanding industries (especially the IT sector) is not enough to counterbalance the declining industries and to accommodate the growing population."

564. Van Den Besselaar, Peter, Andrew Clement, and Pertti Jarvinen, eds. *Proceedings of the IFIP TC9/WG9.1 Working Conference on Information System, Work and Organization Design*. Berlin: Elsevier Science Publishers, 1989.

Keywords: expert systems, computers, work design, general

This volume of papers presented at the 1989 Berlin Working Conference on Information System, Work and Organizational Design covers a broad range of topics related to the design of advanced technological systems in various work environments. Selected article titles include the following: "Expert Systems: Is There Really a Challenge to Industrial Labor?"; "Electronic Monitoring: Worker Reactions and Design Alternatives"; "Decentralized Office Technology and Women's Work"; "Feminist Perspectives on the Design of Computer Communications Networks: An Alternative Design Strategy"; "User Involvement in Requirements Analysis and Specifications: In Theory and in Practice"; and "Human-Computer Interaction and Computer Systems: An Intimate Relationship."

The first article mentioned above is the only one that does not repeat information that is readily available from other sources and is therefore the only one abstracted. The authors examine the actual distribution of expert systems compared with market forecasts—concluding that "the market for expert system technology is still very small" (compared with the whole area of information technology). Two basic questions are considered in relation to expert system technique: "Is it economically profitable and is it acceptable for the quality and structure of work?" Both questions remain open, according to these researchers, but the latter question poses many serious implications for work design.

A number of significant insights arise out of this article. I will note two of them. First, "expert systems are necessarily unsafe, and—even worse—they fail suddenly, unexpectedly, in abrupt ways." In the process of becoming "programmed experts," knowledge-based programs will "occasionally make faults as every expert does." The authors continue: "It is not only the problem of companies, it is as well the problem of science, politics, and society in general whether errors can be accepted as a normal functionality feature of programs."

The second major insight of the authors is a crucial one that concerns the implications of artificial expert systems for areas of human work that are insufficiently understood. "[T]he risks of formal reduction of intelligent work, of rationalization and dequalification are intensified by the security and responsibility risks of erroneous and incomplete programs like expert systems."

565. Vanheule, Stijn, An Lievrouw, and Paul Verhaeghe. "Burnout and Intersubjectivity: A Psychoanalytical Study from a Lacanian Perspective." *Human Relations* 56, no. 3 (March 2003): 321-38.

Keywords: psychological aspects, burnout

This article examines the intersubjective process connected with burnout. On the basis of qualitative research data, this article investigates to what extent Lacan's model of intersubjectivity enables us to understand the burnout process and to differentiate between people who suffer from burnout and those who do not. It first outlines Lacan's theory of intersubjectivity through a discussion of the dialectical master/slave relationship and the difference between imaginary and symbolic interactions. This model is then tested against the interview material of 30 special educators drawn from the results of a wider random sample survey of 765 respondents in response to a burnout questionnaire. It finds that Lacan's distinction between imaginary and symbolic functioning allows us to establish a difference between high and low scorers. High scorers—among whom two subtypes can be distinguished—function mainly in an imaginary way. Among low scorers, two subgroups were similarly found.

566. Van Maanen, John, ed. *Qualitative Studies of Organizations*. Administrative Science Quarterly Series in Organization Theory and Behavior. Thousand Oaks, CA: Sage Publications, 1998.

Keywords: organizational behavior, organizational change

This volume focuses on the areas that have most profoundly shaped the development of organizational theory and behavior by selecting and introducing a compendium of *Administrative Science Quarterly* articles on qualitative research. The grouping of these articles represents a broad range of research styles, methods, topics, and levels of analysis that are spread over four areas of research: groups in organizations, organizational process, the societal and institutional environment, and organizational identity and change. These organizations include factories, churches, engineering groups, universities, voluntary organizations, fisheries, basketball teams, pop music recording firms, and more.

As a result, this work covers a multitude of disciplines, including sociology, political science, management studies, communication, and history.

567. van Veldhoven, Marc, Jan de Jonge, Sjaak Broersen, Michiel Kompier, and Theo Meijman. "Specific Relationships between Psychosocial Job Conditions and Job-Related Stress: A Three-Level Analytic Approach." *Work and Stress* 16, no. 3 (2002): 207-28.

Keywords: psychosocial job demands, job-related strain, job-related well-being, multi-level analysis, negative affectivity

This cross-sectional questionnaire study presents a multi-level analysis on 2,565 workers in 188 departments in 36 organizations in the Netherlands. A three-level model is used in which individual workers are nested within departments, which in turn are nested within organizations. Research questions concern (1) the amount and distribution of variance in job-related stress explained for the three levels in the study (individuals, departments, organizations) and (2) the specificity of relationships between psychosocial job demands and job-related stress in the three-level model. Well-being showed slightly more raw variance to be explained at supra-individual levels than strain. The full regression model explained about 35 percent of the total variance in both work-related strain and well-being. Psychosocial job conditions did not exceed the expected amount of 10 to 15 percent contribution to this explained variance. These results do not differ from comparable studies that do not use multi-level analysis. The variance distribution in the full model, however, showed unexplained variance to be located at the individual level for both strain and well-being, and at the departmental level only for well-being. This last finding shows a direction for possible improvement of work stress models. Specificity of relationships was also shown: psychological job demands were more strongly related to strain, whereas job content variables (i.e., job variety, job control) were more strongly related to well-being. Results also suggested that social support was more strongly associated with well-being than with strain. Well-being appeared to have a more widely varying range of predictors than strain.

568. Various. *Conditions of Work Digest.*

Keywords: work resources

This is an annual listing of research projects on work giving annotations, information on who to contact, etc.

569. Various. *Human Relations.*

Keywords: work resources

This journal from the Tavistock Institute usually contains a range of articles pertinent to healthy work.

570. Various. *Social Science and Medicine.*

Keywords: work resources

This journal sometimes contains relevant articles.

571. Various. "Social Science and Workplace Reform." Special issue, *Human Relations* 51, no. 3 (1998): 215-448.

Keywords: sociotechnical systems, lean production, neo-Taylorism, industrial relations, group work, working life, work design, sociology

The theme examined in this special volume of the journal *Human Relations* is the nature of the social scientific contribution to the improvement of workplaces as both social and economic entities. The first article by J. H. Smith offers a reevaluation of the life and work of probably the most eminent pre-Tavistock Institute workplace social scientist, Elton Mayo. Smith describes Mayo's concern with establishing a connection between social collaboration and workplace efficiency, as well as his particular agenda in regard to workplace reform. In "Work Design Issues in Lean Production from a Sociotechnical Systems Perspective: Neo-Taylorism or the Next Step in Sociotechnical Design?" the authors assess the design principles of "lean production" in light of the principles of sociotechnical systems design. They conclude that there are some areas of compatibility but also of difference, particularly concerning systems for management control and the importance of local autonomy and decentralized decision making.

In "The Three Waves of Industrial Group Work: Historical Reflections on Current Research on Group Work" by Manfred Moldaschl and Wolfgang Weher, the authors offer a critique of how three successive ways of theorizing about the nature and benefits of group-based work—the "human relations" school, STS, and lean production—need to be understood in terms of the changing contexts of economic and political interests.

See also "Making Sense of 'Quality'? Toward a Review and Critique of Quality Initiatives in Financial Services," "Social Defenses against Organizational Learning," and "From Experiments to Network Building: Trends in the Use of Research for Reconstructing Working Life" for useful discussions.

572. Vischer, Jacqueline C. *Workspace Strategies: Environment as a Tool for Work.* New York: Chapman and Hall, 1996.

Keywords: work environment

Jacqueline Vischer is the founder of the Buildings-in-Use (BIU) assessment system, a diagnostic tool based on information provided by users about their workspaces. The BIU system has grown to become a user-manager communication tool as well as a decision making tool for managers. The BIU seeks to determine what office workers think of the lighting, noise, temperature, odors, furniture and other physical aspects of their working environments, as well as the convenience of the building in terms of the location and/or availability of bathrooms, elevators, parking, security and maintenance services. The BIU system, Vischer argues, helps to solve workspace problems and facilitates the reengineering of work. Furthermore, the results of many BIU assessments reveal, according to Vischer, the nature of the relationship between workers and their workspaces. These findings are noted in the book. It serves as a reference guide for managers, property owners and building professionals who seek to help make people more effective at their jobs by improving office planning. The chapters only reveal a hint of a preventive orientation; reengineering is encouraged for the sake of increased efficiency.

573. Voss, Chris, and David Clutherbuck. *Just-in-Time: A Global Status Report.* Berlin: IFS Publications/Springer-Verlag, 1989.

Keywords: just-in-time production, participation, management, comparative, waste reduction

This is a comprehensive treatment of just-in-time (JIT) production. It identifies time-based competition as the critical dimension in competitive manufacturing. The fundamental tenets of JIT, its history, its economic background, and its deployment around the world are described. Waste reduction is identified as a core philosophy of JIT. In this case, waste can refer to wasted time, movement, or material, or wastes resulting from defective products, returned goods, manufacturing readjustments, or overproduction.

574. Wall, Toby D., Chris W. Clegg, and Nigel J. Kemp, eds. *The Human Side of Advanced Manufacturing Technology*. Wiley Series in Psychology and Productivity at Work. Chichester, UK: John Wiley and Sons, 1987.

Keywords: human resources, technological change, advanced manufacturing technology

This is another volume in the Wiley Series in Psychology and Productivity at Work. Written by applied psychologists, engineers, and management specialists, this collection examines the human implications of advanced manufacturing technology (AMT). A wide range of human issues are covered, including: "the planning and implementation of AMT; work systems design; selection and training; supervisory roles; organization design; industrial relations; societal implications; and research and development needs for the future."

The basic aim of the book is "to debate some of the questions about the social and psychological dimensions of information technology" with a particular focus on AMT. The perspective of the authors "ranges from . . . implications for the individual at the level of the job through to . . . organizational ramifications."

See chapter 1 "The Nature and Implications of Advanced Manufacturing Technology" for a discussion of the diffusion of AMT, the deskilling process, and early views of the human side of AMT. Chapter 3 considers "AMT and Work Design." Topics include computer-aided design, group technology, flexible manufacturing systems, and work design (personal and environmental factors, self-regulating work groups, etc.). Case studies that assess the introduction of such technologies are also provided. See chapter 7 for "Industrial Relations Issues in AMT." Topics include the following: types of innovation; union organization and bargaining structure; and implementation. See also chapter 8 "Societal Implications of AMT" for a discussion of the skilling process (for management and workers) and a general assessment of social trends as they relate to AMT. See chapter 9 "Research and Development into Humanizing Advanced Manufacturing Technology" for additional case studies, research and development practices, and cost-benefit outcomes.

575. Wall, Toby D., Paul R. Jackson, and Sean Mullarkey. "Further Evidence on Some New Measures of Job Control, Cognitive Demand and Production Responsibility." *Journal of Organizational Behavior* 16 (1995): 431-55.

Keywords: work design, stress

The authors summarize their work as follows: "Current approaches to job design and job stress, and their application in the context of new manufacturing technologies and practices, call for new widely applicable measures of job properties. In response to this need, Jackson, Wall, Martin, and Davids (1993) described the development of new scales of timing control, method control, monitoring demand, problem-solving demand and production responsibility. This article provides further evidence concerning these measures, based on the responses of nearly 1700 employees from five separate samples. The evidence includes: investigation through confirmatory factor analysis of the applicability of the underlying five-factor measurement model on two new samples; improvement of the problem-solving demand scale; a test of the replicability of the measurement model by formal factorial invariance tests across four samples; additional information on scale reliability and construct validity; and normative data for a wide range of shopfloor and related jobs."

576. Wall, Toby D., Paul R. Jackson, Sean Mullarkey, and Sharon K. Parker. "The Demands-Control Model of Job Strain: A More Specific Test." *Journal of Occupational and Organizational Psychology* 69 (1996): 153-66.

Keywords: stress

The article seeks to clarify and retest Karasek and Theorell's theory. More specifically, the decision latitude variable is operationalized more clearly. In Karasek and Theorell's model, this variable encompasses factors such as control, task variety, and learning opportunities. However, Karasek and Theorell state *control*, not the other factors, as the important variable in their theory. Thus when these authors conducted a study of 1,451 manufacturing employees, with more clearly defined measures of demand and control, results congruent with Karasek and Theorell's theory were obtained. However, when the variable of decision latitude was replaced with the control variable, the results were not as expected.

577. Walton, R. "How to Counter Alienation in the Plant." *Harvard Business Review*, November-December 1972: 72-81.

Keywords: participation, alienation, productivity, case study

A plant where work teams perform without supervisors, where decisions are based on employee consensus, and where most of the staff functions are assigned to line operators—in what future organization would such a phenomenon exist? "Probably in most," says this author, "because such radical innovations are part of the emerging answer to alienation in the workplace." He argues that total "systemic" restructuring of the way work is done is required to both meet the changing expectations of employees and increase productivity. Some companies, in fact, have already used this approach with considerable success—and they have the productivity and high morale to prove it. After analyzing the employee dissatisfaction that dictates the innovations he recommends, the author draws lessons from a redesign effort implemented in a pet-food plant by a particularly forward-looking organization.

578. Walton, R. E. "Improving the Quality of Work Life." *Harvard Business Review*, May-June 1974: 12, 16, 155.

Keywords: QWL, productivity, alienation

This is a very short article on QWL that tries to redress the imbalance between work and other aspects of life.

579. Walton, R. E. "Work Innovations in the United States." *Harvard Business Review*, July-August 1979: 88-98.

Keywords: QWL, work design

What have ten years of work innovations taught us? For one thing, these efforts are usually neither extreme successes nor extreme failures. For another, people who sponsor these projects are neither villains nor saints. Also, the quality of work life projects may add to productivity but not necessarily. In other words, work innovations are not absolute solutions to any set of problems; rather, they represent an approach to looking at problems. In this article, the author, a well-known authority in the area of work innovation, sets out to examine some of the myths that surround it. To do this, he puts forth his own three-level conception of work innovation showing how techniques, outcomes, and culture relate to each other. Using this conception, managers can better approach improving work in their own operations. One of his main conclusions from looking at the past ten years of experience is that work improvement efforts that have both productivity and quality of work life as goals are more likely to succeed on both counts than projects that stress one goal to the exclusion of the other.

580. Walton, R. E. "From Control to Commitment in the Workplace." *Harvard Business Review*, March-April 1985: 77-84.

Keywords: participation

The symptoms are familiar: a good strategy is not executed well, costs rise out of all proportion to gains in productivity, high rates of absenteeism persist, and a disaffected work force, taking little pride or pleasure in what it does, retards innovation and quality improvements. To those at the top of the corporate ladder, it seems as if they are the captains of a ship in which the wheel is not connected to the rudder. Whatever decisions get made, little happens down below. Only lately have managers themselves begun to take responsibility for these symptoms and for the approach to work-force management out of which they grow. Only lately have they begun to see that workers respond best—and most creatively—not when they are tightly controlled by management, placed in narrowly defined jobs, and treated like an unwelcome necessity, but, instead, when they are given broader responsibilities, encouraged to contribute, and helped to take satisfaction in their work. It should come as no surprise that eliciting worker commitment—and providing the environment in which it can flourish—pays tangible dividends for the individuals and for the company. The author describes these opposing approaches to a company's human capital and points out the key challenges in moving from one to another.

581. Walton, R. E., and G. I. Susman. "People Policies for the New Machines." *Harvard Business Review*, March-April 1987: 98-106.

Keywords: work design, skill, deskilling, advanced manufacturing technology, policy

When advanced manufacturing technology is introduced in a firm, it faces various labor policy options. By examining these options through the use of case studies, the authors conclude that AMT invariably leads to greater interdependence and that jobs designed with higher skill requirements become essential. They believe that managers are making a mistake when they lower skill requirements and decouple activities.

582. Waluyo, Lieke, Kerstin Ekberg, and Jörgen Eklund. "Assembly Work in Indonesia and in Sweden: Ergonomics, Health and Satisfaction." *Ergonomics* 39, no. 2 (1996): 199-212.

Keywords: job satisfaction, work load, stress, ergonomics

The authors summarize their work as follows: "Work conditions in industrial production vary substantially between different cultures. In the present study the aims were to identify differences between Swedish and Indonesian assembly industry workers regarding work environment factors, health and job satisfaction, and to find associations between work environment factors, and the health measures. Data were collected by a questionnaire from 326 Swedish and 136 Indonesian assembly industry workers, interviews, and from company documents. The prevalence of musculoskeletal symptoms was high in both groups. Stress and psychosomatic symptoms had higher prevalence in the Swedish group, that also rated their work conditions as worse in most respects. Work tasks were physically heavier in Indonesia, but less monotonous and with lower demands on productivity. The Indonesians were more satisfied with their jobs. Physical job demands were associated with musculoskeletal symptoms. Competence development was associated with increased job satisfaction. Conflicts and harassment at work were associated with stress and psychosomatic symptoms. Job pressure, especially deficient planning of the jobs was associated with lower job satisfaction, psychosomatic and stress symptoms in the Swedish group. Implications for job design in the two cultures are presented."

583. Wardell, Mark, Thomas L. Steiger, and Peter Meiksins, eds. *Rethinking the Labor Process*. Albany: State University of New York Press, 1999.

Keywords: industrial sociology, division of labor, effect of technological innovations on employees, industrial relations, sex roles in the work environment, management, social conflict, equality, organizational change

This book takes stock of the field known as labor process by using both quantitative and qualitative methodologies to demonstrate ideas such as the sociology of work, organizations, and stratification. This venue serves as an opportunity for both American and British authors to rethink and reinvigorate the labor process field. They focus on aspects central to the labor process perspective including management strategies, innovations in the workplace, the value of labor, technology, and control and resistance.

584. Warner, Malcolm, Werner Wobbe, and Peter Brödner, eds. *New Technology and Manufacturing Management: Strategic Choices for Flexible Production Systems*. New Technologies and Work. Chichester: John Wiley and Sons, 1990.

Keywords: technological change, manufacturing, flexible manufacturing

The authors of this collection of papers argue that the basic determinants in future manufacturing are the organizational and human resource aspects—that "these are the key strategic resources . . . technology design has to adapt to this given potential." This viewpoint is rather different from the one usually expressed by managers who are responsible for coordinating the introduction of highly-advanced, automated and computer integrated technological systems. All too often, management is preoccupied with the question of how human resources can be best adapted to the technological potential.

This book criticizes "the technologically dominated view of production systems for being too narrow." Instead, the contributors prefer to start the debate about the "future of the factory" from "a fresh consideration of what kind of products and what types of manufacturing might be demanded, and what manufacturing means should be considered in making a strategic choice."

The authors also explore how the technocentric view of manufacturing management (referred to above) is now often "manifest in the CIM factory, with the result of very restricted flexibility, rather than a genuine flexibility and adaptability." The "promises involving high-tech flexibility, computer integration, and large scale automation have yet to prove themselves," according to the authors.

The book strongly advocates the increased use of flexible manufacturing systems but contends that "the means for this are not to be found in technology, division of labor, and automation . . . but rather in skill-oriented organization."

See especially chapter 4 "Changing Concepts of Work and Qualifications," chapter 8 "Technocentric-Anthropocentric Approaches: Toward Skill-Based Manufacturing," and chapter 9 "'Design for Human-Machine Interfaces."

585. Warr, Peter, and Toby Wall. *Work and Well-Being*. Harmondsworth, UK: Penguin Books, 1975.

Keywords: QWL, psychology, job satisfaction

Although written back in 1975, this book remains an important one today. The topic of quality of working life is approached from a psychological study of work satisfaction and mental health of individuals. But, perspectives from sociology, industrial relations, organizational behavior, and management theory are also included. Based on studies of various occupations and workplaces, the book seeks to determine both what the quality of working life is like and how workplaces can be altered to improve their quality.

The opening chapter provides an outline of the field of research to date, and this is put into an historical context in the second chapter. Chapters 3 through 6 deal with the following issues respectively: systems and levels of pay, interpersonal relations, participation in decision making and designing jobs for people. The following chapter, entitled "Work Stress," focuses on stress arising from social organization. The concluding chapter integrates the findings of the preceding chapters in order to move from theory to the practice of promoting well-being at work.

586. Wastell, David G., and Michael Newman. "Stress, Control and Computer System Design: A Psychophysiological Field Study." *Behavior & Information Technology* 15, no. 3 (1996): 183-92.

Keywords: computers, stress

The authors summarize their work as follows: "The stressful nature of computer-based work is often highlighted in the research literature. In this study, we argue that a well designed computer system should realize the twin aims of enhancing performance and lowering stress. This paper reports on a psychophysiological field study of the implementation of a command-and-control system in an ambulance service. The evaluation revealed both improvements in operator performance and a reduction in stress levels. In particular, it was found that computer support reduced both systolic blood pressure and subjective anxiety during conditions of peak workload. These findings are discussed in terms of Turner and Karasek's integrated model of the relationships between computer system design, task performance, and well-being. The success of the computer system was attributed to the support that it gave operators; by enhancing their degree of control it enabled them to cope better in a highly demanding work environment. The study shows that psychophysiological techniques have a valuable role to play in system design/evaluation; and more generally, that systems development methodologies should take greater account of applied psychological research, especially in areas such as stress."

587. Watson Fritz, Mary Beth. "Communication and Coordination in the Virtual Office." *Journal of Management Information Systems* 14, no. 4 (Spring 1998): 7-28.

Keywords: telecommuting, job satisfaction

In this article, the authors examine the relationships between organizational factors and individual satisfaction with office communication among telecommuters and traditional office workers. It is noted that as information technology becomes more pervasive, the structure of the traditional work environment is changing. As more work is performed at remote locations, it is found that "existing work practices and managerial strategies are often not appropriate in this environment. In particular, traditional office communication with coworkers and management, that is often dependent on physical proximity, is disrupted. In this study, individual satisfaction with office communication in the telecommuting and conventional work environments is compared through a study of telecommuters and a comparison group of non-telecommuters in nine firms."

The researchers investigate the influence of certain organizational factors, such as job characteristics, IT support, and coordination methods, on satisfaction with office communication in the two work environments. It is reported that telecommuters indicate higher satisfaction with office communication than do non-telecommuters. However, organizational factors including task predictability and electronic coordination are found to have similar influences on satisfaction with communication for both groups. The authors conclude that managers should develop strategies for managing a network of distributed workers (i.e., workers in a variety of different geographical locations) and suggest a number of different managerial actions. In addition, they suggest a number of areas for future research.

588. Webster, Juliet. *Office Automation: The Labor Process and Women's Work in Britain*. New York: Harvester Wheatsheaf, 1990.

Keywords: women, computers

The author of this volume examines "whether the introduction of computerized office technology has had the impact and effects predicted of it, and whether such developments herald the end of women's office work or a radical shift in the sexual division of labor." In the process of attempting to answer these questions, Webster "compares the design of secretarial jobs before and after the introduction of word processing and assesses specific changes in task content and use of different work skills, placing her analysis firmly in the broader context of the organization of the office, the historical use of managerial control practices, the wider labor market and women's position within it, thereby raising key questions about how the role of technological change is conceptualized."

The author's sociological investigation demonstrates that it is not always productive to become preoccupied with the technology in use. It is concluded that the introduction of office automation has no simple effect on office labor processes. "More important determinants are the principles of job design in the organization that are in turn related to the control of female labor power in particular labor markets."

Webster also suggests that preliminary evidence would seem to indicate that "deskilling (as a computer or other technologically-induced effect) is an outdated managerial strategy and is being replaced by the use of labor as an 'all-round' and flexible resource to meet the specialized demands of niche markets."

Essentially, the case studies in this book suggest overwhelmingly that there is great variability in the application of new technologies with little evidence of an overarching managerial strategy for the organization of work.

589. Webster, Juliet. "Advanced Manufacturing Technologies: Work Organization and Social Relations Crystallised." 192-222 in *A Sociology of Monsters*, edited by John Law. New York: Routledge, 1991.

Keywords: AMT, JIT

This paper considers the ways in which technologies are underpinned by patterns of work organization and power relations in the manufacturing industry. It takes as a starting point the emergence of manufacturing technologies during the Industrial Revolution, showing how these were imbued with the methods of factory organization that were then gaining currency—the visions of industrial entrepreneurs, engineers and political economists. Technologies have continued to be associated with particular patterns of work organization, both actual and envisioned. The major concern of the paper is with a contemporary manufacturing technology, Computer-Aided Production Management (CAPM). It shows how CAPM has developed according to the dominant templates of manufacturing organization—first American and now Japanese.

It charts the growth of the "enterprise" culture in the West—a discourse that stresses flexibility and prescribes production methods, such as just-in-time, that mimic those of the Japanese. It looks at the promotion of CAPM as a technology that can assist in this process and at the incorporation within CAPM of facilities for doing so. Finally, the paper shows that these manufacturing agendas are not easily implemented. CAPM user organizations find the technology inappropriate to their existing patterns of work, and so modify systems to fit these. CAPM technology therefore embodies patterns of work organization at several levels. It incorporates both the dreams and programs for work organization that are promoted by the industrially powerful at any one time, and the actual practices of work organization that pertain in the sphere of use.

590. Webster, Juliet. *Shaping Women's Work: Gender, Employment and Information Technology*. London: Longman, 1996.

Keywords: women, gender relations, information technology, sociology, technology, computers, feminism, sexual division of labor

This text, written from a sociological perspective, provides a broad overview of the current debates about technologies (particularly computer-based information technologies) and gender relations at work in a range of occupational areas. Both conceptual and empirical material is presented. Consideration is given to "gender relations both in terms of the ways in which they influence the design and development of technologies, and in terms of the ways in which relations themselves are in turn shaped by technologies."

This volume, intended primarily for undergraduate students in industrial sociology, technological change, women's studies, and social policy, draws heavily on the social shaping of technologies' theoretical perspective; the text "explores the ways in which sexual divisions of labor and gender relations in the workplace profoundly affect the direction and pace of technological change and trace the development of certain technologies, showing how, throughout their evolution, they embody these social relations." It also considers the prospect of feminist work design initiatives that attempt to invoke women in the construction of the computer systems they use.

See especially chapter 2 "Perspectives on Women's Work and Technology," chapter 4 "Information and Communication Technologies and the Shaping of Women's Employment," and chapter 6 "Women in Systems Design—Values, Methods, and Artefacts."

591. Weeks, James L., Barry S. Levy, and Gregory R. Wagner. *Preventing Occupational Disease and Injury*. Washington, DC: American Public Health Association, 1991.

Keywords: occupational health and safety, industrial hygiene

The subject of this volume is public health in the workplace. The authors' sole aim is the prevention or reduction of occupational disease and injury. They argue that the issue of workplace health holds out a significant promise: "Because the workplace is a wholly human invention, virtually everything that happens there can be changed. It is therefore possible to eliminate or control—to a degree unmatched in other environments—conditions in the workplace that are harmful, thus significantly reducing the incidence of occupational disease and injury." It is further argued that prevention depends on four fundamental tasks: "1) anticipation of the potential for disease or injury; 2) surveillance: accurate identification, reporting, and recording of occupational disease and injury; 3) analysis of collected data; and 4) control."

Part 1 presents an integrated and multidisciplinary approach to prevention. The authors suggest that "good public health practice requires a technical understanding of the problem as well as an appreciation of the social, economic, and political context in which the problem occurs" (i.e., the social environment of work). The role of health professionals is also discussed. Part 2 provides the basis for occupational disease prevention. This section includes a compendium of adverse health outcomes caused by work; the format consists of identification, occurrence, causes, pathophysiology, and prevention. Part 3 offers an overview of occupational musculoskeletal and infectious diseases as well as of occupational cancers.

592. Weil, Michelle M., and Larry D. Rosen. *Technostress: Coping with Technology @ Work @ Home @ Play*. New York: John Wiley and Sons, 1997.

Keywords: technology, stress

This volume addresses the issue of technology-related stress. Particular attention is given to computer technologies, fax machines, voice mail, the Internet and electronic mail, as well as other commonly used technologies such as automatic teller machines, VCRs and cellular phones.

The authors acknowledge the contribution of Dr. Craig Brod in coining the term "technostress" in 1984. Brod (a clinical psychologist) defined technostress as "a modern disease of adaptation caused by an inability to cope with the new computer technologies." The authors of this volume, however, do not see technostress as a disease. Rather, they think of it as "any negative impact on attitudes, thoughts, behaviors, or body physiology that is caused either directly or indirectly by technology."

The authors argue that "the proliferation of increasingly sophisticated technology at home and in the workplace has spawned unprecedented use of machines by men, women, and children. Although each individual machine was devised to make our lives easier, or to provide entertainment, collectively the mass of modern technology tends to alienate us from one another, increase daily stress levels, and leave many of us feeling dependent, inadequate, and incompetent."

Topics discussed in the book include the following: computerphobia; overcoming technostress; the myth of technological ease; the learning process; the boundaries in a virtual world; machine machismo; problems of identity and emotional health; technocommunication etiquette; on-line stresses; technological stress and family health; the speed of technological change; and problems of human adaptation.

593. Weisbord, Marvin R. *Productive Workplaces: Organizing and Managing for Dignity, Meaning and Community*. Jossey-Bass Management Series. San Francisco: Jossey-Bass Publishers, 1991.

Keywords: QWL, industrial relations, sociotechnical systems

The author of this volume attempts to provide a comprehensive analysis of the concept of "productive workplaces" from a management perspective. It is suggested that "productive workplaces are those where people learn and grow as they cooperate to improve an organization's performance. The 'bottom line,' in this way of looking at things, is dignity, meaning, and community in work. The tools—conceptual and practical—exist to build more productive workplaces." Well versed in quality of working life (QWL) programs and sociotechnical systems design, the author provides a history of various QWL strategies, gives a number of illustrative case studies, and offers new guidelines for effective action. The basic theme presented in this book is that "we hunger for community in the workplace and are a great deal more productive when we find it." Weisbord is convinced that "to feed this hunger in ways that preserve democratic values of individual dignity, opportunity for all, and mutual support is to harness energy and productivity beyond imagining."

Part 1 of the book elaborates the theme that deep human strivings underlie the search for productive workplaces. The author presents new interpretations of how the founder of "scientific management," Frederick W. Taylor, and four social scientists, Eric Trist, Fred Emery, Kurt Lewin, and Douglas McGregor, "have translated values into action and why their innovations are important today." Weisbord explores how Taylor's scientific management lost credibility in the face of unexamined human processes, and how inappropriately applied "scientific" knowledge can conflict with the preservation of democratic values and effective dialogue.

Part 2 takes up the practice of management and consultation based on participative methods. Six case studies are offered. Part 3 offers a new "third wave practice theory" for managing productive workplaces and also discusses participative work design and work team development strategies.

594. Wellins, Richard S., William C. Byham, and Jeanne M. Wilson. *Empowered Teams: Creating Self-Directed Work Groups That Improve Quality, Productivity, and Participation*. San Francisco: Jossey-Bass Publishers, 1991.

Keywords: work groups, self-directed teams

Self-directed work groups are small groups of people who are empowered to manage their own work. They usually have control over scheduling and production-related decisions and they share leadership responsibilities. Although the perspective is not a preventive one, the book is nevertheless useful as a practical guide for implementing and maintaining self-directed teams. The guidelines were developed based on surveys of 500 organizations that use self-directed teams, interviews with people in 28 such organizations, review of the literature and experience from assisting companies with setting up teams.

Part 1 "How Teams Work" introduces readers to what empowered teams are and how they work. "A Day in the Life of a Self-Directed Team: A Case Study" is also included. Part 2 "Preparing for Teams" gives instructions on work team implementation. Creating an organizational culture that is conducive to team development, the role of leaders, hiring and training are also discussed. The four stages of teams: "Getting Started," "Going in Circles," "Getting on Course" and "Full Speed Ahead" and the "feel" of teams at each stage are the subjects of part 3 "Building Strong Teams." The book also contains an annotated bibliography of the team concept.

595. Wells, Don. *Soft Sell: "Quality of Working Life" Programs and the Productivity Race.* Ottawa: Canadian Centre for Policy Alternatives, 1986.

Keywords: QWL, productivity, industrial relations, personnel management

The outspoken trade unionist Don Wells espouses the premise that quality of working life (QWL) programs do not live up to their promises. They promise workplace improvements for workers such as changes necessary for greater job satisfaction and more control over their work. However, Wells contends that QWL is used by management only to increase productivity, profits, and even their control over employees. He sees QWL as a threat to the union movement that undermines worker solidarity.

Included in this short, readable, and confrontational book are two case studies that tell the story of implementation of QWL in two plants. The workers were at first excited about the management's promises of QWL, but became disappointed and disillusioned when they failed to see most of the promised improvements.

Also contained in this book are chapters regarding management's goals, impact on workers and unions, "hollow" promises and strategies for attaining real worker control. These chapters all emphasize the point that QWL shapes workers to the job, instead of redesigning jobs for workers.

596. Wells, Don. *Empty Promises: Quality of Working Life Programs and the Labor Movement.* New York: Monthly Review Press, 1987.

Keywords: QWL, unions

Quality of Working Life (QWL) programs promise better working conditions for employees and higher productivity for the organization. While these ideals are a welcome addition to the workplace, QWL programs do not deliver what they claim to. This is the thesis forwarded by Wells, a trade unionist. Two case studies of companies that implemented QWL programs demonstrate the three-part thesis. Firstly, QWL programs arose out of the desire for higher productivity. Secondly, QWL efforts give management more power and workers less power by undermining workers' solidarity. The last chapter entitled "Union Counter-Strategies" reveals the third part of the thesis that states that workers can fight QWL programs by attempting to realize the true ideals of QWL programs.

597. Werneke, Diane. *Microelectronics and Office Jobs: The Impact of the Chip on Women's Employment.* Geneva: International Labor Office, 1983.

Keywords: women, computers, technological change, general

This volume focuses specifically on the implications for women of changes in office technology. The study begins with a brief description of the new computer technology in offices, provides an overview of the issues, and gives an analytical survey of the recent literature on the subject. The second section discusses the relationship between technological change and employment. The author assesses the question of whether technical changes in the way goods and services have been produced recently have led to rising living standards and a broadening of employment opportunities. Also questioned is the prospect for new job creation in light of the labor-saving features of new computer technology. The vulnerability of women to changes in office work is the subject of the third section. The book suggests that women generally are found to be in those occupations that are "at risk" to a greater extent than men, with regard to the new technology. Section 4 looks at the North American experience of technological change and labor displacement; case studies in banking, insurance, and general office work are presented. Job content and the organization of work in the context of computerization is the subject of section 5. Topics discussed here include deskilling, job satisfaction, home work (i.e., telecommuting) and health and safety concerns. Section 6 considers the European experience of office work and changing technology, again with a focus on the problems posed for women in particular. The final chapter summarizes the trends and recent developments and draws a number of general conclusions for policy making. The need for a broader concept of training is emphasized along with the humanization of jobs through redesign of work.

598. Wessells, Michael G. *Computer, Self and Society*. Englewood Cliffs, NJ: Prentice-Hall, 1990.

Keywords: computers, general

This volume presents a large body of basic research on a diverse set of issues related to computer technology, society, and the individual. The author begins by acknowledging that computers have become indispensable for managing information and problem solving in a variety of contexts—but quickly adds that recognition of computers as powerful instruments of social change has been less apparent.

This book examines many of the fundamental social changes that have accompanied the introduction of computer technology, as well as the ethical issues that are raised by them. For example, "should governments be allowed to keep extensive computer files on private citizens, or would this place too much power in the hands of the government? Are the huge amounts of money being spent on computers in the schools justified by the gains in the quality of education? . . . How does reliance on computers in the military affect our security? Who benefits from the use of computers?"

Topics considered are "Computers, Technology, and Culture," "Work Transformed," "Management and Labor," "The Global Economy," "National

Security," "Crime and Security," "The Challenge to Privacy," "Artificial Intelligence," "Minds and Selves," and "Education."

599. West, Michael A., ed. *Handbook of Work Group Psychology*. Chichester: John Wiley and Sons, 1996.

Keywords: work groups, psychology

This comprehensive volume offers "a clear overview of psychological knowledge about groups at work, drawing principally from the literatures of social and industrial/organizational psychology." It also presents the ideas of researchers in this field about alternative perspectives on work group development for future research and application. All of the major factors influencing work group effectiveness are considered: "group development, group structure, group limits, group innovation, inter-group processes, and relationships between groups and their wider organizations."

The various chapters "focus primarily on formal groups, in work contexts that vary across manufacturing and service industries, and represent many types of work groups" (including research and development, operational innovation, and multiprofessional groups). See especially section 3 of the book on "Group Pressures." Topics explored here include: an analysis of decision making and interaction processes (with practical insights for the promotion of effective work groups), group leadership and its role in facilitating productive group operations, work group autonomy and decision making, and autonomous work groups and quality circles (chapter 10). This last topic is given an extensive critical assessment, along with the suggestion that quality circles may often give a sense of "false empowerment" to participants. This chapter also contains practical strategies for effective implementation of autonomous work groups within organizations.

600. Westlander, Gunnela. *People at Work: Investigating Social-Psychological Contexts*. Goteborg, Sweden: Gunnela Westlander and Studentlitteratur, 1999.

Keywords: social psychology, work psychology, organizational psychology, self-evaluation, self-esteem, leadership, ideals and practice

Above all, this book provides a topical and theoretically-grounded overview of social psychology as it is relevant to the elucidation and understanding of social conditions in working life. In order to provide a coherent picture of the social reality of working life, the emphasis and approaches shift in stages from the individual to the organizational frames that determine the nature of interaction between different persons. Thus, the complexities of working life are reflected by the perspectives and themes of social psychology.

601. Westwood, Sallie. *All Day, Every Day: Factory and Family in the Making of Women's Lives*. London: Pluto Press, 1984.

Keywords: women

Patriarchal relations play a central role in defining the lives of working class women, not only at work but at home as well. However, the workplace exerts the greatest pressure to subordinate women and to produce gender identities. This is the thesis forwarded by Westwood that evolved out of her working in a British hosiery factory from March 1980 to May 1981 as a participant observer. She links the oppression of women at home with their oppression at the factory.

The book begins with observations of women's factory work and how it is constrained by capitalism and patriarchy. The rich drama of everyday life on the shop floor is conveyed engagingly to reveal how the women domesticate production, rebel against the measured day-work system and take part in union movements. The contradictory nature of shop-floor culture that the author observes is "oppositional in terms of the demands of their employers; [and] collusive in its emphasis upon women's traditional roles in the home and the family."

The later chapters probe the women's home lives and how they are related to their working lives. Interestingly, Westwood shows how factory life leads to traditional romantic and subordinate notions of womanhood. Marriage and motherhood are actually seen as liberating events; womanhood is defined by the workers as being a wife and a mother. Their marriage rituals are examined first through the stories of white women, then those of Indian women. Since one third of the female factory workers were women of color, race issues are investigated along with gender and class matters.

602. Wiggenhorn, William. "Motorola U: When Training Becomes an Education." *Havard Business Review*, July-August 1990: 71.

Keywords: case study, worker education, skill

This article highlights the major features of the Motorola Corporation's training and education programs for its employees. The author notes that in the past the company was content with having most of its workers and managers learn their jobs by observation, experience, and trial and error. However, in the new economic environment of global competition, Motorola found that the rules of manufacturing changed profoundly. "We had to rewrite the rules of corporate training and education. . . . We learned that line workers had to actually understand their work and their equipment, that senior management had to exemplify and reinforce new methods and skills if they were going to stick, that change had to be continuous and participative, and that education—not just instruction—was the only way to make all this occur."

Motorola began its basic education program with literacy training and skill instruction and gradually moved on to new concepts of work, quality, community, learning and leadership. The monetary investment in developing such progress was quickly seen to be well worthwhile, both in production terms and in human resource terms.

This article points out the methods used by the company to enable workers to carry out their own problem solving, to analyze those problems and learn to communicate them. Quality, for the company, is seen as a pervasive concept that involves all aspects of the manufacturing process, including the human factor. Details are also provided in the article regarding the setting up of the Motorola Training and Education Center (MTEC)—essentially an education service department for company employees.

603. Willcocks, Leslie, and David Mason. *Computerising Work: People, Systems Design and Workplace Relations*. London: Paradigm, 1987.

Keywords: computers, organizational change, organizational design

This volume explores the human aspects of computer systems—in all areas of computer system design, implementation, and operation. The authors take a very practical, applied approach to the subject and endeavor to break down the traditional barriers between sociology, psychology, economics, and technology in the process of reviewing extensive case research.

Chapter 1 provides "a detailed overview of a broadened understanding of human aspects of computer-based systems and places the politics of computerization at its core." Chapter 2 considers "Resistance to Change" (computerphobia, organizational factors, group resistance, etc.). Chapter 3 discusses the importance of human resource planning in the early stages of computer projects, and chapter 4 reviews "a range of different systems analysis and design perspectives and methodologies." Chapter 5 extends this approach into job work organization design and chapter 6 examines the immediate computer environment (psychological and biological factors, workstation design, etc.). Chapter 7 analyzes the role of industrial relations in the successful implementation of computer systems, and the final chapter 8 focuses on organizational and political aspects of the design process.

604. Williams, Joan. *Unbending Gender: Why Family and Work Conflict and What to Do about It*. New York: Oxford University Press, 2000.

Keywords: family, sexual division of labor, mothers, employment, economic aspects, forecasting

The modern economy has separated mothers from their families and their job potential. Having children has had a very negative effect on women's income despite the fact that women have become better educated since the 1980s. The pay gap that has existed for many years has lessened over the past several years, however for mothers, especially single mothers, it has increased: they earn only sixty cents for every dollar earned by full-time fathers. This means that in an age where gender biased pay is decreasing, mothers are tremendously disadvantaged, and since ninety percent of women will become mothers during their working lives, something must be done in order to ensure gender equality. Mothers have also failed to achieve equality at home. Despite our gender equality, women still do eighty percent of the child raising and two-thirds of the housework. In short, women still specialize in family work and men in market work. Thus, domesticity did not die, it simply mutated. It is this topic that is the main focus of the book.

605. Williams, Trevor A. *Computers, Work and Health: A Sociotechnical Approach*. London: Taylor and Francis, 1989.

Keywords: computers, health, video display terminal

The focus of this book is on office work, and particularly on how computer technology may affect clerical and keyboard work and the people performing it. The implications of computerization for office work are placed in the context of a larger technological transformation that is affecting increasing areas of working life. The book is intended primarily for occupational health and safety specialists, computer systems analysts and designers, managers, unionists, and for workers involved in the application of computer technology to work. The author uses an integrative sociotechnical approach to examine the relationships between computerized office technology, health and work organization. Emphasis is given to the role of work computerization in the trend toward the increasing subdivision of labor, the fractionation of tasks allocated to people on the job, and the imposition of organizational control over workers.

The first chapter offers an overview of how information technology generally affects work both directly and through the mediating influence of work design. This chapter also summarizes concerns about the occupational health and safety implications of new technology. Chapter 2 examines an important class of health problems known as musculotendinous disorders—long associated with the widespread adoption of visual display technology by office workers. Once again, work redesign issues are considered. Chapter 3 develops a theoretical basis for sociotechnical approaches to new office technology, and chapter 4 presents important case studies of different strategies for the design of information systems and work organization. Chapter 5 focuses specifically on the actual processes of designing and implementing new technology in organizations. Finally, chapter 6 raises some general implications for practice as these bear upon the roles of managers, information systems designers, and occupational health and safety specialists in technological and organizational innovation.

606. Wirth, Arthur G. *Productive Work—In Industry and Schools: Becoming Persons Again*. Lanham, MD: University Press of America, 1983.

Keywords: technology, education

This well-researched book is an investigation of "parallel tensions in both education and industry, between two major value orientations in American life: values of technocratic efficiency and values of the democratic tradition." The author begins by bemoaning the fact that during the 1970s and early 1980s "schools were being brought under the grip of the values and techniques of technocratic ideology that were prevalent in industry." On the positive side, though, he notes "the emergence of significant instances of democratic redesign of work . . . as a response to economic crisis."

The basic premise of the text is that "if technocratic values from industry can exert powerful influences on schools, countermovements toward industrial democracy might support different ideas about learning and school life."

See especially chapter 2 "Industry and Education in America" for a literature review of technique-based vs. humanistic learning methods and industrial strategies. Chapter 3 discusses democratic sociotechnical theory in Scandinavia and Norway, and QWL in the United States case study material is provided.

Chapter 5 examines "John Dewey's Philosophy on the Relation of Education and Industrial Democracy." Chapter 7 offers a critique of "Technocratic Ideology." Chapter 8 considers sociotechnical theory and learning at work and in school. In chapter 9 "Beyond Good Work: Social Renewal" the author explores the way in which democratic sociotechnical theory could become a "leading edge" for wider social change. The case of Lucas Aerospace Industries is also considered.

607. Wirth, Arthur G. "Issues in the Reorganization of Work: Implications for Education." *Theory into Practice* 30, no. 4 (1991): 280-7.

Keywords: work design, skill, deskilling, democracy, education, sociotechnical systems

"Which philosophy of work design shall prevail—the technical control model or the democratic sociotechnical design of work"? Wirth contemplates this important question and its implications for education. He theorizes that conventional approaches to work design and education will prove to be handicaps as we move into a post-industrial electronic/computer era. He recognizes that new approaches are necessary to deal with the coming changes. We must also, he observes, end our reliance on quantitative measures of our quality of life.

The first section presents the changes in work that have taken place since the late 1700s in the United States. The introduction of Taylor's scientific management, automation, the shortage of skilled labor and the enormous gap between the rich and the poor are addressed. Will the skill level of work be increased by high technology, or will the deskilling of work extend into middle level technical and managerial jobs? Will more jobs be created than lost by technology? Wirth reports that "a formula to bring together inventive technology with flexible, intelligent response by a committed, engaged work force" is required.

This statement serves as a transition to the next section that describes how democratic sociotechnical design for work can help achieve this requirement. It traces the origins of and arguments for the move toward sociotechnical design. Semi-autonomous work teams who determine their own workspace, are involved in hiring and firing, and perform their own quality controls are emerging and succeeding. The freedom to learn and to apply their learning seem to be the keys. This is also precisely what is important for students in schools. Wirth asserts that the problems with industry and with schools are comparable. The "rationalization of instruction" organizes material into unrelated subject areas and treats education as a production system.

The author next ponders possible alternatives to the education system, based on the sociotechnical approaches similar to those used in the redesign of work. The restructuring of schools should involve more hands-on learning, more freedom over curricula, more group work, and students and teachers who are personally engaged in their learning.

608. Wiseman, Henry, et al., eds. *Critical Choices! Ethics, Science and Technology*. Toronto: Thompson Educational Publishing, 1991.

Keywords: technology, ethics

This volume contains original essays on ethics, science, and technology by international authors. The book is based on the presentations made at the World Conference on Ethical Choices in the Age of Pervasive Technology, held at the University of Guelph, October 25-29, 1989. The editors have included the main plenary sessions, summaries of conference workshops, the edited transcript of the final roundtable debate, and action proposals for governments, industry, professionals, and the general public.

See especially "Workshop 4: Technology and Ethical Choice in Computers and Information Systems—From Poetry to Practicalities: Ethical Choices in an Information Age." The particular issues raised here speak to three key themes: "1) The potential control which communications and computer technologies can exercise over our daily lives; 2) the way in which human activities are being both enriched and ensnared in a variety of global information networks; 3) the growing disparities between the information-rich and the information-poor whether these be defined in socio-economic, regional or North-South terms." Also see "Technology: A Labor Perspective," "Ethical Issues in an Age of Pervasive Technology," "Ethical Concerns in the Relationship between the State and Technology," and "Workshop 11—Technology and Ethical Choice in Labor Relations."

One of the central realizations to emerge from the conference essays presented here is the overall recognition that "ethical considerations must become an integrated part of the decision-making process as it affects society as a whole."

609. Wolf, S., and A. Finestone, eds. *Occupational Stress*. Littleton, MA: PSG Publishing Co., 1986.

Keywords: stress, job satisfaction, alienation

Wolf and Finestone document the importance of personal fulfillment and job satisfaction to the health of the worker. They provide a good treatment of ulcers, blood pressure, and myocardial infarction due to work stress. Worker alienation, absenteeism, alcoholism, and drug use are also discussed, as is the historical perspective.

610. Wood, Ellen Meiksins, Peter Meiksins, and Michael Yates, eds. *Rising from the Ashes? Labor in the Age of "Global" Capitalism*. New York: Monthly Review Press, 1998.

Keywords: labor movement, capitalism, international trade

Questions such as, Can workers regain the initiative against the tidal wave of corporate downsizing and government cutbacks? Can unions revive their ranks and reignite the public imagination? and Is labor rising from the ashes? have arisen to the forefront of worldwide labor movements. These questions are set in a global context, connecting and contrasting new developments in the United States to recent trends abroad—from Mexico to Asia, and from Canada to Eastern Europe. Key issues such as the changing composition of the international working class, patterns of work under contemporary capitalism, the relationship of race and gender to class, the promise and limitations of recent eruptions of labor militancy, and the strategic options available to working people in an age of globalization are addressed.

611. Wood, S. "The Deskilling Debate, New Technology and Work Organization." *Acta Sociologica* 30, no. 1 (1987): 3-24.

Keywords: Taylorism, labor process, skill, tacit knowledge, knowledge embedded in experience

Taking as its starting point what has become known as the British labor process debate, this paper discusses some of the developing ideas within what the author characterizes as its third wave. In particular it focuses on the question of alternatives to Taylorism and the concept of skill. Rather than assuming the dominance of Taylorism (or superiority of flexible forms of organization), it is more useful to start from an appreciation of the limits of and contradictions within scientific management. A central problem that has bedeviled the post-Braverman debate about both new forms of work organization and the concept of skill is the centrality accorded to a unidimensional concept of control. The paper points to the need to get away from this and for a broader discussion of skill that includes consideration of the "social construction of skill," tacit knowledge, and the sexual division of labor. The author links this discussion to the question of "new" technologies, showing for example that the notion of tacit skills cautions against assuming they deskill most jobs, because such existing skill may be vital for their successful implementation. An examination of both the effects of recession on work organization and Japanese management further highlights some of the issues raised by the third wave of the labor process debate.

612. Wood, Stephen. *The Degradation of Work? Skill, Deskilling and the Labor Process*. London: Hutchison and Co., 1989.

Keywords: skill, deskilling, knowledge embedded in experience

This book on the role and importance of skill in work asks a number of fundamental questions such as "Has there been a general deskilling and routinization of jobs? Are 'skilled' jobs really any different from semi- or unskilled ones? Is the skill of the skilled worker essentially artificial, socially constructed in order to maintain differentials in wages and status? Have particular groups been able to resist encroachment by management into their traditional craft autonomy? Has working-class pressure itself been able to reverse or counter the 'deskilling trend' or has it influenced management to do so? Are attempts to humanize work simply cosmetic. . . ? And what of the new technology—computers, micro-processors, numerically controlled machines: do they deskill jobs further?"

The theoretical foundation of the book is Braverman's deskilling and degradation thesis, which the author uses as a starting point for his own analysis of capitalist rationalization and the labor process. Topics examined in the text include the sexual division of labor and deskilling, craft work, skills and the "politics" of the workplace, the role of Taylorism in the deskilling of workers, deskilled jobs versus deskilling of the individual, and computer-related work and the deskilling process. See especially chapters 2, 4, 6, and 10.

613. Wood, Stephen, ed. *The Transformation of Work? Skill, Flexibility and the Labor Process*. London: Unwin Hyman, 1989.

Keywords: QWL, technological change, division of labor

This extensive collection of essays explores the theoretical, methodological, and empirical questions surrounding the debate on flexible specialization, skill, and work organization. Major themes covered in the text include the following: "technological development and the limits of automation; . . . Japanese management and developments in concepts of management; gender relations and occupational segregation; developments in skill requirements and focus of work organization; the service sector" and the labor process in the context of capitalist enterprise.

See especially chapter 2 "When Certainty Fails: Inside the Factory of the Future" for information on the question of workerless factories, total managerial control and workers' on-the-job knowledge. See chapter 5 for a discussion of key features of the Japanese production system. Topics considered here include the historical context of Japanese management techniques, work segregation and lifetime employment. Chapter 8 explores "how the transformation of training has been an important element in the increased flexibility in the labor market and workplace." Chapters 9 and 10 focus on developments in the automobile industry. Worker participation programs and other forms of work reorganization are analyzed. Other chapters in the text concentrate on the microelectronics industry and its implications for skilling of workers; flexible manufacturing systems, case studies of computerization in the insurance industry, and technological changes in the service and administration sectors.

614. Worthy, James C. *Lean but Not Mean: Studies in Organizational Structure.* Chicago: University of Illinois Press, 1994.

Keywords: organizational behavior, industrial relations

James C. Worthy wrote over four hundred papers and speeches about management and organization from the late 1930s to the 1980s. He discussed these topics from the perspective of business, government, politics, and academia. This book, edited by David G. Moore and Ronald G. Greenwood, represents a collection of Worthy's best works on organization theory. Most of these papers were written in the 1940s and '50s when Worthy worked at Sears. Sears at this time was a successful enterprise that was very lean, but not mean. The importance of this is emphasized throughout the book.

Part 1 is concerned with providing background information on Sears under the rule of CEO General Robert E. Wood and especially the human relations research that Worthy started up. Part 2 delves into this research program and its results. Worthy's concepts of organizational structure are presented in part 3. Finally, part 4 looks into Worthy's view of management values and their effects on employees and organizations. The editors proudly announce that "the papers represent a significant contribution to management theory and practice."

615. Yalnizyan, Armine, T. Ran Ide, and Arthur J. Cordell. *Shifting Time: Social Policy and the Future of Work.* Toronto: Between the Lines Press, 1994.

Keywords: technological change, human resources, policy

This volume is written by a labor market analyst, a teacher, and a researcher of the social impact of technology. The authors offer a Canadian perspective on "the real world of work, wealth, and technology" by questioning the values and ethics of a society and economy based on the maximization of wealth and the worship of technological progress. Yalnizyan analyzes "a labor market which is increasingly incapable of producing anything but a two-tier society where the poor and the rich will see each other across a great unbridgeable divide." Ide and Cordell focus their attention on "the technological imperative and the accompanying secular religion of economic growth at whatever cost—including unsustainable costs to the environment." Instead, these analysts propose a future free from today's idolatry of market ideology.

The authors make it clear that the kind of full employment envisioned in the decades after World War II is no longer possible. "What's needed is a redistribution of work and wealth, of time and money. It is time to rethink the almost automatic equation of work with employment and in this way seek a real solution to the unsolved riddle of social justice." The authors also believe that we have to rethink the dominant approaches to dealing with "the wrenching changes wrought by globalization, automation, and the apparent end of employment—at least as we have known it."

The book offers solid evidence (statistics, policy analysis, case after case of the new realities of production and distribution) of the bankruptcy of old ideas about progress. The alternative advocated by the authors hinges on a new approach to productivity. For example, they suggest: "Why not institute a 'productivity tax' on the new computer and information technologies that are replacing so many jobs?"

616. Zeytinoglu, Isik Urla, ed. *Changing Work Relationships in Industrialized Economies*. Advances in Organization Studies 1. Amsterdam: John Benjamins Publishing Co., 1999.

Keywords: hours of labor, flexible, part-time employment, work environment, effect of technological innovations on employees

Throughout, this work examines the experiences of industrialized economies in dealing with changing work relationships and the policy implications of creating such work relationships. The central thesis was that nonstandard employment forms in restructuring economies affected all workers, especially females and the youth. However, the research demonstrates both positive and negative effects of changing work relationships on workers, though there is no conclusive result whether one or the other affect is stronger. A variety of experts of different backgrounds are used to delve into issues such as part-time/temporary/casual and self-employment work, and how these are affected by gender, age, race, education level, and economic class.

617. Zuboff, Shoshana. *In the Age of the Smart Machine: The Future of Work and Power*. New York: Basic Books, 1988.

Keywords: automation, technological change, case study, sociology

This masterfully researched volume stands as one of the most insightful recent books on the subject of the transformation of work. The author provides a powerful framework for evaluating the impact of computer technology in the workplace. Through "in-depth interviews over several years with workers and managers in . . . high-tech paper-making plants, bank and insurance offices, a telecommunications enterprise, and a pharmaceutical manufacturer," the author conveys workers' deepest personal experiences and feelings as their work lives are radically changed by the introduction of new technologies.

Zuboff's research approach combines participant observations with formal and informal interviews and small group discussions. She uses her considerable clinical skills "to help people articulate their still-implicit experiences in the new work settings." The data obtained from this method of research become the foundation for the book's central insights.

This volume's greatest strength is its success in going beyond mere sociological observations. As Zuboff states: "I wanted to discover the flesh and blood behind the concepts, the interior texture rather than the external form."

See especially part 1, entitled "Knowledge and Computer-Mediated Work." This section examines the transformation in the knowledge base used in the modern workplace via computer technology—as implicit, tacit knowledge embedded in experience is increasingly replaced by abstract knowledge separated from experience.

In the summary, Zuboff demonstrates that "computers may merely further automate blue- and white-collar jobs, achieving unprecedented speed and consistency, robbing workers of whatever skill and gratification they may retain and increasing the impersonality and remoteness of management. That same technology, however, may "informate," empowering ordinary working people with overall knowledge of the production process."

Author Index

Note: This index is to annotation numbers.

Keyword Index

Note: This index is to annotation numbers.

About the Authors

Willem H. Vanderburg is the founding director of the Centre for Technology and Social Development in the Faculty of Applied Science and Engineering at the University of Toronto and holds cross-appointments in the Institute for Environmental Studies and the Department of Sociology. He is editor-in-chief of the *Bulletin of Science, Technology & Society* and the author of *Perspectives on Our Age: Jacques Ellul Speaks of His Life and Work* (House of Anansi Press, 1997), *The Growth of Minds and Cultures* (University of Toronto Press, 1985), and *The Labyrinth of Technology* (University of Toronto Press, 2000).

Namir Khan is a lecturer at the Centre for Technology and Social Development in the Faculty of Applied Science and Engineering at the University of Toronto. He is the coauthor of several annotated bibliographies including *Sustainable Production* (Scarecrow Press, 2001), *Sustainable Energy* (Scarecrow Press, 2001), and *Healthy Cities* (Scarecrow Press, 2001).

Nina Nakajima is a postdoctoral fellow at the Centre for Technology and Social Development in the Faculty of Applied Science and Engineering at the University of Toronto. She is the acting managing editor of the *Bulletin of Science, Technology & Society.*

www.ingramcontent.com/pod-product-compliance
Ingram Content Group UK Ltd.
Pitfield, Milton Keynes, MK11 3LW, UK
UKHW041142300926
15471UKWH00011B/106

9 780810 852853